Pancreatic Neoplasms

Editor

NIPUN B. MERCHANT

SURGICAL ONCOLOGY CLINICS OF NORTH AMERICA

www.surgonc.theclinics.com

Consulting Editor
NICHOLAS J. PETRELLI

April 2016 • Volume 25 • Number 2

ELSEVIER

1600 John F. Kennedy Boulevard • Suite 1800 • Philadelphia, Pennsylvania, 19103-2899

http://www.theclinics.com

SURGICAL ONCOLOGY CLINICS OF NORTH AMERICA Volume 25, Number 2
April 2016 ISSN 1055-3207, ISBN-13: 978-0-323-41775-4

Editor: John Vassallo (j.vassallo@elsevier.com)
Developmental Editor: Meredith Clinton

Surgical Oncology Clinics of North America (ISSN 1055-3207) is published quarterly by Elsevier Inc., 360 Park Avenue South, New York, NY 10010-1710. Months of publication are January, April, July, and October. Business and Editorial Offices: 1600 John F. Kennedy Blvd., Ste. 1800, Philadelphia, PA 19103-2899. Customer Service Office: 3251 Riverport Lane, Maryland Heights, MO 63043. Periodicals postage paid at New York, NY and additional mailing offices. Subscription prices are $290.00 per year (US individuals), $471.00 (US institutions) $100.00 (US student/resident), $330.00 (Canadian individuals), $596.00 (Canadian institutions), $205.00 (Canadian student/resident), $410.00 (foreign individuals), $596.00 (foreign institutions), and $205.00 (foreign student/resident). Foreign air speed delivery is included in all *Clinics* subscription prices. All prices are subject to change without notice. **POSTMASTER**: Send address changes to *Surgical Oncology Clinics of North America*, Elsevier Health Science Division, Subscription Customer Service, 3251 Riverport Lane, Maryland Heights, MO 63043. **Customer Service: 1-800-654-2452 (US and Canada). 314-447-8871 (outside US and Canada). Fax: 314-447-8029. E-mail: journalscustomerservice-usa@elsevier.com (for print support); journalsonline support-usa@elsevier.com (for online support).**

Reprints. For copies of 100 or more, of articles in this publication, please contact the Commercial Reprints Department, Elsevier Inc., 360 Park Avenue South, New York, New York 10010-1710. Tel. 212-633-3874; Fax: 212-633-3820; E-mail: reprints@elsevier.com.

Surgical Oncology Clinics of North America is covered in *MEDLINE/PubMed (Index Medicus)* and *EMBASE/Excerpta Medica, Current Contents/Clinical Medicine, and ISI/BIOMED.*

Contributors

CONSULTING EDITOR

NICHOLAS J. PETRELLI, MD, FACS
Bank of America Endowed Medical Director, Helen F. Graham Cancer Center and Research Institute, Christiana Care Health System, Newark, Delaware; Professor of Surgery, Thomas Jefferson University, Philadelphia, Pennsylvania

EDITOR

NIPUN B. MERCHANT, MD, FACS
Alan S. Livingstone Professor of Surgery, Vice Chair of Surgical Oncology Services, Chief, Division of Surgical Oncology, Chief Surgical Officer, Sylvester Comprehensive Cancer Center, University of Miami Medical Center, Miami, Florida

AUTHORS

MOHAMMAD AL EFISHAT, MD
Department of Surgery, Research Fellow, Memorial Sloan Kettering Cancer Center, New York, New York; Senior General Surgery Resident, Department of Surgery, Johns Hopkins Hospital, Baltimore, Maryland

MAHMOUD M. AL-HAWARY, MD
Associate Professor, Department of Radiology, University Hospital, University of Michigan, Ann Arbor, Michigan

PETER J. ALLEN, MD
Department of Surgery, Professor of Surgery, Memorial Sloan Kettering Cancer Center, New York, New York

CARINNE W. ANDERSON, MD
Department of Surgery, Helen F. Graham Cancer Center, Newark, Delaware

JI YOUNG BANG, MD, MPH
Advanced Endoscopy Fellow, Division of Gastroenterology-Hepatology, Indiana University, Indianapolis, Indiana

JOSEPH J. BENNETT, MD
Department of Surgery, Helen F. Graham Cancer Center, Newark, Delaware

VINCENT BERNARD, MS
Sheikh Ahmed Pancreatic Cancer Research Center, University of Texas MD Anderson Cancer Center; The University of Texas Graduate School of Biomedical Sciences at Houston, Houston, Texas

PRIYA BHOSALE, MD
Associate Professor, Diagnostic Radiology, University of Texas MD Anderson Cancer Center, Houston, Texas

JENNIFER A. CHAN, MD, MPH
Department of Medical Oncology, Dana-Farber Cancer Institute, Assistant Professor of Medicine, Harvard Medical School, Boston, Massachusetts

AMARESHWAR CHIRUVELLA, MD
Chief Surgical Resident, Department of Surgery, Winship Cancer Institute, Emory University School of Medicine, Atlanta, Georgia

CRISTINA R. FERRONE, MD
Associate Professor, Department of Surgery, Massachusetts General Hospital, Harvard Medical School, Boston, Massachusetts

JASON FLEMING, MD
Sheikh Ahmed Pancreatic Cancer Research Center, Department of Surgical Oncology, University of Texas MD Anderson Cancer Center, Houston, Texas

ISAAC R. FRANCIS, MD
Professor, Department of Radiology, University Hospital, University of Michigan, Ann Arbor, Michigan

JONATHAN B. GREER, MD
Resident, General Surgery, Department of Surgery, Massachusetts General Hospital, Harvard Medical School, Boston, Massachusetts

BETH A. HELMINK, MD, PhD
Division of Surgical Oncology, Vanderbilt University Medical Center, Nashville, Tennessee

MELISSA HOGG, MD
Division of GI Surgical Oncology, University of Pittsburgh Medical Center, Pittsburgh, Pennsylvania

KAMRAN IDREES, MD
Division of Surgical Oncology, Vanderbilt University Medical Center, Nashville, Tennessee

RAVI K. KAZA, MD
Associate Professor, Department of Radiology, University Hospital, University of Michigan, Ann Arbor, Michigan

DAVID A. KOOBY, MD, FACS
Professor of Surgery, Department of Surgery, Winship Cancer Institute, Emory University School of Medicine, Atlanta, Georgia

MATTHEW H. KULKE, MD, MMSc
Department of Medical Oncology, Dana-Farber Cancer Institute, Associate Professor of Medicine, Harvard Medical School, Boston, Massachusetts

JEFFREY H. LEE, MD
Professor, Department of Gastroenterology, Hepatology and Nutrition, University of Texas MD Anderson Cancer Center, Houston, Texas

DANENG LI, MD
Department of Medicine, Memorial Sloan Kettering Cancer Center, New York, New York

DEEPA MAGGE, MD
Division of GI Surgical Oncology, University of Pittsburgh Medical Center, Pittsburgh, Pennsylvania

ANIRBAN MAITRA, MBBS
Sheikh Ahmed Pancreatic Cancer Research Center; Department of Pathology, University of Texas MD Anderson Cancer Center, Houston, Texas

NIPUN B. MERCHANT, MD, FACS
Alan S. Livingstone Professor of Surgery, Vice Chair of Surgical Oncology Services, Chief, Division of Surgical Oncology, Chief Surgical Officer, Sylvester Comprehensive Cancer Center, University of Miami Medical Center, Miami, Florida

EILEEN M. O'REILLY, MD
Associate Director, Clinical Research David M. Rubenstein Center for Pancreatic Cancer; Attending Physician, Member Memorial Sloan Kettering Cancer Center; Professor of Medicine, Weill Cornell Medical College, New York, New York

ALEXANDER A. PARIKH, MD, MPH
Division of Surgical Oncology, Vanderbilt University Medical Center, Nashville, Tennessee

KATHERINE E. PORUK, MD
Department of Surgery, The Sol Goldman Pancreatic Cancer Research Center, Johns Hopkins University School of Medicine, Baltimore, Maryland

ERIC M. ROHREN, MD, PhD
Professor, Department of Nuclear Medicine, University of Texas MD Anderson Cancer Center, Houston, Texas

REBECCA A. SNYDER, MD, MPH
Department of Surgical Oncology, University of Texas MD Anderson Cancer Center, Houston, Texas

ERIC P. TAMM, MD
Professor, Diagnostic Radiology, University of Texas MD Anderson Cancer Center, Houston, Texas

SHYAM VARADARAJULU, MD
Medical Director, Center for Interventional Endoscopy, Florida Hospital, Orlando, Florida

CHRISTOPHER L. WOLFGANG, MD, PhD
Department of Surgery, The Sol Goldman Pancreatic Cancer Research Center, Johns Hopkins University School of Medicine, Baltimore, Maryland

HERBERT J. ZEH III, MD, FACS
Associate Professor of Surgery, Division of GI Surgical Oncology, University of Pittsburgh Medical Center, Pittsburgh, Pennsylvania

AMER ZUREIKAT, MD
Division of GI Surgical Oncology, University of Pittsburgh Medical Center, Pittsburgh, Pennsylvania

Contents

Carcinogenic progression in the pancreas arises through a well-established stepwise accumulation of molecular aberrations from a normal cell to an invasive adenocarcinoma. Recent large-scale sequencing efforts have provided insight into novel driver genes as well as enriched core signaling pathways that underlie the inherent heterogeneity found in pancreatic cancer. By exploiting these genomic profiles, we may begin to provide new insights into patient stratification and therapeutic guidance. This review discusses the molecular landscape of pancreatic cancer and its role in tumor progression, clinical prognostication, and the development of novel therapeutic strategies.

Imaging plays a central role in the management of patients with suspected or known periampullary masses, including the initial diagnosis, staging, and follow-up to assess treatment response or recurrence. Use of appropriate imaging tools, application of optimal imaging protocols, and knowledge about imaging findings are essential for the diagnosis and accurate staging of these masses. Structured reporting of the imaging studies offers several advantages over freestyle dictations ensuring completeness of the relevant imaging findings, which would in turn help in deciding the best individual treatment strategy for each patient.

Accurate diagnosis and staging of pancreatic neoplasms is essential for surgical planning and identification of locally advanced and metastatic disease that is incurable by surgery. The ability to position the endoscopic ultrasonography (EUS) transducer close to the pancreas combined with the use of fine-needle aspiration enables the accurate diagnosis of pancreatic cysts and solid masses. EUS is also increasingly being used to procure core tissue for molecular analysis that facilitates personalized treatment of pancreatic cancer. Various therapeutic interventions can be undertaken under EUS guidance. This article focuses on the applications of EUS and endoscopic retrograde cholangiopancreatography in pancreatic neoplasms.

Minimally invasive techniques have the potential to revolutionize the surgical management of pancreatic disease in the setting of benign and malignant processes. Pancreatic surgery, in particular, may be aided significantly by minimal access surgery given the high morbidity associated with traditional open pancreatic procedures. This article presents a review of two minimally invasive techniques for distal pancreatectomy and pancreaticoduodenectomy, focusing on metrics of technique, safety, morbidity, and oncologic outcomes and potential benefits.

Successful surgical resection offers the only chance for cure in patients with pancreatic cancer; however, pancreatic resection is feasible in less than 20% of the patients. In this review, the current state of surgical management of pancreatic cancer is discussed. The definition of resectability based on cross-sectional imaging and the technical aspects of surgery, including vascular resection and/or reconstruction, management of aberrant vascular anatomy and extent of lymphadenectomy, are appraised. Furthermore, common pancreatic resection-specific postoperative complications and their management are reviewed.

Pancreas adenocarcinoma is an aggressive malignancy. The risk of recurrence remains high even for patients with localized disease undergoing surgical resection. Adjuvant systemic therapy has demonstrated the ability to reduce the risk of recurrence and prolong survival. Determination of optimal adjuvant treatment, systemic therapy, and/or combinations to further improve recurrence rates and overall survival are still needed. Neoadjuvant therapy represents an alternative emerging paradigm of investigation with several theoretic advantages over adjuvant therapy. This article summarizes the major adjuvant and neoadjuvant studies for pancreas adenocarcinoma and highlights key areas of ongoing investigation.

Pancreatic adenocarcinoma is the fourth leading cause of cancer death in the United States. Surgical resection offers the best opportunity for prolonged survival but is limited to patients with locally resectable disease without distant metastases. Regrettably, most patients are diagnosed at a point in which curative surgery is no longer a treatment option. In these patients, management of symptoms becomes paramount to improve quality of life and potentially increase survival. This article reviews the palliative management of unresectable pancreatic cancer, including potential palliative resection, surgical and endoscopic biliary and gastric decompression, and pain control with celiac plexus block.

As patients are living longer and axial imaging is more widespread, increasing numbers of cystic neoplasms of the pancreas are found. Intraductal papillary mucinous neoplasms and mucinous cystic neoplasms are the most common. The revised Sendai guidelines provide a safe algorithm for expectant management of certain cystic neoplasms; however, studies are ongoing to identify further subgroups that can be treated nonoperatively. For those patients with high-risk clinical features or symptoms, surgical resection can be performed safely at high-volume pancreatic centers. Accurate diagnosis is critical for accurate decision making.

Management of cystic neoplasms of the pancreas is challenging as it relies on radiologic and cyst fluid markers to discriminate between benign and pre-cancerous lesions; however, their ability to predict malignancy is limited. While asymptomatic serous cystadenomas can be managed conservatively, mucinous cystic neoplasms and intraductal papillary mucinous neoplasms are more difficult to manage. A selective approach, based on the preoperative likelihood of high-grade dysplasia or invasive disease, is the standard of care. Research is focusing on the development of pre-operative markers for identifying high risk lesions, which will spare patients with low-risk or benign lesions the risks of pancreatectomy.

Pancreatic neuroendocrine tumors are a rare group of neoplasms that arise from multipotent stem cells in the pancreatic ductal epithelium. Although they comprise only 1% to 2% of pancreatic neoplasms, their incidence is increasing. Most pancreatic neuroendocrine tumors are nonfunctioning, but they can secrete various hormones resulting in unique clinical syndromes. Clinicians must be aware of the diverse manifestations of this disease, as the key step to management of these rare tumors is to first suspect the diagnosis.

Pancreatic neuroendocrine tumors are rare tumors that present many imaging challenges, from detecting small functional tumors to fully staging large nonfunctioning tumors, including identifying all sites of metastatic disease, particularly nodal and hepatic, and depicting vascular involvement. The correct choice of imaging modality requires knowledge of the tumor type (eg, gastrinoma versus insulinoma), and also the histology (well vs poorly differentiated). Evolving techniques in computed tomography (CT), MRI, endoscopic ultrasonography, and nuclear medicine, such as dual-energy CT, diffusion-weighted MRI, liver-specific magnetic resonance contrast agents, and new nuclear medicine agents, offer new ways to visualize, and ultimately manage, these tumors.

Pancreatic neuroendocrine tumors (pancNETs) are rare neoplasms that comprise 2% to 4% of all clinically detected pancreatic tumors. They are usually indolent, and their malignant potential is often underestimated. The management of this disease poses a challenge because of the heterogeneous clinical presentation and varying degree of aggressiveness. Treatment decisions for this clinical entity are still patient- and/or physician-specific. Optimal clinical management of pancNETs requires a multidisciplinary approach. The only potentially curative treatment option, especially in the early stage disease, remains surgical resection; however, as many as 75% of patients present with advanced disease (nodal and/or distant metastases).

When diagnosed at an early stage, resection of pancreatic neuroendocrine tumors (NETs) is often curative. Unfortunately, curative surgery is rarely an option for patients with metastatic disease. Multiple options are available for the management of patients with advanced pancreatic NETs, including surgery, liver-directed therapy, and systemic therapies. Because of the heterogeneity of disease biology and presentation, a multidisciplinary approach to management is critical. Treatment with somatostatin analogs, sunitinib, everolimus, and alkylating agents provide effective systemic therapeutic options for patients. Future studies to evaluate the optimal timing, sequence, and combination of therapies, as well as to identify predictors of response, are warranted.

SURGICAL ONCOLOGY CLINICS OF NORTH AMERICA

RELATED INTEREST

Surgical Clinics of North America, October 2015 (Vol. 95, Issue 5)
Cancer Screening and Genetics
Christopher L. Wolfgang, *Editor*
Available at: http://www.surgical.theclinics.com/

THE CLINICS ARE AVAILABLE ONLINE!
Access your subscription at:
www.theclinics.com

Foreword

Pancreatic Neoplasms

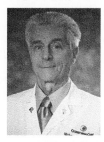

Nicholas J. Petrelli, MD, FACS
Consulting Editor

This issue of the *Surgical Oncology Clinics of North America* is devoted to pancreatic neoplasms. The guest editor is Nipun Merchant, MD. Dr Merchant is the Chief Surgical Officer and Director of the Surgical Oncology Research Programs at the Sylvester Comprehensive Cancer Center at the University of Miami Miller School of Medicine. Dr Merchant was the previous Director of the Vanderbilt Pancreas Center, Chief of Gastrointestinal Surgical Oncology and Co-Leader of the Gastrointestinal Oncology Program at Vanderbilt-Ingram Comprehensive Cancer Center.

This issue of the *Surgical Oncology Clinics of North America* runs the gamut of pancreatic neoplasms. For example, the article by Drs Tamm, Bhosale, Lee, and Rohren, from the MD Anderson Cancer Center, discusses state-of-the-art imaging of pancreatic neuroendocrine tumors. As discussed in this article, knowledge of the type of functional tumor is important in choosing appropriate imaging strategies to identify primary lesions and their metastases. An additional article by Drs Li and O'Reilly, from Memorial Sloan Kettering Cancer Center, discusses both adjuvant and neoadjuvant treatment for pancreatic cancer. This article includes a historic perspective of adjuvant systemic trials in pancreatic cancer and also the use of combination cytotoxic therapy, targeted agents, chemoradiation, and immunotherapy for both adjuvant and neoadjuvant treatment.

Last, there is an excellent article by Drs Helmink, Snyder, Idrees, Merchant, and Parikh on advances in the surgical management of resectable and borderline resectable pancreatic cancer. There is an excellent discussion on the role of minimally invasive surgery and on the complications following pancreaticoduodenectomy.

I would like to thank Dr Merchant for pulling together his colleagues to complete this excellent issue on pancreatic neoplasms. This is an outstanding issue of the

Surg Oncol Clin N Am 25 (2016) xiii–xiv
http://dx.doi.org/10.1016/j.soc.2015.12.004
1055-3207/16/$ – see front matter © 2016 Published by Elsevier Inc.

surgonc.theclinics.com

Surgical Oncology Clinics of North America for attending staff to share with their trainees.

Nicholas J. Petrelli, MD, FACS
Bank of America Endowed Medical Director
Helen F Graham Cancer Center & Research Institute
Christiana Care Health Systems
4701 Ogletown Stanton Road, Suite 1233
Newark, DE 19713, USA

Professor of Surgery
Thomas Jefferson University
Philadelphia, PA

E-mail address:
npetrelli@christianacare.org

Preface

Eat When You Can, Sleep When You Can, and Don't Mess with the Pancreas

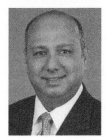

Nipun B. Merchant, MD, FACS
Editor

These three "rules" of surgical training are facetiously instilled into the psyche of all new surgical residents. The third rule was based on the limited understanding of and poor outcomes associated with the management of pancreatic diseases. Since those days, we have made substantial progress in understanding, diagnosing, and treating pancreatic diseases. This issue of *Surgical Oncology Clinics of North America* covers a wide range of topics that represent some of the most important advances in the field of pancreatic neoplasms, and it highlights how we continue to violate rule number three, above.

Pancreatic neoplasms comprise both exocrine and endocrine cancers of the pancreas, as well as pancreatic cystic lesions. Highlighted in this issue are numerous advances in molecular genetics, imaging capabilities, novel therapeutics, and minimally invasive techniques that have significantly changed the practice of pancreatic neoplasms over the past decade. Advances in the molecular genetics of pancreatic cancers have identified key signaling pathways that are critical in the carcinogenesis of most, if not all, pancreatic cancers, providing an opportunity to exploit these targets on a more personalized level.

State-of-the-art imaging capabilities and advances in the endoscopic diagnosis and treatment of both exocrine and endocrine pancreatic tumors are allowing us to better localize and determine the extent of disease prior to surgical intervention, eliminating the morbidity of many unnecessary operations. New definitions of resectable, borderline resectable, and locally advanced pancreas cancers have led to the more appropriate use of neoadjuvant therapies and selection of patients who will benefit most from surgical resection. Expertise in minimally invasive surgery is minimizing the

Surg Oncol Clin N Am 25 (2016) xv–xvi
http://dx.doi.org/10.1016/j.soc.2016.01.001
1055-3207/16/$ – see front matter © 2016 Published by Elsevier Inc.
surgonc.theclinics.com

morbidity of pancreatic surgery, and controversies in the diagnosis and management of cystic lesions of the pancreas are being better delineated.

Articles in this issue are authored by a multidisciplinary group of several national experts across the country in the fields of molecular biology, radiology, surgery, and medical oncology who have been instrumental in the development of many of these recent advances.

Nipun B. Merchant, MD, FACS
Division of Surgical Oncology
Sylvester Comprehensive Cancer Center
University of Miami Medical Center
1120 Northwest 14th Street
Clinical Research Building, Suite 410
Miami, FL 33136, USA

E-mail address:
nmerchant@miami.edu

Molecular and Genetic Basis of Pancreatic Carcinogenesis
Which Concepts May be Clinically Relevant?

Vincent Bernard, MS[a,b], Jason Fleming, MD[a,c],
Anirban Maitra, MBBS[a,d],*

KEYWORDS

- Carcinogenic progression • Pancreatic cancer • Genomic profiling
- Pancreatic ductal adenocarcinoma

KEY POINTS

- Carcinogenic progression of pancreatic cancer involves the stepwise accumulation of molecular aberrations from a normal cell to an invasive adenocarcinoma.
- Recent large-scale sequencing efforts have revealed novel driver genes and enriched core signaling pathways that abridge the inherent heterogeneity found in pancreatic cancer.
- By exploiting these genomic profiles, we may begin to provide new insights into patient stratification and therapeutic guidance.

Although rare (2% of cancer cases), pancreatic ductal adenocarcinoma (PDAC) is the fourth leading cause of cancer-related deaths in this country. In contrast with the decline of cancer-related deaths from other malignancies, the alarming increase in incidence of PDAC is projected to make it the second leading cause of cancer-related death by 2030.[1] With a 5-year survival rate of only 4%, the lethality of this disease is attributed in part to the lack of early detection and a limited armamentarium of effective therapeutic strategies.[2] The main oncogenic driver mutation, observed in greater than 90% of PDAC, *KRAS* (v-Kiras2 Kirsten rat sarcoma viral oncogene homolog) has also compounded its poor survival rate owing to its "undruggability," although

[a] Sheikh Ahmed Pancreatic Cancer Research Center, UT MD Anderson Cancer Center, Houston, TX 77030, USA; [b] The University of Texas Graduate School of Biomedical Sciences at Houston, Houston, TX 77030, USA; [c] Department of Surgical Oncology, The University of Texas MD Anderson Cancer Center, 1515 Holcombe Boulevard, Houston, TX 77030, USA; [d] Department of Pathology, The University of Texas MD Anderson Cancer Center, 6565 MD Anderson Boulevard, Room Z3.3038, Houston, TX 77030, USA
* Corresponding author. Department of Pathology, The University of Texas MD Anderson Cancer Center, 6565 MD Anderson Boulevard, Room Z3.3038, Houston, TX 77030.
E-mail address: amaitra@mdanderson.org

Surg Oncol Clin N Am 25 (2016) 227–238
http://dx.doi.org/10.1016/j.soc.2015.11.003
1055-3207/16/$ – see front matter © 2016 Elsevier Inc. All rights reserved.

chemotherapeutic strategies may exist in certain targetable cases as discussed elsewhere in this paper.

Advances in next-generation sequencing technologies have allowed for a detailed insight into the genomic landscape of PDAC, to better understand how molecular alterations contribute to disease initiation and progression. In particular, dissecting the molecular events involved in the progression of PDAC from pancreatic intraepithelial neoplasia (PanINs) lesions to invasive carcinoma, are being achieved with possible implications to prognosis and targeted therapeutic approaches.

MULTISTEP PROGRESSION OF PANCREATIC DUCTAL ADENOCARCINOMA

The progression of PDAC from a normal cell to an invasive adenocarcinoma involves the accumulation of inherited and/or acquired mutations throughout a span of up to approximately 20 years (**Fig. 1**).[3] This highlights the importance of exploiting this window of progression to develop new screening methods to provide curative surgical approaches. This progression involves the evolution of histologically recognized precursor lesions known as PanINs. As of the date of this publication, the categorization of PanIN is divided into low grade (PanIN-1A and 1B), intermediate (PanIN-2), and high grade (PanIN-3),[4] although there is an emerging consensus in the clinical research community to move to a simplified 2-tiered classification of "low"-grade (PanIn-1 and -2) and "high"-grade PanINs (PanIN-3). This is based on observations that, although PanIN-1 and -2 lesions can be found even in the absence of cancer, PanIN-3 is almost never found without concomitant invasive neoplasia. Genetic alterations can be grouped into those that arise in precursor lesions and are usually, albeit not always, found in the concomitant PDAC, versus those that arise during subclonal evolution of the infiltrating carcinoma resulting in genetic heterogeneity.

One of the earliest genetic events involved in PDAC pathogenesis is an activating point mutation in the *KRAS* oncogene, an oncogenic driver mutation found in more

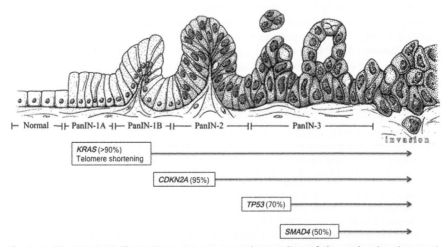

Fig. 1. A "PanINgram" illustrating our current understanding of the molecular changes in the multistep progression model of pancreas adenocarcinomas. (*Adapted from* Maitra A, Adsay NV, Argani P, et al. Multicomponent analysis of the pancreatic adenocarcinoma progression model using a pancreatic intraepithelial neoplasia tissue microarray. Mod Pathol 2003;16(9):909; with permission.)

than 90% of all PDACs. Subsequent genetic aberrations include inactivation of tumor suppressor genes, including *CDKN2A*, *TP53*, and *SMAD4*, which encode for p16^{INK4A}, p53, and Smad4, respectively, and contribute to the histologic evolution of these precursor lesions. Together, these 4 alterations comprise the "big 4" in PDAC, although many other recurrent somatic mutations are found in lower frequencies (5%–10%) of cases, including those that afflict particular functional pathways in the cancer cell, such as DNA damage repair or chromatin regulation.

Among the population of noninvasive precursor lesions, it is also important to recognize intraductal papillary mucinous neoplasms (IPMNs) and mucinous cystic neoplasms. Although histologically distinct from the microscopic PanIN lesions, these cystic precursor lesions share similar diver mutations including point mutations in the KRAS oncogene[5] and inactivating mutations in p53 and p16, with SMAD4 loss typically not being found in IPMNs.[6,7] Among the unique drivers found in both IPMNs and mucinous cystic neoplasms are inactivating mutations in *RNF43*, encoding for an ubiquitin ligase that has a role in WNT signaling inhibition.[5] IPMNs also contain point mutations in the *GNAS* gene, which results in constitutively active guanine nucleotide-binding protein owing to loss of intrinsic GTPase activity preventing hydrolysis of guanosine 5'-triphosphate (GTP).[8]

KRAS

Under physiologic conditions, activation of Ras protein is induced through growth factor receptor signaling, which promotes Ras activity through transitory binding to GTP. This results in the interaction of Ras with a variety of downstream effectors that govern proliferation, cell division, survival, and gene expression such as the RAF-mitogen-activated protein kinase and phosphoinositide 3-kinase pathways.[9] Through an intrinsic GTPase mechanism and GTPase-activating proteins, Ras can then hydrolyze GTP to GDP to inactivate itself. It is this intrinsic GTPase activity that is altered in the activating point mutation of *KRAS*, which results in an inability to hydrolyze GTP, allowing for a constitutively active protein that no longer relies on external stimuli. The most common "hotspot" mutation in the *KRAS* oncogene occurs at codon 12, followed by codon 13, and less frequently codon 61; emerging genomic data suggest that the specific codon involved might have an impact on disease prognosis, underscoring differences in Ras function.[10,11]

TELOMERE SHORTENING

Telomeres are repetitive nucleoprotein complexes found at the end chromosomes that have a role in genomic stability by protecting against chromosomal degradation and chromosome end fusion. In PDAC, shortened telomere lengths that potentially lead to chromosomal abnormalities can be detected in early lesions such as IPMNs and are nearly universally in all PanINs.[12] Genomic instability of this kind typically leads to cell death unless cells are able to inactivate tumor suppressor mechanisms as described elsewhere in this paper.

CDKN2A

The most commonly mutated tumor suppressor in PDAC (~95%) is an inactivation of *cyclin-dependent kinase inhibitor 2A gene* (*CDKN2A*), encoding for the cell cycle checkpoint protein, p16^{INK4A}.[13] Inactivation of CDKN2A in PDAC can occur via several different mechanisms, including mutation, genomic deletions, and promoter hypermethylation, resulting in epigenetic silencing.[14] The encoded protein p16^{INK4A} functions as a cyclin-dependent kinase inhibitor, specifically of CDK4 and CDK6, thereby preventing the phosphorylation of the retinoblastoma protein and blocking G1-S transition.[15] Loss of this protein thus results in unregulated cell cycle transition.

TP53

Aberrations of TP53, which encodes for p53, are typically a later event in the multiprogression of PDAC and is mutated in up to 70% of tumors, often arising in PanIN-3 lesions.[16] As the master guardian of the genome, p53 is involved in cell cycle arrest, DNA repair, blocking of angiogenesis, and induction of apoptosis in response to DNA damage or environmental stressors. Loss of this protein allows for DNA damage and external stressors to go unchecked, thereby promoting genomic instability and aberrant proliferation.

SMAD4

SMAD4 (DPC4, SMAD family member 4 gene), which encodes for the Smad4 protein, is inactivated in approximately 50% of PDACs as a late event in its progression (PanIN-3 – carcinoma).[17] As a downstream effector of transforming growth factor-β, loss of SMAD4 activity leads to tumor promotion by relieving the growth inhibitory effect of transforming growth factor-β signaling.[18]

CLINICAL RELEVANCE OF CORE PANCREATIC DUCTAL ADENOCARCINOMA MUTATIONS

Although pancreatic cancers have been shown to harbor an average of 63 genetic mutations, the genomic landscape of PDAC is faithfully represented by these 4 genomic mutations (KRAS, CDKN2A, TP53, and SMAD4).[10] The high degree of mutational concordance at these 4 loci between primary and metastatic sites of individual cancers[19] suggests these are so-called founder mutations. This term describes a mutation present in all samples from a single patient, thus sharing a common ancestor, which likely originated during PanIN progression.[3,12] Of note, PDACs continue to accumulate genetic alterations through subclonal evolution throughout their natural history, the vast majority of which are so-called passenger mutations that have little functional impact on progression, whereas a minor fraction are so-called progressor mutations, and do have a deleterious consequence on disease progression. In any case, a variable combination of the "big 4" is altered in most PDAC cases, with nearly all cancers showing at least KRAS mutations in conjunction with one or more of the 3 tumor suppressors. Yachida and colleagues[19] describe correlations of the status of these 4 genes to disease progression, metastatic failure, and overall survival, with patients with 3 to 4 of these mutated driver genes demonstrating worse overall survival. When looking at the genes individually, there is no significant difference in outcome in patients with KRAS and CDKN2A mutations, but TP53 and SMAD4 mutations were evidently associated with widespread metastatic disease and worse clinical outcomes.[20,21] In particular, SMAD4 status in PDAC (measured using immunohistochemical expression for the Smad4 protein) is being used to provide guidance toward tailoring treatment with systemic chemotherapy, as patients with Smad4-null tumors are most likely to develop widely metastatic disease.[22]

GERMLINE VARIANTS

With estimates of 10% of PDAC patients having a family history of the disease, elucidation of the PDAC genome has also contributed toward risk assessment and early detection in the context of familial pancreatic cancers.[23,24] Among hereditary pancreatic cancer susceptibility genes, *STK11/LKB1*, which is associated with Peutz–Jegher syndrome, is correlated with one of the highest risks of familial pancreatic cancers with approximately 132 greater relative lifetime risk.[25] *PRSS1* and *SPINK1* germline mutations are seen in hereditary pancreatitis families with a 50× to 80× relative lifetime risk, or 30% to 44% risk, of developing PDAC.[26–28] *P16/CDKN2A* germline mutations, are associated with familial atypical multiple mole melanoma syndrome, which entails a 38× increased risk (17% lifetime risk) of developing PDAC.[29] Additional germline variants associated with increased PDAC risk are clustered into defects of DNA repair pathways. This includes members of the Fanconi anemia pathway such as FANC-C, FANC-G, and PALB2, whose encoded proteins interact with that of BRCA2, and are associated with young onset pancreatic cancer.[30] BRCA1/BRCA2 mutations, which are associated with familial breast and ovarian cancers, have a 3.5× to 10× estimated relative risk.[31–33] Lynch syndrome, caused by mutations in DNA mismatch repair genes, MLH1, MSH2, MSH6, or PMS2, have an estimated 3.68% lifetime risk.[34] Patients with ataxia telangiectasia mutated germline mutations have also demonstrated a predisposition for PDAC.[35] Further elucidation of additional genes associated with familial PDAC may have implications for risk assessment and surveillance in affected family members. Detection of these germline mutations in patients is also important in the context of therapy as a way to exploit synthetic lethal interactions in the case of DNA repair pathways as described elsewhere in this paper.

CORE SIGNALING PATHWAYS IN PANCREATIC CANCER

Large-scale sequencing efforts have uncovered novel mutated genes in PDAC, as well as revealing multiple core signaling pathways that are affected throughout its carcinogenesis. In 2008, Jones and colleagues[10] performed polymerase chain reaction–based exome sequencing of primary and metastatic tumors. Their data supported the role of the 4 main genetic drivers in pancreatic cancer, KRAS, CDKN2A, TP53, SMAD4, and identified genetic alterations in many other critical pathways recognized as "hallmarks of cancer," at least some of which seem to have a prognostic influence in subsequent studies.[11,36] The core "hallmarks of pancreatic cancer" pathways that seem to be targeted in PDAC are highlighted in **Table 1** with some salient examples of genes mutated in each pathway.

Table 1
Core hallmarks of pancreatic cancer pathways

Apoptosis	CASP10, VCP, CAD
DNA damage control	TP53, RANBP2, EP300
Regulation of G1/S phase transition	CDKN2A, FBXW7, APC2
Hedgehog signaling	GLI1, GLI3, BMPR2
Homophilic cell adhesion	CDH1, CDH2, CDH10, PCDH15
Integrin signaling	ITGA4, ITHA9, LAMA1, FN1
C-Jun N-terminal kinase signaling	MAP4K3, TNF, ATF2
KRAS signaling	KRAS, MAP2K4, RASGRP3
Regulation of invasion	ADAM11, ADAM12, DPP6, MEP1A
Small GTPase-dependent	PLXNB1, AGHGEF7, PLCB3, RP1
Transforming growth factor-β signaling	SMAD4, SMAD3, TGFBR2, BMPR2
Wnt/Notch signaling	MYC, GATA6, WNT9A, MAP2, TCF4

The altered genes in these respective pathways varied among separate patient tumors, such as the transforming growth factor-β pathway being altered by a *SMAD4* mutation in 1 patient versus a *BMPR2* mutation in another, but the pathway in itself is often altered among samples. With this new global view of the PDAC genome as a set of a specific and limited number of pathways involved, we can begin to simplify the genetic heterogeneity that is intrinsic to these tumors and develop strategies to target the physiologic effects of the mutations rather than the specific mutations themselves. By targeting key nodes involved in these pathways, such as the impaired ability to repair DNA or altered cell cycle control, we may be able to circumvent the inevitable resistance that these tumors develop after targeted gene therapies.

In 2012, Biankin and colleagues[37] performed next-generation sequencing of whole exomes and copy number analysis of primary resected PDAC from 142 patients, under the umbrella of the International Cancer Genome Consortium (ICGC). This study reaffirmed the core signaling pathways identified by Jones and colleagues[10] and also discovered novel mutated genes in these core signaling pathways including those involved in DNA damage repair (ataxia telangiectasia mutated), which is also shown to have a role in familial PDAC. Novel gene signatures were also identified in axon guidance pathway genes (SLIT/ROBO signaling), which are known to have a role in neuronal migration and positioning during embryogenesis with potential implications in cancer cell survival, growth, invasion, and angiogenesis.[38] Deregulation of these axon guidance genes was shown to have a role in tumor initiation and progression in the context of PDAC. In particular, low ROBO2 or high ROBO3 expression was seen to be associated with poor patient survival. High expression of Semaphorin signaling molecules, specifically SEMA3A and PLXNA1, were also determined to be associated with poor patient survival. The ICGC team's methodology provided them the opportunity to identify potential novel drivers of pancreatic cancer, and new nodal signaling targets involving axon guidance, where therapeutics are being developed currently for neuronal regeneration after injury.[39] Again, we see the importance of developing therapeutics based on molecular phenotypes as further elucidation of genetic heterogeneity provides a cumbersome picture of pancreatic cancer.

In 2015, the next iteration of the ICGC PDAC dataset was published by Waddell and colleagues,[40] who performed whole genome sequencing and copy number variation analysis of 100 PDACs, and demonstrated chromosomal rearrangements that led to genetic aberrations. These structural rearrangements led to gene deletions, amplifications and fusions that are associated with driving carcinogenesis while presenting opportunities for clinical actionability and biomarkers of therapeutic response for platinum based chemotherapies. This led to the classification of PDACs into 4 subtypes based on structural rearrangement profiles (**Table 2**).

In addition to the classic "big 4" and alterations in genes whose products are involved in DNA maintenance, the Waddell and colleagues study highlighted the emerging importance of chromatin regulatory genes in the pathogenesis of PDAC. In particular, mutations of genes whose encoded proteins are involved in histone modification (*MLL2, MLL3, KDM6A*) and SWI/SNF genes that regulate how DNA is packaged in nucleosomes. *ARID1A* and *ARID2* emerged as a family of driver genes with unequivocal significance in PDAC. A recent whole exome study of resected PDAC patients by Sausen and colleagues[36] found strikingly favorable impact of harboring MLL2 or MLL3 mutations in the corresponding tumor, although the functional basis for this observation is still being elucidated. Inactivation of other tumor suppressors such as ROBO1, ROBO2, SLIT2, and RNF43 also demonstrate the role of aberrant WNT signaling in PDAC, as well as the potential for sensitivity that these mutations may confer to WNT inhibitors.[41]

Table 2	
Pancreatic ductal adenocarcinoma structural rearrangement profiles	
Stable	Small number of structural rearrangements (<50) with defects in cell cycle characterized by aneuploidy.
Locally rearranged	Presence of intrachromosomal rearrangements classified as complex: leading to chromothripsis or breakage–fusion–bridge cycles; or focal copy number gains in genes such as KRAS, SOX9, GATA6, and potential therapeutic targets like ERBB2, MET, CDK6, PIK3CA, and PIK3R3.
Scattered	Chromosomal aberrations owing to structural rearrangements (50–200) throughout the genome.
Unstable	Widespread structural rearrangements (>200) with genomic instability pointing toward somatic or germline deleterious mutations in DNA maintenance pathways (eg, BRCA1, BRCA2, and PALB2), which suggest sensitivity to DNA damaging agents. A subset of these patients who were treated with platinum based therapy at tumor recurrence demonstrated robust or exceptional responses.

Overall, the recent series of exome studies in PDAC have suggested that a major mechanism of genomic instability and damage in pancreatic cancer involves structural variations and their potential clinical relevance. This supports the role of platinum based regimens such as FOLFIRINOX in a subgroup of patients that are both able to tolerate the regimen and contain a signature of impaired DNA maintenance pathways owing to an unstable structural rearrangement phenotype within their tumors. It may also provide a model for patient stratification for PARP-1 inhibitor therapy because current clinical trials are predominantly restricted to patient populations with BRCA1 and BRCA2 germline defects. This new model also allows for a surrogate measure of defects in DNA maintenance where there may be a larger population that may benefit from such therapies who have non-BRCA pathway gene mutations, but whose unstable tumor subtype suggests sensitivity to DNA-damaging agents.

More recently, Bailey and colleagues (Bailey P, Chang DK, Nones K, unpublished data, 2016) have used exome and RNA profiling on 450 PDAC samples in the ICGC cohort to define 4 subtypes of PDAC based on differential gene expression signatures with distinct biological underpinnings: squamous, pancreatic progenitor, aberrantly differentiated endocrine exocrine, and immunogenic (Biankin A, personal communication, 2015). Although each of these molecular subtypes is enriched in a particular histologic variant (eg, the nom de plume for squamous subtype arising from its enrichment of adenosquamous carcinomas in this subset), the intent of this expression signature is to tease out biological distinctions that might underlie PDACs that look identical at the morphologic level. Not surprisingly, as is being increasingly noted across pan-cancer profiling datasets, there exists striking molecular similarities between subtypes across cancer types than within subtypes in a single cancer. Thus, the squamous subtype of PDAC has greater similarities to the so-called basal type cancers observed in head and neck and triple negative breast cancers (characterized by an overriding p63-driven signature) than to the other 3 PDAC subtypes.

Among clinical actionability in these subtypes, MYC amplifications have been found to be associated with the adenosquamous subtype and a correlation with poor survival.[11] Also, appreciable differences in roles of the immune system can be identified, which may lead to exploiting immunotherapeutic strategies. In the case of the squamous subtype, a loss of cytotoxic T cells was associated with an increase in Toll-like receptors, $CD4^+$ T cells, and macrophages, as well as high expression of

CTLA4 and PD1 immunosuppressive pathways. Stratification based on these sub-types may thus assist in clinical trial patient selection for therapeutics, such as PD1 and CTLA4 checkpoint inhibitors to decipher their potential role in this disease.

Many of these recent global sequencing efforts provide a biomarker-based approach to identify surrogates for prognostic and therapeutic stratification. Because most of the sequencing of data provided was performed on patients with surgically resectable primary tumors versus those undergoing recurrence or falling into the locally advanced or metastatic category, the complete picture of PDAC remains limited to a small subset of patients (~15%). Still, these efforts provide proof of concept on how measures of aberrant molecular mechanisms may inform clinical actionability using next-generation sequencing techniques.

New and promising strategies involving liquid biopsies are being developed as noninvasive methods of disease detection and monitoring.[42,43] Specifically, through the use of circulating tumor DNA (ctDNA) that is released in the blood by primary and metastatic tumors, one can theoretically obtain a full representation of the tumor heterogeneity that is present within each patient. Sausen and colleagues[36] demon-strated that somatic mutation calling can be made from ctDNA in PDAC patients to determine presence of subclinical, residual, or recurrent disease after surgical resec-tion. Detection of this ctDNA was correlated with disease progression that even pre-dated standard computed tomography imaging by an average of 6 months, suggesting that there may be an ability to treat subclinical disease before it is overtly clinically evident based on imaging. Using ultrasensitive digital polymerase chain re-action techniques, ctDNA was detected in 43% of surgically resectable (ie, lower stage) PDAC patients at the time of diagnosis. Although this study did not examine prediagnostic samples in patients before a clinical manifestation of disease, nonethe-less, it provides a potential screening approach through which high-risk patients, such as those with family history or germline mutations, can undergo noninvasive surveil-lance for the emergence of PDAC in time for curative surgical options.

Liquid biopsy has also shown promise in being able to genomically characterize tu-mors, and predict chemotherapy response and resistance using next generation tech-niques through both ctDNA and circulating tumor cells.[44–46] One can thus begin to imagine how tumor evolution and the emergence of new dominant clones can be iden-tified using these methods to guide therapeutic decisions in real time.

USING GENOMIC SEQUENCING TO GUIDE THERAPY

The genetic heterogeneity of PDAC as presented is unequivocally one of the many sig-nificant contributors to the intrinsic and acquired resistance that is characteristic of these cancers.[47] Targeting of subclonal populations will only lead to transient effects on tumor burden; thus, new strategies are required for therapeutic targeting of core pathways that are induced by founder events. By targeting convergent phenotypes that can be elucidated through genome sequencing of patient tumors, genomic infor-mation has the potential to guide individual patient therapies and outcomes.[48,49]

In patients with familial PDAC, information of deleterious germline variants may pro-vide some success in the cases of gene mutations in double strand break repair path-ways by using therapeutics aimed at compromising additional DNA repair mechanisms such as platinum-based therapies, mitomycin C, and PARP-1 (poly [ADP-ribose] polymerase 1) inhibitors.[50–52] By exploiting synthetic lethal approaches, which result in cancer-specific cell death through exploitation of cancer-specific mo-lecular aberrations, one can target base excision repair through PARP-1 inhibition, leading the accumulation of chaotic DNA damage.[53–55]

The ideal gene target in PDAC is Ras itself because it is the main oncogenic driver in more than 90% of these tumors, although efforts have so far proven ineffective.[56,57] Synthetic lethality screens for KRAS have not been successful, but there have been some data suggesting possible targeting of its downstream effectors such as the MEK-ERK, MAPK, and AKT (protein kinase B) signaling pathway[58]; unfortunately, recent clinical trials have shown unacceptable levels of toxicities in humans when 2 downstream Ras effectors are inhibited.[59] In the small subset of PDAC identified as harboring wild type KRAS, sequencing studies have found mutations in genes encoding RAS effector proteins including PIK3CA and BRAF.[11] In this small subset of cases, targeted therapies using BRAF and PI3 kinase inhibitors may beneficial.

SUMMARY

Further work remains to be done to determine all key components that drive PDAC. Exploiting nodal signaling pathways versus attacking genetic heterogeneity head on may be the best strategy in overcoming the advantages pancreatic cancers have over current treatment regimens. For now, stratification of subsets of patients based on defined molecular markers into clinical trials may prove beneficial in demonstrating the effectiveness of targeted therapies in these populations.

ACKNOWLEDGMENTS

This work was supported by the Cancer Prevention Research Institute of Texas [RP140106 to V.B.].

REFERENCES

1. Rahib L, Smith BD, Aizenberg R, et al. Projecting cancer incidence and deaths to 2030: the unexpected burden of thyroid, liver, and pancreas cancers in the United States. Cancer Res 2014;74(11):2913–21.
2. Siegel R, Ma J, Zou Z, et al. Cancer statistics, 2014. CA Cancer J Clin 2014;64(1): 9–29.
3. Yachida S, Jones S, Bozic I, et al. Distant metastasis occurs late during the genetic evolution of pancreatic cancer. Nature 2010;467(7319):1114–7.
4. Hruban RH, Adsay NV, Albores-Saavedra J, et al. Pancreatic intraepithelial neoplasia: a new nomenclature and classification system for pancreatic duct lesions. Am J Surg Pathol 2001;25(5):579–86.
5. Wu J, Jiao Y, Dal Molin M, et al. Whole-exome sequencing of neoplastic cysts of the pancreas reveals recurrent mutations in components of ubiquitin-dependent pathways. Proc Natl Acad Sci U S A 2011;108(52):21188–93.
6. Iacobuzio-Donahue CA, Klimstra DS, Adsay NV, et al. Dpc-4 protein is expressed in virtually all human intraductal papillary mucinous neoplasms of the pancreas: comparison with conventional ductal adenocarcinomas. Am J Pathol 2000; 157(3):755–61.
7. Iacobuzio-Donahue CA, Wilentz RE, Argani P, et al. Dpc4 protein in mucinous cystic neoplasms of the pancreas: frequent loss of expression in invasive carcinomas suggests a role in genetic progression. Am J Surg Pathol 2000;24(11):1544–8.
8. Wu J, Matthaei H, Maitra A, et al. Recurrent GNAS mutations define an unexpected pathway for pancreatic cyst development. Sci Transl Med 2011;3(92): 92ra66.
9. Jancik S, Drábek J, Radzioch D, et al. Clinical relevance of KRAS in human cancers. J Biomed Biotechnol 2010;2010:150960.

10. Jones S, Zhang X, Parsons DW, et al. Core signaling pathways in human pancreatic cancers revealed by global genomic analyses. Science 2008;321(5897): 1801–6.

11. Witkiewicz AK, McMillan EA, Balaji U, et al. Whole-exome sequencing of pancreatic cancer defines genetic diversity and therapeutic targets. Nat Commun 2015; 6:6744.

12. Campbell PJ, Yachida S, Mudie LJ, et al. The patterns and dynamics of genomic instability in metastatic pancreatic cancer. Nature 2010;467(7319):1109–13.

13. Caldas C, Hahn SA, da Costa LT, et al. Frequent somatic mutations and homozygous deletions of the p16 (MTS1) gene in pancreatic adenocarcinoma. Nat Genet 1994;8(1):27–32.

14. Schutte M, Hruban RH, Geradts J, et al. Abrogation of the Rb/p16 tumor-suppressive pathway in virtually all pancreatic carcinomas. Cancer Res 1997; 57(15):3126–30.

15. Sharpless NE. INK4a/ARF: a multifunctional tumor suppressor locus. Mutat Res 2005;576(1–2):22–38.

16. Scarpa A, Capelli P, Mukai K, et al. Pancreatic adenocarcinomas frequently show p53 gene mutations. Am J Pathol 1993;142(5):1534–43.

17. Maitra A, Adsay NV, Argani P, et al. Multicomponent analysis of the pancreatic adenocarcinoma progression model using a pancreatic intraepithelial neoplasia tissue microarray. Mod Pathol 2003;16(9):902–12.

18. Siegel PM, Massague J. Cytostatic and apoptotic actions of TGF-beta in homeostasis and cancer. Nat Rev Cancer 2003;3(11):807–21.

19. Yachida S, White CM, Naito Y, et al. Clinical significance of the genetic landscape of pancreatic cancer and implications for identification of potential long-term survivors. Clin Cancer Res 2012;18(22):6339–47.

20. Biankin AV, Morey AL, Lee CS, et al. DPC4/Smad4 expression and outcome in pancreatic ductal adenocarcinoma. J Clin Oncol 2002;20(23):4531–42.

21. Bardeesy N, Cheng KH, Berger JH, et al. Smad4 is dispensable for normal pancreas development yet critical in progression and tumor biology of pancreas cancer. Genes Dev 2006;20(22):3130–46.

22. Iacobuzio-Donahue CA, Fu B, Yachida S, et al. DPC4 gene status of the primary carcinoma correlates with patterns of failure in patients with pancreatic cancer. J Clin Oncol 2009;27(11):1806–13.

23. Shi C, Hruban RH, Klein AP. Familial pancreatic cancer. Arch Pathol Lab Med 2009;133(3):365–74.

24. Permuth-Wey J, Egan KM. Family history is a significant risk factor for pancreatic cancer: results from a systematic review and meta-analysis. Fam Cancer 2009; 8(2):109–17.

25. Su GH, Hruban RH, Bansal RK, et al. Germline and somatic mutations of the STK11/LKB1 Peutz-Jeghers gene in pancreatic and biliary cancers. Am J Pathol 1999;154(6):1835–40.

26. Witt H, Luck W, Hennies HC, et al. Mutations in the gene encoding the serine protease inhibitor, kazal type 1 are associated with chronic pancreatitis. Nat Genet 2000;25(2):213–6.

27. Lowenfels AB, Maisonneuve P, DiMagno EP, et al. Hereditary pancreatitis and the risk of pancreatic cancer. International Hereditary Pancreatitis Study Group. J Natl Cancer Inst 1997;89(6):442–6.

28. Lowenfels AB, Maisonneuve P, Whitcomb DC, et al. Cigarette smoking as a risk factor for pancreatic cancer in patients with hereditary pancreatitis. JAMA 2001;286(2):169–70.

29. Rutter JL, Bromley CM, Goldstein AM, et al. Heterogeneity of risk for melanoma and pancreatic and digestive malignancies: a melanoma case-control study. Cancer 2004;101(12):2809–16.
30. van der Heijden MS, Yeo CJ, Hruban RH, et al. Fanconi anemia gene mutations in young-onset pancreatic cancer. Cancer Res 2003;63(10):2585–8.
31. Goggins M, Schutte M, Lu J, et al. Germline BRCA2 gene mutations in patients with apparently sporadic pancreatic carcinomas. Cancer Res 1996;56(23):5360–4.
32. Lynch HT, Deters CA, Snyder CL, et al. BRCA1 and pancreatic cancer: pedigree findings and their causal relationships. Cancer Genet Cytogenet 2005;158(2): 119–25.
33. Hruban RH, Canto MI, Goggins M, et al. Update on familial pancreatic cancer. Adv Surg 2010;44:293–311.
34. Kastrinos F, Mukherjee B, Tayob N, et al. Risk of pancreatic cancer in families with Lynch syndrome. JAMA 2009;302(16):1790–5.
35. Roberts NJ, Jiao Y, Yu J, et al. ATM mutations in patients with hereditary pancreatic cancer. Cancer Discov 2012;2(1):41–6.
36. Sausen M, Phallen J, Adleff V, et al. Clinical implications of genomic alterations in the tumour and circulation of pancreatic cancer patients. Nat Commun 2015;6:7686.
37. Biankin AV, Waddell N, Kassahn KS, et al. Pancreatic cancer genomes reveal aberrations in axon guidance pathway genes. Nature 2012;491(7424):399–405.
38. Mehlen P, Delloye-Bourgeois C, Chedotal A. Novel roles for Slits and netrins: axon guidance cues as anticancer targets? Nat Rev Cancer 2011;11(3):188–97.
39. Kikuchi K, Kishino A, Konishi O, et al. In vitro and in vivo characterization of a novel semaphorin 3A inhibitor, SM-216289 or xanthofulvin. J Biol Chem 2003; 278(44):42985–91.
40. Waddell N, Pajic M, Patch AM, et al. Whole genomes redefine the mutational landscape of pancreatic cancer. Nature 2015;518(7540):495–501.
41. Jiang X, Hao HX, Growney JD, et al. Inactivating mutations of RNF43 confer wnt dependency in pancreatic ductal adenocarcinoma. Proc Natl Acad Sci U S A 2013;110(31):12649–54.
42. Bettegowda C, Sausen M, Leary RJ, et al. Detection of circulating tumor DNA in early- and late-stage human malignancies. Sci Transl Med 2014;6(224):224ra24.
43. Newman AM, Bratman SV, To J, et al. An ultrasensitive method for quantitating circulating tumor DNA with broad patient coverage. Nat Med 2014;20(5):548–54.
44. Ting DT, Wittner BS, Ligorio M, et al. Single-cell RNA sequencing identifies extracellular matrix gene expression by pancreatic circulating tumor cells. Cell Rep 2014;8(6):1905–18.
45. Murtaza M, Dawson SJ, Tsui DW, et al. Non-invasive analysis of acquired resistance to cancer therapy by sequencing of plasma DNA. Nature 2013; 497(7447):108–12.
46. Yu KH, Ricigliano M, Hidalgo M, et al. Pharmacogenomic modeling of circulating tumor and invasive cells for prediction of chemotherapy response and resistance in pancreatic cancer. Clin Cancer Res 2014;20(20):5281–9.
47. Misale S, Yaeger R, Hobor S, et al. Emergence of KRAS mutations and acquired resistance to anti-EGFR therapy in colorectal cancer. Nature 2012;486(7404): 532–6.
48. Barrett MT, Lenkiewicz E, Evers L, et al. Clonal evolution and therapeutic resistance in solid tumors. Front Pharmacol 2013;4:2.
49. Haeno H, Gonen M, Davis MB, et al. Computational modeling of pancreatic cancer reveals kinetics of metastasis suggesting optimum treatment strategies. Cell 2012;148(1–2):362–75.

50. Xia B, Sheng Q, Nakanishi K, et al. Control of BRCA2 cellular and clinical functions by a nuclear partner, PALB2. Mol Cell 2006;22(6):719–29.

51. Villarroel MC, Rajeshkumar NV, Garrido-Laguna I, et al. Personalizing cancer treatment in the age of global genomic analyses: PALB2 gene mutations and the response to DNA damaging agents in pancreatic cancer. Mol Cancer Ther 2011;10(1):3–8.

52. van der Heijden MS, Brody JR, Dezentje DA, et al. In vivo therapeutic responses contingent on Fanconi anemia/BRCA2 status of the tumor. Clin Cancer Res 2005; 11(20):7508–15.

53. Farmer H, McCabe N, Lord CJ, et al. Targeting the DNA repair defect in BRCA mutant cells as a therapeutic strategy. Nature 2005;434(7035):917–21.

54. McCabe N, Lord CJ, Tutt AN, et al. BRCA2-deficient CAPAN-1 cells are extremely sensitive to the inhibition of Poly (ADP-Ribose) polymerase: an issue of potency. Cancer Biol Ther 2005;4(9):934–6.

55. McLornan DP, List A, Mufti GJ. Applying synthetic lethality for the selective targeting of cancer. N Engl J Med 2014;371(18):1725–35.

56. Marcotte R, Brown KR, Suarez F, et al. Essential gene profiles in breast, pancreatic, and ovarian cancer cells. Cancer Discov 2012;2(2):172–89.

57. Ward AF, Braun BS, Shannon KM. Targeting oncogenic ras signaling in hematologic malignancies. Blood 2012;120(17):3397–406.

58. Collisson EA, Trejo CL, Silva JM, et al. A central role for RAF–>MEK–>ERK signaling in the genesis of pancreatic ductal adenocarcinoma. Cancer Discov 2012;2(8):685–93.

59. Shimizu T, Tolcher AW, Papadopoulos KP, et al. The clinical effect of the dual-targeting strategy involving PI3K/AKT/mTOR and RAS/MEK/ERK pathways in patients with advanced cancer. Clin Cancer Res 2012;18(8):2316–25.

Optimal Imaging Modalities for the Diagnosis and Staging of Periampullary Masses

Mahmoud M. Al-Hawary, MD[a],*, Ravi K. Kaza, MD[b],
Isaac R. Francis, MD[c]

KEYWORDS

- Pancreas • Periampullary • Tumor • Staging • MDCT • MRI • MRCP

KEY POINTS

- High-quality cross-sectional diagnostic imaging has a central pivotal role in evaluation of patients with known or suspected periampullary masses.
- The most commonly used imaging tools include contrast-enhanced multidetector computed tomography and contrast-enhanced MRI with MR cholangiopancreatography.
- The role of imaging is to identify periampullary masses, assess the presence or absence of tumor extension to surrounding vessels and organs, and identify distant metastasis.
- Accurate and complete reporting of relevant imaging findings should be done through the use of template reporting ensuring proper staging and optimal treatment strategies.

INTRODUCTION

Diagnostic imaging is the first step in the evaluation of patients presenting with clinical signs and symptoms referred to the pancreatobiliary system. The most common indications for imaging include painless obstructive jaundice, epigastric pain (suspected of pancreatic or biliary origin), or unexplained pancreatitis in patients older than 40.[1] The most commonly used imaging modalities include transabdominal ultrasound, contrast-enhanced multidetector computed tomography (MDCT), and contrast-enhanced MRI with MR cholangiopancreatography (MRCP).[2] The role of each imaging

Disclosures: Non relevant.
[a] Department of Radiology, University Hospital, University of Michigan, Room B1 D502, 1500 East Medical Center Drive, Ann Arbor, MI 48109, USA; [b] Department of Radiology, University Hospital, University of Michigan, Room B1 D501, 1500 East Medical Center Drive, Ann Arbor, MI 48109, USA; [c] Department of Radiology, University Hospital, University of Michigan, Room B1 D540, 1500 East Medical Center Drive, Ann Arbor, MI 48109, USA
* Corresponding author.
E-mail address: alhawary@med.umich.edu

Surg Oncol Clin N Am 25 (2016) 239–253
http://dx.doi.org/10.1016/j.soc.2015.12.001
1055-3207/16/$ – see front matter © 2016 Elsevier Inc. All rights reserved.

surgonc.theclinics.com

modality varies depending on the clinical presentation and if malignancy is highly suspected or already known from prior imaging.

Transabdominal ultrasound examination can serve as a screening test to detect the presence of biliary dilatation in patient presenting with jaundice and can be helpful in identifying gallbladder stones and/or choledocholithiasis as the cause of the biliary dilatation. However, often the distal common bile duct and pancreatic head region are poorly visualized owing to shadowing from overlying gas limiting the overall sensitivity of ultrasound in screening for pancreatic head or periampullary masses. In patients presenting with painless jaundice, suspected distal common bile duct obstruction, unexplained pancreatitis, or a high suspicion of a pancreatic head mass, the most commonly obtained imaging study is either MDCT or MRI/MRCP. Both examinations provide high contrast and spatial resolutions and can help in assessing the presence of biliary or pancreatic duct dilatation, identifying the level of the biliary or pancreatic duct obstruction, and frequently diagnosing the etiology of the obstruction accurately. A detailed description of these imaging techniques and imaging findings in patients presenting with periampullary masses are discussed.

PERIAMPULLARY MASSES

Masses that can affect the periampullary region can arise either from the pancreatic head, duodenum, Ampulla of Vater or distal common bile duct. These include but are not limited to pancreatic ductal adenocarcinoma (PDA), pancreatic neuroendocrine tumors, cystic pancreatic neoplasms, ampullary adenoma or adenocarcinoma, duodenal adenocarcinoma, and extrahepatic cholangiocarcinoma.[3,4] PDA represent the most common tumor detected on cross-sectional imaging for painless jaundice. It is a very aggressive malignancy with a reported survival rate as low as 4% at 5 years after diagnosis.[5] Despite its low incidence comprising only 3% of the estimated new cases of cancer in the United States, PDA is currently the fourth most common cause of cancer-related death in both males and females.[6] Currently, complete surgical resection without microscopic residual disease or positive margins (R0 resection) offers the best hope of improved survival and potential cure in newly diagnosed patients. Unfortunately, this cannot be achieved in the majority of cases because no more than 15% to 20% of patients have potentially resectable disease at the time of presentation.[7,8] Patients with margin-positive resection at surgery have been shown to have similar survival rates to patients with unresectable disease.[9] Accordingly, these patients would not benefit from the surgical resection and should be spared major surgery with its associated mortality and significant morbidity. Staging of periampullary masses and assessment of the feasibility of complete surgical resection by imaging remains of paramount importance in determining the therapeutic plan. The most relevant determinant of surgical resection in almost all cases is the presence or absence of peripancreatic vessel involvement by the tumor and the absence of distant metastasis.

CROSS-SECTIONAL IMAGING TECHNIQUES
Multidetector Computed Tomography

MDCT is the most commonly used cross-sectional imaging modality in the evaluation and staging of periampullary lesions owing to its widespread availability and high spatial resolution, making it a favorable first choice modality in most institutions. Performance of high-quality MDCT examination in high-volume referral centers specialized in imaging and treating pancreatic diseases has been shown to improve preoperative staging and alter management in a significant proportion of patients.[10] A dedicated pancreatic protocol MDCT includes dual phase acquisition through the upper abdomen including the liver and the pancreas in the pancreatic and the portal venous phases of iodinated intravenous contrast enhancement.[11] The first phase of acquisition (pancreatic phase) is obtained around 40 to 50 seconds after the start of the intravenous contrast administration. This phase provides several important advantages in assessing pancreatic pathologies and the adjacent vasculature. During this phase, there is maximal enhancement of the pancreatic parenchyma, which provides the best visual contrast between hypoattenuating masses and the enhancing pancreatic parenchyma (eg, PDA). Arterially enhancing lesions such as neuroendocrine tumors are better depicted on this phase owing to their early contrast enhancement (**Fig. 1**). A second advantage is the assessment of the peripancreatic vessels, including the common hepatic artery, celiac artery, and superior mesenteric artery. The second phase of acquisition is obtained around 65 to 70 seconds after the start of intravenous contrast administration, which coincides with the portal venous phase. This phase also provides several important advantages including assessment of solid intraabdominal organs for metastasis, most importantly the liver, in addition to evaluation of the peripancreatic venous system including the main portal vein, splenic vein and superior mesenteric vein for possible involvement with tumor.

Thin slice acquisition with subcentimeter slice selection is currently widely available on almost all multidetector CT scanners and should be obtained in every case for optimal evaluation and staging. The thin slices offer significant improvement in the spatial resolution with the acquisition of near isotropic voxels, which offer similar resolution in any plane of image reformation (ie, sagittal, coronal, or oblique)[11,12] (**Fig. 2**). This significant increase in the spatial resolution can help to identify small focal pancreatic lesions and assess the contour of the peripancreatic vessels for possible involvement.

A minimum of 300 mg iodine per milliliter concentration of iodine for the nonionic intravenous contrast medium should be used to improve the contrast to noise ratio profile in assessing the degree of parenchymal organ enhancement and the vascular structures. Reduced scan kilovolts peak setting (<120 KVp) has been shown to lead to increased attenuation of enhancing structures containing high concentration of the iodinated contrast without degrading the diagnostic imaging quality.[13,14] This can potentially help to identify small enhancing structures or lesions such as neuroendocrine tumors and can also potentially help in reducing the amount of intravenous contrast administered.

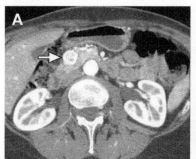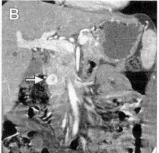

Fig. 1. Pancreatic neuroendocrine tumor. (*A*) Axial and (*B*) coronal contrast-enhanced multidetector computed tomography images in the pancreatic phase show an enhancing pancreatic tumor in the pancreatic head (*arrow*), which is enhancing more than the background pancreatic parenchyma consistent with a neuroendocrine tumor.

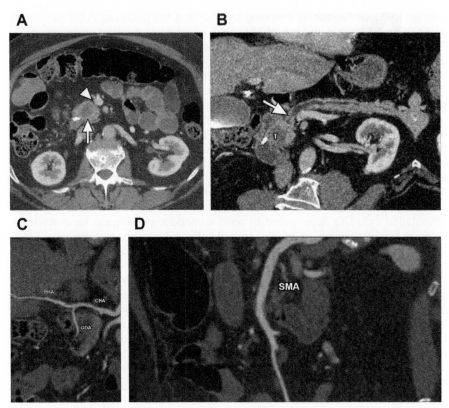

Fig. 2. High-quality dedicated multidetector computed tomography (MDCT) evaluation of pancreatic head adenocarcinoma. (*A*) Axial contrast-enhanced MDCT image through the pancreatic head demonstrate an ill-defined hypodense mass (*arrow*) consistent with pancreatic adenocarcinoma. There is no contact with the adjacent superior mesenteric vein or artery (*arrowhead*), suggesting a resectable tumor. (*B*) Curved reformatted image through the pancreas demonstrate the level of pancreatic duct obstruction (*arrow*) and outlines the edge of the tumor (T). (*C*) High-resolution curved reformatted image through the celiac axis branches improves the assessment of the peripancreatic vessels confirming the lack of tumor contact with the common hepatic artery (CHA), gastroduodenal artery (GDA), and proper hepatic artery (PHA). (*D*) Additional curved reformat through the superior mesenteric artery (SMA) demonstrate lack of tumor contact.

Neutral or low-density oral contrast (such as water or low-density barium suspension) should be used instead of the high attenuation or positive oral contrast used in routine CT examinations. The main role of the neutral or low-density oral contrast is to adequately distend the stomach and duodenum, which helps in assessing local tumor invasion. The neutral contrast agent also avoids streak artifacts associated with the high density positive oral contrast on the 3-dimensional vascular reconstructed images.

MRI

Contrast-enhanced MRI with MRCP has been shown to be of equal accuracy to MDCT for the staging of periampullary masses s[15–17] (**Fig. 3**). However, MRI examinations are not commonly obtained as first-line imaging studies in most institutions,

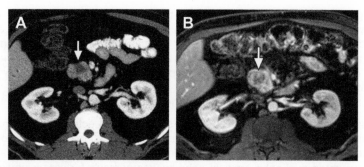

Fig. 3. Pancreatic head mass on multidetector computed tomography (MDCT) and MRI. (*A*) Axial contrast-enhanced MDCT and (*B*) T1-weighted gradient echo with fat suppression images through the pancreatic head demonstrate a focal mass (*arrow*) completely surrounded by pancreatic parenchyma with no extension beyond the contour of the pancreas suggesting a resectable tumor. Both imaging modalities have comparable accuracy for staging pancreatic adenocarcinoma.

mostly owing to their limited availability, higher cost, and the more challenging technical component of performing the examination. Both 1.5- and 3-T magnet systems can be used to obtain high-resolution images of the pancreas and upper abdomen after the administration of gadolinium containing contrast agents (**Fig. 4**). The main

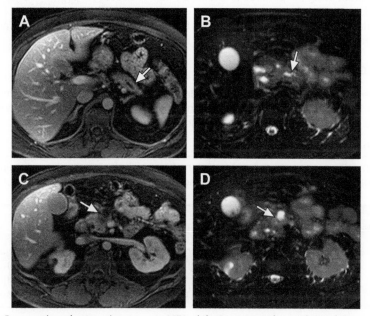

Fig. 4. Pancreatic adenocarcinoma on MRI. (*A*) Contrast-enhanced axial T1-weighted gradient echo with fat suppression and (*B*) axial T2-weighted fast spin echo with fat suppression images through the pancreas demonstrate dilated pancreatic duct in the distal body (*arrow*) concerning for proximal obstructing lesion. (*C, D*) Similar images at a lower level demonstrate a focal mass in the pancreatic head showing low signal intensity on the T1-weighted images (*arrow* in *C*) and high signal intensity on the T2-weighted images (*arrow* in *D*).

advantages of MRI include the higher signal-to-noise ratio compared with the MDCT, which would be most useful in evaluating focal pancreatic masses that are not detected on CT examination and in better evaluation of the biliary or pancreatic duct for assessment of localized stricture. An additional advantage of MRI is the specificity in characterizing indeterminate or suspicious liver lesions identified on the CT examinations to exclude metastasis.

MRI protocol includes the acquisition of the following sequences:

- Axial and coronal T2-weighted single shot fast spin echo images, which are mainly used as localizers to generally assess the location of the pathology and established different planes of acquisition.
- T1-weighted dual echo gradient echo images primarily for assessing lipid and fat-containing lesions (**Fig. 5**).
- T2-weighted fast spin echo with fat saturation to highlight the high signal intensity noted frequently in most periampullary malignant lesions.
- Precontrast and dynamic multiphasic acquisition postcontrast T1-weighted gradient echo with fat saturation after gadolinium administration, which helps to evaluate the enhanced pancreatic parenchyma and hypoenhancing or hyperenhancing focal periampullary lesions. Assessment of the peripancreatic arterial and venous structures can also be assessed during this acquisition.
- MRCP protocol includes the acquisition of heavily T2-weighted 3-dimensional fast recovery fast spin echo images with thin axial or thick slab single shot fast spin echo images. These heavily T2-weighted images highlight the endogenous contrast using the pancreatic and biliary fluid to assess for presence and level of strictures (**Fig. 6**).
- Diffusion-weighted imaging can also be obtained, which can help in the assessment of extrapancreatic metastasis, in particular within the liver.

IMAGING FINDINGS

The role of cross-sectional imaging modalities is to detect the focal periampullary masses, assess for the presence or absence of tumor extension to surrounding vessels and organs, and to identify distant metastasis.

Tumor Detection

PDA typically is seen as a focal low density or signal intensity mass against the background of the enhancing normal pancreatic parenchyma and is best visualized

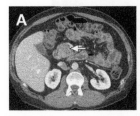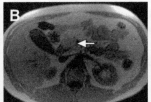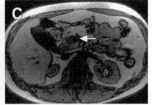

Fig. 5. Role of MRI in evaluating suspected lesions in the pancreas. (*A*) Axial contrast-enhanced multidetector computed tomography (MDCT) image through the pancreatic head demonstrate an ill-defined hypodense masslike area (*arrow*) concerning for pancreatic adenocarcinoma. Lack of secondary findings such as distal parenchymal atrophy and biliary/pancreatic duct dilatation prompted further evaluation with MRI. (*B*) In-phase and (*C*) out-of-phase T1-weighted gradient echo images demonstrate loss of signal in the same region on the out of phase images (*arrows*) consistent with a benign area of focal fat replacement.

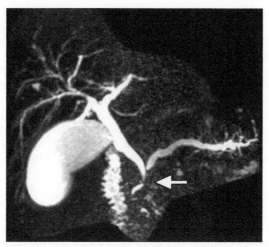

Fig. 6. Maximum intensity projection (MIP) image from T2-weighted 3-dimensional fast recovery fast spin echo sequence shows focal stricture in the distal common bile duct and proximal pancreatic duct at the same level (*arrow*) consistent with double duct sign, which is a common sign of obstruction secondary to a malignant mass in the pancreatic head.

on the pancreatic phase of acquisition (**Fig. 7**). A small percentage of small PDAs are isoattenuating on CT and cannot be discriminated readily from the surrounding pancreatic parenchyma.[18,19] Indirect signs such as mass effect, contour change, distal pancreatic parenchymal atrophy, and abruptly interrupted main pancreatic duct, despite the lack of visualization of mass, are important indicators for the presence of tumor.[20] These small isoattenuating tumors are best assessed with either MRI examination or endoscopic ultrasonography. Pancreatic neuroendocrine tumors on the other hand typically demonstrate increased enhancement compared

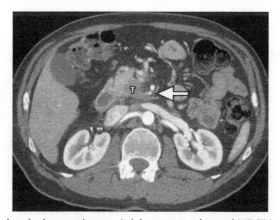

Fig. 7. Pancreatic head adenocarcinoma. Axial contrast-enhanced MDCT image through the pancreatic head demonstrate an ill-defined hypodense mass (T) consistent with pancreatic adenocarcinoma. There is less than 180° tumor contact with the adjacent superior mesenteric artery (*arrow*), suggesting a borderline resectable tumor.

with the background pancreas on the pancreatic phase imaging.[21,22] The pattern of enhancement of pancreatic neuroendocrine tumors can be either homogenous, particularly in small lesions, or heterogeneous with areas of central necrosis, especially in larger lesions. The presence of calcification in these lesions helps in differentiating them from other pancreatic tumors, particularly PDA. Extrahepatic cholangiocarcinomas demonstrate delayed progressive enhancement and are best assessed on MR examinations.[23,24] Ampullary masses are usually difficult to assess on cross-sectional imaging owing to their endoluminal location and are not routinely visualized; however, cross-sectional imaging evaluation remains of value in these cases to assess for extension beyond the ampulla or duodenal wall and to assess vascular involvement as well as the presence of metastasis.[25,26]

Assessment of Tumor Extension

Once a periampullary mass is identified, the next step in the assessment is appropriate staging of the disease and determination of tumor extent to evaluate for potential resectability. This is primarily achieved by assessing whether there is invasion of surrounding vessels including the common hepatic artery, celiac axis, superior mesenteric artery, main portal vein, and superior mesenteric vein, and excluding presence of distant metastasis (**Fig. 8**). Tumor involvement of the adjacent vessels is classified based on the degree of contact between the tumor and the circumference of the involved vessel and is primarily divided into less than or equal to 180° or greater than 180° (**Fig. 9**). Masses with greater than 180° contact with the adjacent vessels indicate high specificity for vascular invasion and consequently tumor unresectability.[27,28] Additional findings of contour deformity and change in the vessel caliber are also considered signs of vascular invasion. Less than 180° contact with the involved vessel would be generally classified as borderline resectable, which have less likelihood of vascular invasion however could benefit from neoadjuvant therapy to decrease tumor size and improve the chances of complete R0 resection at the time of surgery. The NCCN Clinical Practice Guidelines in Oncology (NCCN Guidelines®) provide a classification scheme of resectable, borderline resectable or unresectable tumor depending on the location of the tumor and extent of vascular contact[29] (**Table 1**). Additional advantages of imaging include the identification of vascular anatomic variants that can both affect the staging and the surgical approach to tumor resection (**Fig. 10**).

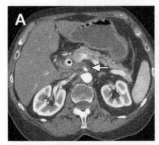
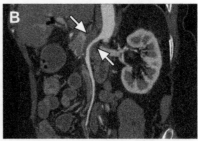

Fig. 8. Superior mesenteric artery (SMA) tumor contact. (*A*) Axial contrast-enhanced multidetector computed tomography (MDCT) image through the pancreatic head demonstrate an ill-defined mass surrounding the SMA (*arrow*) surrounding more than 180° of the vessel circumference. (*B*) Curved reformatted image through the SMA displays the entire length of the vessel and confirms the circumferential contact between the tumor and the vessel (*arrows*) and the mild narrowing in the vessel caliber.

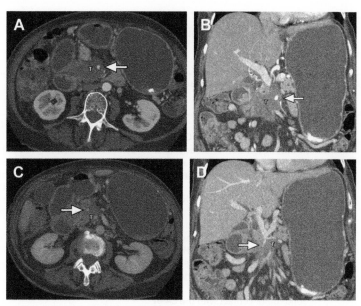

Fig. 9. Unresectable pancreatic head adenocarcinoma. (*A*) Axial and (*B*) coronal contrast-enhanced multidetector computed tomography (MDCT) images in the pancreatic phase through the pancreatic head demonstrate an ill-defined hypodense mass arising from the pancreatic head (T) consistent with pancreatic adenocarcinoma. There is circumferential tumor contact with the adjacent superior mesenteric artery (SMA) (*arrow* in A), which can be seen on both views. There is tumor involvement of the jejunal branches of the SMA (*arrow* in image B). (*C*) Axial and (*D*) coronal contrast-enhanced MDCT images in the portal venous demonstrate the circumferential contact of the tumor (T) with the superior mesenteric vein (*arrow*). The coronal view better displays the level of SMV involvement and level of occlusion.

Distant Metastasis

Frequent sites of the metastasis from PDA include peripancreatic lymph nodes, liver, peritoneal cavity and lung. Typically metastatic lesions to the liver seem to be hypodense on MDCT and may demonstrate a targetlike appearance (**Fig. 11**). Metastatic disease can develop in a relatively short time interval and therefore repeat imaging before surgery should be considered if there is a significant interval since the initial staging (**Fig. 12**). Small subcentimeter lesions detected on CT examination are often too small to characterize by CT examination and cannot be characterized accurately as cystic or benign and would be therefore considered indeterminate. These lesions can be further evaluated with MRI examination and/or biopsy for definite characterization and to confirm or exclude metastasis.

For lymph node assessment, generally enlarged lymph nodes measuring more than 1 cm in short axis diameter and with the presence of central necrosis are highly suggestive of metastatic involvement. Regional lymph node involvement at the site of the tumor are not a contraindication to surgery because these lymph nodes can be resected with the primary tumor; however, nonregional lymph node involvement (ie, retroperitoneal lymph nodes) would be considered as metastatic disease and would exclude the patient from curative intent (**Fig. 13**). In the postoperative setting,

Table 1
Criteria for classification of tumors resectability status

Resectability Stage	Arterial Contact	Venous Contact
Resectable	No arterial tumor contact present	No tumor contact of the SMV or PV or solid tumor contact of $\leq 180°$ without vein irregularity

Borderline	• Pancreatic head:
	  ○ Solid tumor contact with CHA without extension to celiac axis or hepatic artery bifurcation allowing for safe and complete resection and reconstruction
	  ○ Solid tumor contact with the SMA of $\leq 180°$
	  ○ Presence of variant arterial anatomy with tumor contact (eg, accessory RHA, replaced RHA, replaced CHA and the origin of replaced or accessory artery)
	• Pancreatic body/tail:
	  ○ Solid tumor contact with the CA of $\leq 180°$
	  ○ Solid tumor contact with the CA of $>180°$ without involvement of the aorta and with intact and uninvolved GDA
		• Solid tumor contact $>180°$ with the SMV or PV
		• Solid tumor contact $\leq 180°$ with contour irregularity of the vein and or thrombosis but with suitable vessel proximal and distal to the site of involvement allowing for safe and complete resection and vein replacement
		• Solid tumor contact with the IVC

Unresectable	Distant metastasis (including nonregional lymph node metastasis)
	• Pancreatic head:
	  ○ Solid tumor contact with SMA $>180°$
	  ○ Solid tumor contact with the CA $>180°$
	  ○ Solid tumor contact with the first SMA branch
	• Pancreatic body/tail:
	  ○ Solid tumor contact of $>180°$ with the SMA or CA
	  ○ Solid tumor contact with the CA and aortic involvement
		• Pancreatic head:
		  ○ Unreconstructable SMV/PV tumor involvement or occlusion (can be owing to tumor or bland thrombus)
		  ○ Solid tumor contact with the most proximal draining jejunal vein into SMV
		• Pancreatic body/tail:
		  ○ Unreconstructable SMV/PV tumor involvement or occlusion (can be owing to tumor or bland thrombus)

Abbreviations: CA, celiac axis; CHA, common hepatic artery; GDA, gastroduodenal artery; IVC, inferior vena cava; PV, portal vein; RHA, right hepatic artery; SMA, superior mesenteric artery; SMV, superior mesenteric vein.

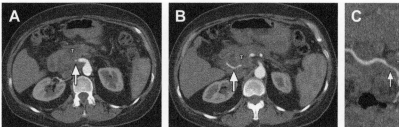

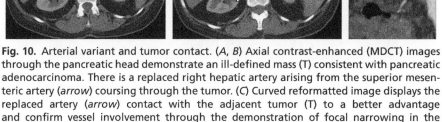

Fig. 10. Arterial variant and tumor contact. (*A, B*) Axial contrast-enhanced (MDCT) images through the pancreatic head demonstrate an ill-defined mass (T) consistent with pancreatic adenocarcinoma. There is a replaced right hepatic artery arising from the superior mesenteric artery (*arrow*) coursing through the tumor. (*C*) Curved reformatted image displays the replaced artery (*arrow*) contact with the adjacent tumor (T) to a better advantage and confirm vessel involvement through the demonstration of focal narrowing in the vessel caliber.

cross-sectional imaging is also helpful in evaluating for tumor recurrence locally or in the pancreatic remnant (**Fig. 14**).

STRUCTURED REPORTING

Using a structured report, instead of freestyle dictations, ensures an accurate, detailed, and comprehensive radiology report to optimize patient care and thus outcome.[30,31] This can be achieved through the use of reporting templates, which requires the entry of imaging findings into defined fields pertaining to all the information that is needed in the staging of tumor. An additional advantage of the structured report is facilitating the use of standardized lexicon that is mutually accepted, understood, and used by the various medical specialties involved in the care of these

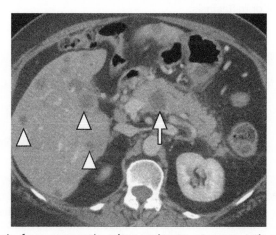

Fig. 11. Metastasis from pancreatic adenocarcinoma at presentation. Axial contrast-enhanced multidetector computed tomography (MDCT) image at the level of the liver obtained at the time of diagnosis demonstrate focal mass in the pancreatic body (*arrow*) corresponding to the primary pancreatic tumor. Multiple hypodense masses with enhancing rim are present in the liver (*arrowheads*) corresponding with metastatic deposits.

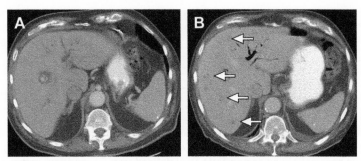

Fig. 12. Metastasis from pancreatic adenocarcinoma. (*A*) Axial contrast-enhanced multidetector computed tomography (MDCT) image at the level of the liver obtained at the time of pancreatic adenocarcinoma diagnosis (tumor not shown) demonstrates no focal hepatic lesions. (*B*) Follow-up examination after 4 weeks demonstrates multiple hypodense lesions with enhancing rim in the liver (*arrows*) corresponding with interval development of metastatic deposit.

patients. Structured reporting in patients with PDA has been shown to provide superior evaluation of the tumor and facilitate surgical planning.[32] Several professional organizations such as the Society of Abdominal Radiology, American Pancreatic Association, American College of Radiology, and Radiological Society of North America have introduced several standardized structured templates for reporting into radiology practice. One of these templates developed by the Society of Abdominal Radiology and American Pancreatic Association, which was adopted by the National Comprehensive Cancer Network, has been published recently.[33] The template includes all pertinent imaging findings including tumor characteristics (ie, size, location, biliary or pancreatic ductal dilatation, and presence of calcifications), vascular contact with the peripancreatic arteries and veins (including description of vascular variants) and whether there are pathologic lymph nodes (regional or nonregional), surrounding organ involvement or metastasis.

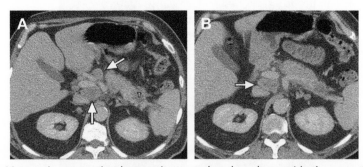

Fig. 13. Metastatic pancreatic adenocarcinoma to lymph nodes outside the operative field. (*A*, *B*) Axial contrast-enhanced multidetector computed tomography (MDCT) images in the portal venous phase demonstrates a hypodense lesion (T) in the pancreatic tail consistent with pancreatic adenocarcinoma. Enlarged porta hepatis and portocaval lymph nodes are seen (*arrows*). The primary pancreatic would have been classified as resectable, but the presence of the metastatic lymph nodes outside the operative field (distal pancreatectomy) changes the classification to metastatic disease.

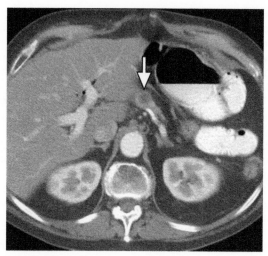

Fig. 14. Tumor recurrence after resection. Axial contrast-enhanced multidetector computed tomography (MDCT) image through the pancreatic body after a Whipple procedure and resection of previously diagnosed pancreatic adenocarcinoma in the pancreatic head demonstrate a new focal ill-defined hypodense mass (*arrow*) in the proximal remaining portion of the pancreas consistent with recurrent tumor.

SUMMARY

Cross-sectional diagnostic imaging including MDCT and MRI/MRCP play an essential role in the evaluation of patients with known or suspected periampullary masses. Both imaging modalities can accurately identify and localize the focal periampullary masses establishing the diagnosis. Moreover, these imaging modalities play a critical role in the assessment of the patient for treatment allocation based on the local staging of the tumor and excluding the presence of distant metastasis. MDCT is the most frequently obtained modality owing to widespread availability and familiarity of most radiologists with the technique and imaging findings. MRI with MRCP can be used interchangeably with CT where access and expertise is available.

REFERENCES

1. Mujica VR, Barkin JS, Go VL. Acute pancreatitis secondary to pancreatic carcinoma. Study group participants. Pancreas 2000;21(4):329–32.
2. Lalani T, Couto CA, Rosen MP, et al. ACR appropriateness criteria jaundice. J Am Coll Radiol 2013;10(6):402–9.
3. Nikolaidis P, Hammond NA, Day K, et al. Imaging features of benign and malignant ampullary and periampullary lesions. Radiographics 2014;34(3):624–41.
4. Katabathina VS, Dasyam AK, Dasyam N, et al. Adult bile duct strictures: role of MR imaging and MR cholangiopancreatography in characterization. Radiographics 2014;34(3):565–86.
5. Vincent A, Herman J, Schulick R, et al. Pancreatic cancer. Lancet 2011; 378(9791):607–20.
6. Siegel R, Naishadham D, Jemal A. Cancer, statistics, 2012. CA Cancer J Clin 2012;62(1):10–29.

7. Conlon KC, Klimstra DS, Brennan MF. Long-term survival after curative resection for pancreatic ductal adenocarcinoma. Clinicopathologic analysis of 5-year survivors. Ann Surg 1996;223(3):273–9.

8. Varadhachary GR, Tamm EP, Abbruzzese JL, et al. Borderline resectable pancreatic cancer: definitions, management, and role of preoperative therapy. Ann Surg Oncol 2006;13(8):1035–46.

9. Bilimoria KY, Talamonti MS, Sener SF, et al. Effect of hospital volume on margin status after pancreaticoduodenectomy for cancer. J Am Coll Surg 2008;207(4): 510–9.

10. Walters DM, Lapar DJ, de Lange EE, et al. Pancreas-protocol imaging at a high-volume center leads to improved preoperative staging of pancreatic ductal adenocarcinoma. Ann Surg Oncol 2011;18(10):2764–71.

11. Ichikawa T, Erturk SM, Sou H, et al. MDCT of pancreatic adenocarcinoma: optimal imaging phases and multiplanar reformatted imaging. AJR Am J Roentgenol 2006;187(6):1513–20.

12. Tamm EP, Balachandran A, Bhosale P, et al. Update on 3D and multiplanar MDCT in the assessment of biliary and pancreatic pathology. Abdom Imaging 2009; 34(1):64–74.

13. Kalva SP, Sahani DV, Hahn PF, et al. Using the K-edge to improve contrast conspicuity and to lower radiation dose with a 16-MDCT: a phantom and human study. J Comput Assist Tomogr 2006;30(3):391–7.

14. Clark ZE, Bolus DN, Little MD, et al. Abdominal rapid-kVp-switching dual-energy MDCT with reduced IV contrast compared to conventional MDCT with standard weight-based IV contrast: an intra-patient comparison. Abdom Imaging 2015; 40(4):852–8.

15. Sheridan MB, Ward J, Guthrie JA, et al. Dynamic contrast-enhanced MR imaging and dual-phase helical CT in the preoperative assessment of suspected pancreatic cancer: a comparative study with receiver operating characteristic analysis. AJR Am J Roentgenol 1999;173(3):583–90.

16. Tamm EP, Bhosale PR, Lee JH. Pancreatic ductal adenocarcinoma: ultrasound, computed tomography, and magnetic resonance imaging features. Semin Ultrasound CT MR 2007;28(5):330–8.

17. Koelblinger C, Ba-Ssalamah A, Goetzinger P, et al. Gadobenate dimeglumine-enhanced 3.0-T MR imaging versus multiphasic 64-detector row CT: prospective evaluation in patients suspected of having pancreatic cancer. Radiology 2011; 259(3):757–66.

18. Kim JH, Park SH, Yu ES, et al. Visually isoattenuating pancreatic adenocarcinoma at dynamic-enhanced CT: frequency, clinical and pathologic characteristics, and diagnosis at imaging examinations. Radiology 2010;257(1):87–96.

19. Yoon SH, Lee JM, Cho JY, et al. Small (</= 20 mm) pancreatic adenocarcinomas: analysis of enhancement patterns and secondary signs with multiphasic multidetector CT. Radiology 2011;259(2):442–52.

20. Prokesch RW, Chow LC, Beaulieu CF, et al. Isoattenuating pancreatic adenocarcinoma at multi-detector row CT: secondary signs. Radiology 2002;224(3): 764–8.

21. Manfredi R, Bonatti M, Mantovani W, et al. Non-hyperfunctioning neuroendocrine tumours of the pancreas: MR imaging appearance and correlation with their biological behaviour. Eur Radiol 2013;23(11):3029–39.

22. Semelka RC, Custodio CM, Cem Balci N, et al. Neuroendocrine tumors of the pancreas: spectrum of appearances on MRI. J Magn Reson Imaging 2000; 11(2):141–8.

23. Gore RM, Shelhamer RP. Biliary tract neoplasms: diagnosis and staging. Cancer Imaging 2007;7 Spec No A:S15–23.
24. Kim MJ, Choi JY, Chung YE. Evaluation of biliary malignancies using multidetector-row computed tomography. J Comput Assist Tomogr 2010;34(4): 496–505.
25. Hennedige TP, Neo WT, Venkatesh SK. Imaging of malignancies of the biliary tract- an update. Cancer Imaging 2014;14:14.
26. Raman SP, Fishman EK. Abnormalities of the distal common bile duct and ampulla: diagnostic approach and differential diagnosis using multiplanar reformations and 3D imaging. AJR Am J Roentgenol 2014;203(1):17–28.
27. Wong JC, Lu DS. Staging of pancreatic adenocarcinoma by imaging studies. Clin Gastroenterol Hepatol 2008;6(12):1301–8.
28. Lu DS, Reber HA, Krasny RM, et al. Local staging of pancreatic cancer: criteria for unresectability of major vessels as revealed by pancreatic-phase, thin-section helical CT. AJR Am J Roentgenol 1997;168(6):1439–43.
29. Referenced with permission from the NCCN Clinical Practice Guidelines in Oncology (NCCN Guidelines®) for Pancreatic Adenocarcinoma V.2.2015. © National Comprehensive Cancer Network, Inc 2015. All rights reserved. Accessed October 27, 2015. To view the most recent and complete version of the guideline, go online to NCCN.org. NATIONAL COMPREHENSIVE CANCER NETWORK®, NCCN®, NCCN GUIDELINES®, and all other NCCN Content are trademarks owned by the National Comprehensive Cancer Network.
30. Kee D, Zalcberg JR. Radiology reporting templates in oncology: a time for change. J Med Imaging Radiat Oncol 2009;53(6):511–3.
31. Sistrom CL, Honeyman-Buck J. Free text versus structured format: information transfer efficiency of radiology reports. AJR Am J Roentgenol 2005;185(3): 804–12.
32. Brook OR, Brook A, Vollmer CM, et al. Structured reporting of multiphasic CT for pancreatic cancer: potential effect on staging and surgical planning. Radiology 2015;274(2):464–72.
33. Al-Hawary MM, Francis IR, Chari ST, et al. Pancreatic ductal adenocarcinoma radiology reporting template: consensus statement of the society of abdominal radiology and the American Pancreatic Association. Gastroenterology 2014; 146(1):291–304.e291.

Role of Endoscopic Ultrasonography and Endoscopic Retrograde Cholangiopancreatography in the Clinical Assessment of Pancreatic Neoplasms

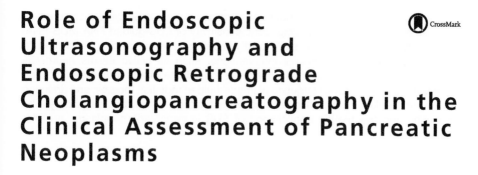

Shyam Varadarajulu, MD[a],*, Ji Young Bang, MD, MPH[b]

KEYWORDS

- Endoscopic ultrasonography • Fine-needle aspiration
- Endoscopic retrograde cholangiopancreatography • Pancreatic cancer
- Pancreatic cyst neoplasm • Biliary decompression

KEY POINTS

- Endoscopic ultrasonography (EUS)–guided fine-needle aspiration is an accurate technique for establishing tissue diagnosis in patients with pancreatic mass lesions.
- There has been growing interest in evaluating core tissue specimens procured by EUS for molecular markers that may serve as prognostic predictors and targets for focused therapy in pancreatic cancer.
- Endoscopic retrograde cholangiopancreatography (ERCP) with biliary stent placement relieves obstructive jaundice and is widely practiced both as a palliative measure and for preoperative biliary decompression in pancreatic cancer.
- EUS-guided drainage is becoming an effective rescue therapy for relief of obstructive jaundice in patients who fail ERCP, and it may be superior to percutaneous transhepatic biliary drainage.

ENDOSCOPIC ULTRASONOGRAPHY IN PANCREATIC NEOPLASMS

Endoscopic ultrasonography (EUS) is a sensitive technology for detecting pancreatic lesions and for performing fine-needle aspiration (FNA). Although computed tomography (CT) and magnetic resonance cholangiopancreatography are excellent modalities

Disclosure: S. Varadarajulu is a consultant for Olympus Medical Systems Corporation and Boston Scientific Corporation. J.Y. Bang is a consultant for Olympus Medical Systems Corporation.
[a] Center for Interventional Endoscopy, Florida Hospital, 601 East Rollins Street, Orlando, FL 32803, USA; [b] Division of Gastroenterology-Hepatology, Indiana University, 702 Rotary Circle, Suite 225, Indianapolis, IN 46202, USA
* Corresponding author.
E-mail address: svaradarajulu@yahoo.com

for imaging the pancreas, neuroendocrine tumors and pancreatic cyst lesions are better characterized by EUS. The diagnostic sensitivity of EUS-guided FNA (EUS-FNA) exceeds 85% to 90% and it is significantly superior to percutaneous techniques. In addition, EUS enables additional interventions, such as celiac plexus neurolysis (CPN) for palliation of pain, fiducial placements to facilitate intraoperative identification of small tumors or improved targeting of image-guided radiation therapy, and drainage of well-encapsulated pancreatic fluid collections after a distal pancreatectomy. The diagnostic and therapeutic applications of EUS in pancreatic neoplasms are discussed here.

Pancreatic Cancer

Staging endoscopic ultrasonography

Staging of pancreatic malignancy is performed according to the American Joint Committee for Cancer Staging TNM (tumor, node, metastasis) classification. Reported accuracies of EUS range from 63% to 94% for T classification and 41% to 86% for N classification.[1] Although early studies found that EUS was superior to conventional CT for T and N[2–4] staging, recent studies report that EUS is not superior to CT and MRI for T and N staging of pancreatic tumors.[5] The initial advantages shown by EUS compared with the other imaging modalities for staging of pancreatic tumors were not confirmed in subsequent studies.

The sensitivity and specificity of EUS for malignant vascular invasion are 42% to 91% and 89% to 100%, respectively.[5–7] Although some studies show that EUS is more accurate than CT for vascular invasion,[8–10] other investigators have reported that the accuracy of CT is superior to that of EUS.[5,6,11] The overall accuracy of MRI is reportedly equivalent or superior to that of EUS.[5,6] The overall sensitivity and accuracy of EUS for arterial invasion are 56%[12] and 50%,[2] respectively. The sensitivity of EUS for tumor invasion of the portal vein or portal vein confluence is 60% to 100%, with most studies showing sensitivities of more than 80%[1] (**Fig. 1**). The sensitivity of EUS for portal vein invasion is also consistently superior to that of CT.[4,13,14] For the superior mesenteric vein (SMV), superior mesenteric artery (SMA), and celiac artery, the sensitivity of EUS is only 17% to 83%, 17%, and 50%,[9,15,16] respectively. The sensitivity and specificity of EUS for determining resectability of pancreatic cancer in a pooled analysis of 377 patients was 69% (range, 23%–91%) and 82% (63%–100%), respectively.[1] The overall EUS accuracy for tumor resectability was reported at 77%. Thus, more cost and decision analysis and comparative

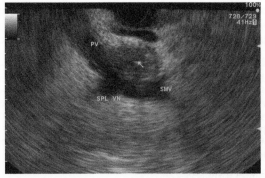

Fig. 1. EUS reveals a 2-cm hypoechoic pancreatic head mass (*arrow*) invading the confluence of the portal vein. PV, portal vein; SMV, superior mesenteric vein; SPL, splenic vein; VN, vein.

studies of EUS with state-of-the-art CT and MRI are required to make definitive recommendations on the precise role of EUS in staging pancreatic cancer.

Endoscopic ultrasonography fine-needle aspiration

Two recently published meta-analyses totaling more than 8400 patients and 67 studies reported pooled sensitivities for the diagnosis of malignancy based on cytology of 85% and 89% and pooled specificities of 98% and 99%.[17,18] However, the negative predictive value of EUS-FNA for pancreatic tumors remains limited at 65%.[19] Therefore a negative or nondiagnostic biopsy does not exclude the possibility of malignancy. Fritscher-Ravens and colleagues[20] found that, in a series of 207 consecutive patients with focal pancreatic lesions, the sensitivity of EUS-FNA for the diagnosis of malignancy in patients with normal parenchyma (89%) was superior to the sensitivity in those with chronic pancreatitis (54%). The presence of chronic pancreatitis may also hinder cytologic interpretation of pancreatic biopsy, thus decreasing the sensitivity of EUS-FNA of pancreatic masses. In a meta-analysis of 34 studies that evaluated the diagnostic accuracy of EUS-FNA for pancreatic cancer in 3644 patients with solid pancreatic mass lesions, rapid on-site evaluation (ROSE) was a significant determinant of EUS-FNA accuracy.[18] Also, at least 5 to 7 EUS-FNA passes should be performed when sampling pancreatic masses to maximize diagnostic yield (**Fig. 2**) and this information may prove helpful to endosonographers performing EUS-FNA when ROSE is not available.

Occasionally, ROSE may be inconclusive because of tumor necrosis, fibrosis, or hypervascularity. The diagnostic yield may be increased by fanning the lesion, in which different angles of scope deflection are used in order to sample the peripheral parts of the lesion. In a recent randomized study by these authors, the fanning technique was superior to the standard approach, with fewer passes being required to establish a diagnosis.[21]

The most commonly used commercially available EUS-FNA needle sizes are 19, 22, and 25 gauge. In a recent meta-analysis of 8 studies comprising 1292 patients, 25-gauge needles were associated with higher sensitivity but comparable specificity with 22-gauge needles.[22] In general, 25-gauge needles are associated with lower technical failures compared with 19-gauge and 22-gauge needles when sampling pancreatic head and uncinate process lesions.

Postprocedure adverse events following EUS-FNA are rare. In a recent systematic review that included 8246 patients with pancreatic lesions, 7337 of those being solid masses, minor adverse events after EUS-FNA occurred in 60 patients (0.82%), which included pancreatitis, abdominal pain, bleeding, fever, and infection.[23]

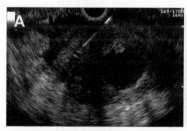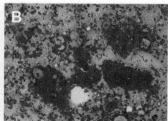

Fig. 2. (*A*) EUS-FNA of a 3-cm pancreatic head mass. (*B*) Rapid on-site evaluation reveals atypical ductal cells consistent with pancreatic adenocarcinoma. (Diff-Quik, original magnification ×100)

Pancreatic Neuroendocrine Tumors

Pancreatic neuroendocrine tumors (PNETs) represent less than 10% of pancreatic tumors. In a series of studies that compared EUS with other imaging modalities, the sensitivity of EUS for detection of PNETs was 77% to 94%.[24,25] EUS seems especially useful for detection of small PNETs (<2.5 cm) missed by other imaging studies. In a study of 30 patients with 32 insulinomas, the sensitivity of EUS was 94% compared with 29% for nonhelical CT and 57% for dual-phase multidetector CT.[24] In another study of 217 patients,[25] CT was more likely than EUS to miss insulinomas and PNETs less than 2 cm. These investigators also found that the overall sensitivity of EUS (91%) was greater than that of CT (63%). In recent studies, the reported sensitivity of MRI for PNET detection is 85% to 100%[26,27] with positive predictive value of 96%.[28]

In a series of patients with histologically proven insulinomas (n = 20) or gastrinomas (n = 21), the sensitivity and positive predictive value of EUS were 77% and 94%, respectively.[29] For the same patients, the sensitivity and positive predictive value of somatostatin receptor scintigraphy (SRS) for insulinoma and gastrinoma detection were 60% and 100%, and 25% and 100%, respectively. When both tests were combined and a subgroup analysis was performed, the overall sensitivity of combined EUS and SRS was 89% for insulinomas and 93% for gastrinomas. It seems that the combination of EUS and SRS may optimize preoperative identification of PNETs and limit the need for more invasive tests such as angiography. As with pancreatic cancer, EUS-FNA seems to be an excellent modality for establishing tissue diagnosis in PNETs (**Fig. 3**). In a recent meta-analysis of 13 studies comprising 456 patients, the pooled sensitivity of EUS for detecting PNET was 87% and the pooled specificity was 98%.[30]

Pancreatic Cyst Lesions

When a cystic lesion has been identified in the pancreas, the size, location, relation to adjacent vessels and organs, and the presence of locoregional or distant metastases should be noted. The cyst should be examined to determine the wall thickness, presence of a mural nodule, or associated mass. The size of the main pancreatic duct, whether it communicates with the cyst, the presence of mucin or a mural nodule within the pancreatic duct, or any focal dilatation should also be noted.

There are several features on EUS that are worrisome for malignant transformation of the cyst and these include thick wall or septum, an associated solid mass, or a mural nodule (**Fig. 4**). The presence of focal dilatation of the main pancreatic duct, pancreatic duct measuring greater than or equal to 10 mm, or mural nodules are features associated with malignant transformation (See Greer JB, Ferrone CR: Spectrum and classification of cystic neoplasms of the pancreas, in this issue).

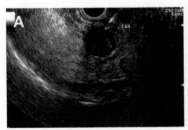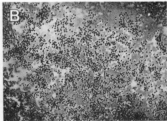

Fig. 3. (*A*) EUS-FNA of a well-circumscribed 1.2-cm hypoechoic mass in the pancreatic tail region. (*B*) Rapid on-site evaluation of the pancreatic tail mass is suggestive of a neuroendocrine tumor. (Diff-Quik, original magnification ×200)

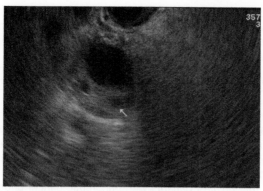

Fig. 4. EUS reveals an anechoic cyst in the pancreatic head with thick peripheral rim walls (*arrow*). EUS-FNA proved the lesion to be a cystic neuroendocrine tumor.

The risk of adverse events from EUS-FNA of pancreatic cysts is slightly higher than that resulting from EUS-FNA of a solid lesion. In a recent review of adverse events associated with EUS-FNA,[23] the most common adverse event was pancreatitis, which occurred in 1.1% of patients, followed by pain (0.77%), bleeding (0.33%), fever (0.33%), and infection (0.22%). Antibiotic prophylaxis is therefore recommended, usually with intravenous ciprofloxacin before the procedure. If FNA is performed, the aspirate must be sent for carcinoembryonic antigen (CEA) and/or cytology.

The specificity of cytology for malignancy is excellent and approaches 100%, but the sensitivity varies considerably in reported series. This finding reflects the difficulty in interpreting these lesions, especially when the cellularity of the samples is low. Brandwein and colleagues[31] and Brugge and colleagues[32] reported sensitivities of 55% and 59%, respectively, for differentiating benign from malignant or potentially malignant pancreatic cysts. The CEA levels are higher in mucinous than in nonmucinous cysts, with a reference value of 192 ng/mL for mucinous cysts. In a large study, the diagnostic accuracy of this reference level for differentiating mucinous from nonmucinous cysts was 79%.[32] Although molecular markers such as KRAS and GNAS are being studied as indicators of malignant transformation, data are limited and further research is needed before they can be incorporated into clinical practice.

The Concept of Core Biopsy

Although considerable progress has been made in the treatment of breast and lung cancers in which the delivery of chemotherapy is guided by the expression of molecular markers in the tumor, which can in turn help prognosticate the tumor and guide treatment algorithms, data on personalized therapy in pancreatic cancer are scant. There is growing evidence that immune cells in pancreatic ductal adenocarcinoma produce immune suppressive signals that allow tumors to evade the immune response. Also, the stromal fibroblasts provide a protective environment that not only supports and promotes pancreatic adenocarcinoma tumor growth and progression but also likely suppresses the development of and/or access to the antitumor immune responses. Strategies to deplete the desmoplastic stroma before institution of immune therapy could promote robust response against tumor cells. Therefore, it is increasingly apparent that the evaluation of fibrous stroma for molecular markers may be an integral part of cancer therapy.[33] Preliminary evidence in our laboratory suggests that specimens procured using a 19-gauge or 22-gauge FNA needle and fixed in formalin have preserved microcores that enable detailed assessment of the histologic architecture with neoplastic glands embedded in the stroma. Randomized trials are in progress to identify the best technique for core tissue procurement. We believe that the results of these trials will be of significant help in advancing personalized therapy in pancreatic cancer.

Therapeutic Applications of Endoscopic Ultrasonography in Pancreatic Neoplasms

Endoscopic ultrasonography–guided celiac plexus neurolysis

At EUS, after identifying the celiac artery take-off from the aorta, the FNA needle is positioned adjacent and anterior to the lateral aspect of the aorta at the level of the celiac trunk (**Fig. 5**). The FNA needle is then aspirated to rule out vessel penetration before injection. For CPN in patients with pancreatic cancer, 10 mL of 0.25% bupivacaine are injected followed by 10 mL of dehydrated (98%) alcohol. A recent meta-analysis reported that 80% of patients with pancreatic cancer undergoing CPN had pain relief.[34] Also, patients who had injections on both sides of the celiac artery had a higher rate of pain relief than those who received injections only on 1 side (85% vs 46%). In a randomized trial, 96 patients with inoperable pancreatic cancer were assigned to either CPN or conventional pain management.[35] At 3 months, patients treated with CPN had significantly greater pain relief, with a trend toward lower morphine consumption. There was no difference between the two groups in quality-of-life scores or survival.

Endoscopic ultrasonography–guided implantation therapy

PNETs are small and tumor localization at laparoscopic surgery can be challenging. EUS-guided fiducial placement is a new technique for intraoperative localization of pancreatic tumors (**Fig. 6**). At EUS, once a tumor is localized, a small gold fiducial (2–3 mm × 0.8 mm) is back-loaded to a 19-gauge FNA needle (after stylet retraction) and the lumen of the needle is sealed with bone wax. After puncturing the lesion, the stylet is advanced to facilitate deployment of gold fiducials within the tumor. At surgery, using fluoroscopy, the tumor is identified to facilitate laparoscopic resection.[36] Likewise, fiducial placement enables better targeting of pancreatic cancers by image-guided radiation therapy.[37]

Endoscopic ultrasonography–guided pancreatic cyst ablation

Ethanol and chemotherapeutic agents such as paclitaxel are used for EUS-guided ablation of pancreatic cyst lesions under EUS guidance. In a systematic review,[38] the pooled proportion of patients with complete cyst resolution was 56.2%

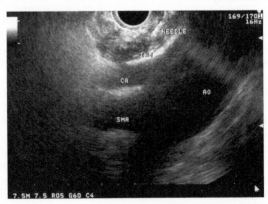

Fig. 5. EUS-CPN undertaken with a 19-gauge FNA needle. AO, aorta; CA, celiac artery; INJ, injection.

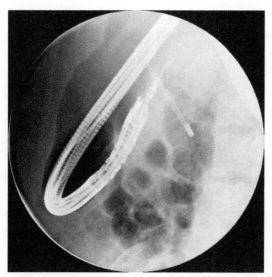

Fig. 6. EUS-guided fiducial placement within a pancreatic head mass. A plastic stent is seen within the bile duct for biliary decompression.

(95% confidence interval [CI], 48.2%–64.1%) and partial cyst resolution was 23.7% (95% CI, 17.2%–30.9%). Postprocedural adverse events included abdominal pain in 6.5% (95% CI, 3.1%–11.0%) and pancreatitis in 3.9% (95% CI, 1.4–7.6).

Endoscopic ultrasonography–guided drainage of postoperative pancreatic fluid collections

Development of a postoperative pancreatic fluid collection is a common complication after distal pancreatectomy and is usually managed by percutaneous drainage. Major disadvantages of percutaneous drainage include fistula formation, infection, skin excoriation, and accidental dislodging of the catheter. At EUS, the pancreatic fluid collection can be easily accessed using a 19-gauge needle. After dilating the transmural tract to 6 to 10 mm, multiple internal stents can be deployed for transgastric drainage (**Fig. 7**). The treatment success rate for this approach exceeds 90% and it yields faster symptom relief and resolution of the pancreatic fluid collection compared with percutaneous drainage or transpapillary stenting.[39,40]

ENDOSCOPIC RETROGRADE CHOLANGIOPANCREATOGRAPHY IN PANCREATIC NEOPLASMS

The main objective of endoscopic retrograde cholangiopancreatography (ERCP) in patients with pancreatic neoplasm is to provide drainage for obstructive jaundice by placement of self-expandable metal or polyethylene stents. Despite the indispensable role of EUS in tissue acquisition, ERCP presents a unique opportunity to establish a diagnosis of malignancy during a drainage procedure, thereby saving the patient subsequent unnecessary and expensive procedures. The outcomes of different techniques adopted at ERCP for tissue sampling are reviewed here, and an objective assessment is provided of the role of various endoprostheses in both preoperative and palliative biliary decompression.

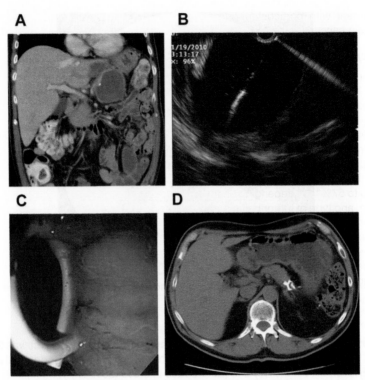

Fig. 7. (*A*) CT of the abdomen revealing a pancreatic fluid collection after distal pancreatectomy measuring 7 × 6 cm in the lesser sac. (*B*) The pancreatic fluid collection is accessed using a19-gauge needle under EUS guidance. (*C*) Transesophageal stent was deployed for drainage of the fluid collection. (*D*) Follow-up CT of the abdomen at 8 weeks reveals near-complete resolution of the pancreatic fluid collection.

Rationale for Tissue Sampling

Although EUS-FNA is currently the technique of choice for tissue acquisition in pancreatic cancer, most patients with malignant biliary obstruction require ERCP for relief of jaundice. In addition, only 15% of patients presenting with malignant obstructive jaundice undergo an attempt at surgical curative resection. Therefore, it is logical to attempt tissue sampling before biliary stent placement in this patient cohort because it obviates an additional procedure, namely EUS.

The diagnostic yield of tissue sampling is influenced by tumor cellularity and its differentiation. Pancreatic cancer stimulates a desmoplastic and fibrotic reaction making the tumor very dense and low in cellularity. Establishing a definitive diagnosis in these patients therefore requires sampling of layers deeper than the surface epithelium via a biliary biopsy and superficial sampling of the tumor by techniques such as brush cytology often yields an acellular or false-negative specimen. Well-differentiated tumors can also be difficult to diagnose by cytology and large histologic specimens are often necessary to enable pathologists to differentiate cancer from normal tissue. When the clinical suspicion for malignancy remains high, but cytology is inconclusive, it may be necessary to perform a biopsy for histologic confirmation. There is increasing recognition of autoimmune pancreatitis, a condition that can cause obstructive jaundice and mimic pancreatic cancer. This benign disorder responds well to treatment with corticosteroids and hence must be reliably distinguished from pancreatic cancer.

Endoscopic Techniques

The 3 most common tissue acquisition techniques adopted at ERCP are fluoroscopy-guided biliary brushing, fluoroscopy-guided biliary biopsy, and cholangioscopy-guided biopsy.

Biliary brushings are performed using an 8-Fr cytology brush that is advanced over a guidewire that bypasses the stricture (**Fig. 8**). Because most endoscopists negotiate a guidewire through the stricture as the first major step in the therapeutic goal of biliary stent placement, brushings for tissue sampling can be done at the same time without interrupting this sequence. The reported overall sensitivity for biliary brushings ranges from 8% to 57%[41–44] depending on the length of the brush, type of bristles, duration of brushing, and type of tumor being sampled. In a recent review, the overall sensitivity of biliary brushings in 837 patients was reported to be 42%.[45] In general, the yield of biliary brushings for pancreatic adenocarcinoma is lower than that for cholangiocarcinoma because the interior of a biliary stricture resulting from pancreatic cancer is composed of benign epithelium that is compressed by surrounding neoplastic tissue. Biliary brushes only scrape the superficial layers of the stricture and therefore are low in yield.

The technique of fluoroscopy-guided forceps biopsy involves the insertion of 5-Fr to 10-Fr devices to the lower edge of the stricture (**Fig. 9**). Under fluoroscopy, multiple biopsies can be obtained from the lower margin of the apparent tumor. The biopsy forceps are available in several designs: straight, angled, freehand, and over-the-wire devices. In a recent review, the overall sensitivity of forceps biopsy in 502 patients was reported to be 56%.[45]

Given the disappointing results of single sampling techniques, endoscopists currently combine multiple techniques during an ERCP procedure to improve the diagnostic yield. In clinical practice, a cytology brushing is first performed, followed by biopsy of the stricture site. In a study by Ponchon and colleagues,[46] biliary brushing

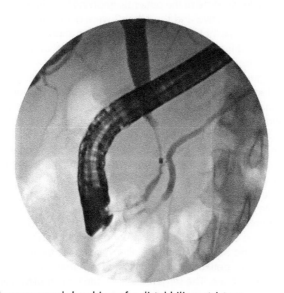

Fig. 8. Cholangiogram reveals brushing of a distal biliary stricture.

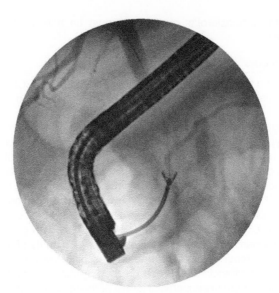

Fig. 9. Biopsy of a distal biliary stricture performed at ERCP.

had a sensitivity of 43% and forceps biopsy 30%, but when both of these techniques were combined the yield increased to 63%.

Some investigators combine intraductal FNA during an ERCP procedure. In this technique, a 22-gauge intraductal FNA needle is able to sample deeper layers of a lesion than are afforded by a biliary brush or biopsy forceps. In one study at Indiana University, the combination of all 3 of these techniques (brushing, biopsy, and intraductal FNA), resulted in successful diagnosis in 82% of patients during a single ERCP session.[2] When the results were analyzed, each technique contributed to making the diagnosis in at least some of the patients, implying that, in many patients, only 1 of the 3 techniques was positive and the other 2 were negative or equivocal. Despite the results of this study, this method of triple sampling is impractical because it is time consuming, technically difficult, and ancillary to the main goal of placing a biliary endoprostheses for biliary decompression.

Cholangioscopy-guided biopsy is a novel technique that is gaining increasing acceptance. This technique involves the use of a so-called mother-daughter scope to sample the biliary lesion. While one endoscopist controls the mother duodenoscope, the second endoscopist maneuvers the daughter cholangioscope, which is advanced from within the biopsy channel of the duodenoscope into the bile duct for tissue sampling. The advantage of this technique is that it enables sampling of the biliary stricture under direct visualization. The disadvantage is that it is cumbersome because it involves 2 endoscopists, requires careful coordination, and the equipment is fragile and expensive. A novel single-operator system called SpyGlass is currently available and being increasingly used for tissue acquisition in the bile duct (**Fig. 10**). This system uses a disposable high-definition probe with an inbuilt camera and separate miniature channels for passage of biopsy forceps and water for irrigation of the bile duct, and advancement of laser probes for fragmentation of stones. The probe has a 4-way deflection capability that enables movement in both updown and left-right directions. The targeted lesion can be sampled using mini–biopsy forceps and, if cytopathology support is available, an on-site diagnosis can be

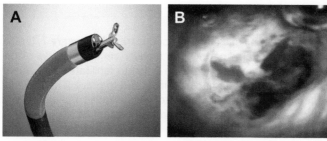

Fig. 10. (*A*) The SpyGlass cholangioscope for evaluating the bile duct at ERCP. (*Courtesy of Boston Scientific, Marlborough, MA*). (*B*) A malignant lesion is identified at SpyGlass cholangioscopy in the bile duct.

established rapidly. The diagnostic accuracy of the SpyGlass system when evaluating biliary strictures exceeds 75%.[47] A simplified algorithm for tissue acquisition is proposed in **Fig. 11**.

Biliary Stenting

Indications for biliary stenting at ERCP include jaundice, fever, and pruritus. Compared with percutaneous and surgical drainage, endoscopic biliary stenting is associated with lower morbidity and mortality.[48,49] The procedure has also been shown to improve symptoms such as anorexia and patient quality of life. In a randomized trial of 201 patients with pancreatic head cancer who underwent surgery or preoperative stent placement, the overall rate of adverse events was significantly higher in the endoscopy cohort, mainly owing to stent-related complications.[50] Despite these findings, preoperative drainage is indicated when surgical resection is not imminent.

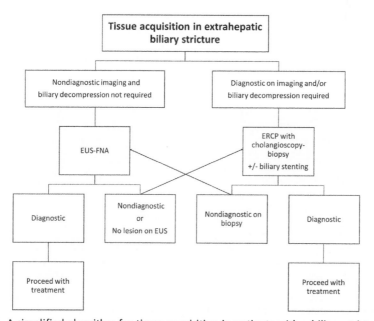

Fig. 11. A simplified algorithm for tissue acquisition in patients with a biliary stricture.

Types of Biliary Stents

Plastic stents

The most common sizes of plastic stents placed in the bile duct are 7, 8.5, and 10 Fr. Larger diameter stents perform better than smaller stents because of better flow rates and less stasis. Most stents have side holes to facilitate biliary drainage and are designed with either pigtails or flaps at either end to prevent migration. Different materials have been used for stent construction, including polyethylene, polyurethane, and Teflon. Teflon stents have the lowest friction coefficient and the best potential for preventing stent clogging. The stents also range in length from 4 to 15 cm.

The choice of stent depends on the location and length of the biliary stricture. Whenever feasible, a 10-Fr plastic stent must be placed in lieu of small-caliber stents given their longer patency. Plastic stents are deployed over a guidewire using a push-catheter and a biliary sphincterotomy is not a prerequisite to stent placement. The stent is positioned with the proximal and distal ends bridging the stricture so as to facilitate free flow of bile into the duodenum. Compared with metal stents, plastic endoprostheses have shorter durations of patency and hence require elective stent exchanges (**Fig. 12**). The usual time to perform a stent exchange is 10 to 12 weeks. However, plastic stents are much cheaper than metal stents.

Self-expanding metal stents

Metal stents differ in the manner in which they are braided, the size of the mesh, composition, length, width, rigidity, and degree of covering. The usual diameter of the stent is 8 to 10 mm and the length varies between 4 and 12 cm. After deployment, some stents can expand and also shorten by up to 30%. Given their large diameter, metal stents remain patent for longer durations than plastic stents. However, that does not eliminate the risk of stent obstruction (**Fig. 13**), and the average duration of stent patency is between 6 and 9 months. The mechanism of stent dysfunction differs from that seen in plastic stents and includes tumor ingrowth through the stent interstices, overgrowth at both ends, and intimal hyperplasia. To overcome the problem of tumor ingrowth, self-expandable metal stents have been fully or partially covered with a polyurethane or silicone membrane. Although some studies have shown that stent occlusion caused by tumor ingrowth occurs less frequently

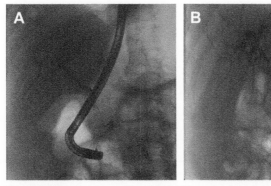

Fig. 12. (A) Cholangiogram reveals a distal biliary stricture in a patient with a pancreatic head mass. (B) Successful deployment of a 10-Fr plastic stent in the bile duct for biliary decompression.

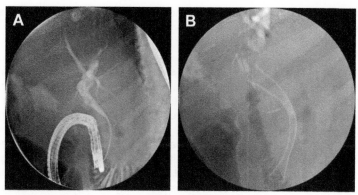

Fig. 13. (*A*) Cholangiogram reveals a distal biliary stricture in a patient with pancreatic cancer of the uncinate region (partial stent deployment). (*B*) Successful deployment of a 10-mm self-expandable metal stent for biliary decompression.

with covered than with uncovered metal stents, these data have been disputed by others.[51,52] Although data on adverse events are scarce, stent migration, cholecystitis, and pancreatitis seem to occur at a higher rate with covered stents.[51,52] Covered stents should not be used intrahepatically because of occlusion of the hepatic side branches by the covering membrane. In addition, placement of metal stents can be technically challenging and uncovered metal stents cannot be removed after deployment. Furthermore, metal stents are more expensive than plastic stents.

Choice of Stent Placement

Inoperable cancer
In a recent randomized trial of 219 patients with extrahepatic biliary obstruction from inoperable cancer, the mean functional time for plastic stents was 172 days and for metal stents was 288 days (*P*<.005).[53] Given the longer duration of patency, self-expanding metal stents should ideally be placed in all patients but their high costs have limited their use to specific settings. In a cost-effective approach, the choice of stent depends mainly on an estimate of patient survival. Patients with liver metastases and poor functional status have a short survival time (<3 months) and should preferably be treated with plastic stents. In contrast, patients with longer life expectancy (>3 months; ie, patients with no liver metastasis, good functional status, and/or undergoing chemotherapy) should preferably be treated with metal stents. Also, patients who present with early obstruction of plastic stents (ie, within 1 month) should receive a self-expandable metal stent.

Preoperative biliary decompression
Based on the findings of a recent randomized trial in which patients undergoing preoperative ERCP had poor clinical outcomes, biliary stenting should not be performed routinely in all operable patients.[50] However, in patients with intractable pruritus or cholangitis, biliary stent placement can be performed after interdisciplinary consultation. Also, some surgeons prefer placement of biliary stents in patients with obstructive jaundice before performing a Whipple procedure because of concerns of metabolic derangement. In such instances, we have shown that the placement of a fully covered metal stent 2 cm below the liver hilum

provides symptomatic relief and does not adversely affect clinical or surgical outcomes.[54]

Technical Outcomes

The technical success rate for biliary stenting at ERCP exceeds 85% and approaches 95% to 99% in expert hands.[55] Although standard cannulation techniques facilitate biliary access in most patients, advanced techniques, such as precut sphincterotomy, transpapillary pancreatic sphincterotomy, fistulotomy, and cannulation over a pancreatic duct stent, may be required when standard techniques fail. Advanced cannulation techniques confer higher risks and are associated with a 5% to 10% rate of adverse events that include pancreatitis, bleeding, perforation, pneumoperitoneum, and abdominal pain.[56,57] Patients with failed biliary access using standard cannulation techniques preferably should be referred to tertiary centers with advanced expertise for a repeat ERCP procedure. Several studies have shown that the technical success rate for repeat ERCP at expert centers exceeds 90%.[55,58]

Endoscopic Treatment Alternatives

Although percutaneous transhepatic biliary drainage and surgical biliary bypass are considered the main treatment alternatives following a failed ERCP, EUS-guided biliary drainage is becoming increasingly popular as a rescue technique. At EUS, the dilated extrahepatic bile duct or intrahepatic duct radicle is identified and punctured using a 19-gauge needle. After the passage of a stiff guidewire, the transmural tract is dilated and a fully covered metal stent is deployed for biliary drainage. The technical success rate for EUS-guided biliary drainage exceeds 90% and is associated with 5% to 10% risk of adverse events that include bile leak, perforation, and infection.[59] The procedure requires advanced technical expertise and is best performed at tertiary-level endoscopy units (**Fig. 14**).

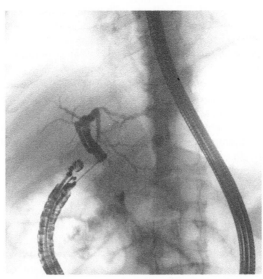

Fig. 14. EUS-guided cholangiogram reveals a long-segment biliary stricture in a patient with locally advanced pancreatic cancer. The patient underwent successful EUS-guided choledochoduodenostomy.

SUMMARY

EUS-FNA is the cornerstone of pancreatic tissue acquisition and is associated with excellent operating characteristics. The ability to reliably procure core tissue enables personalization of chemotherapy and improves clinical outcomes. In addition, EUS facilitates palliation of pain in pancreatic cancer and ablation of pancreatic cyst neoplasms. Biliary decompression at ERCP is successful in greater than 95% of patients with obstructive jaundice. However, EUS-guided biliary drainage is also becoming an effective rescue technique for palliation of jaundice when access to the bile duct is unsuccessful at ERCP.

REFERENCES

1. Luz L, Al-Haddad M, DeWitt J. EUS and pancreatic tumors. Endosonography. In: Hawes R, Fockens P, Varadarajulu S, editors. Chapter 15. 3rd edition. Elsevier; p. 187–208.
2. Palazzo L, Roseau G, Gayet B, et al. Endoscopic ultrasonography in the diagnosis and staging of pancreatic adenocarcinoma. Results of a prospective study with comparison to ultrasonography and CT scan. Endoscopy 1993; 25:143–50.
3. Müller MF, Meyenberger C, Bertschinger P, et al. Pancreatic tumors: evaluation with endoscopic US, CT, and MR imaging. Radiology 1994;190:745–51.
4. Rösch T, Braig C, Gain T, et al. Staging of pancreatic and ampullary carcinoma by endoscopic ultrasonography. Comparison with conventional sonography, computed tomography, and angiography. Gastroenterology 1992;102:188–99.
5. Soriano A, Castells A, Ayuso C, et al. Preoperative staging and tumor resectability assessment of pancreatic cancer: prospective study comparing endoscopic ultrasonography, helical computed tomography, magnetic resonance imaging, and angiography. Am J Gastroenterol 2004;99:492–501.
6. Ramsay D, Marshall M, Song S, et al. Identification and staging of pancreatic tumors using computed tomography, endoscopic ultrasound and mangafodipir trisodium-enhanced magnetic resonance imaging. Australas Radiol 2004;48: 154–61.
7. Tierney WM, Francis IR, Eckhauser F, et al. The accuracy of EUS and helical CT in the assessment of vascular invasion by peripapillary malignancy. Gastrointest Endosc 2001;53:182–8.
8. Gress FG, Hawes RH, Savides TJ, et al. Role of EUS in the preoperative staging of pancreatic cancer: a large single-center experience. Gastrointest Endosc 1999;50:786–91.
9. Mertz HR, Sechopoulos P, Delbeke D, et al. EUS, PET, and CT scanning for evaluation of pancreatic adenocarcinoma. Gastrointest Endosc 2000;52:367–71.
10. Rivadeneira DE, Pochapin M, Grobmyer SR, et al. Comparison of linear array endoscopic ultrasound and helical computed tomography for the staging of periampullary malignancies. Ann Surg Oncol 2003;10:890–7.
11. Dufour B, Zins M, Vilgrain V, et al. Comparison between spiral x-ray computed tomography and endosonography in the diagnosis and staging of adenocarcinoma of the pancreas. Clinical preliminary study. Gastroenterol Clin Biol 1997; 21:124–30 [in French].
12. Marty O, Aubertin JM, Bouillot JL, et al. Prospective comparison of ultrasound endoscopy and computed tomography in the assessment of locoregional invasiveness of malignant ampullar and pancreatic tumors verified surgically. Gastroenterol Clin Biol 1995;19:197–203 [in French].

13. Sugiyama M, Hagi H, Atomi Y, et al. Diagnosis of portal venous invasion by pancreatobiliary carcinoma: value of endoscopic ultrasonography. Abdom Imaging 1997;22:434–8.

14. Midwinter MJ, Beveridge CJ, Wilsdon JB, et al. Correlation between spiral computed tomography, endoscopic ultrasonography and findings at operation in pancreatic and ampullary tumours. Br J Surg 1999;86:189–93.

15. Buscail L, Pages P, Berthelemy P, et al. Role of EUS in the management of pancreatic and ampullary carcinoma: a prospective study assessing resectability and prognosis. Gastrointest Endosc 1999;50:34–40.

16. Rösch T, Dittler HJ, Lorenz R, et al. The endosonographic staging of pancreatic carcinoma. Dtsch Med Wochenschr 1992;117:563–9 [in German].

17. Hewitt MJ, McPhail MJ, Possamai L, et al. EUS-guided FNA for diagnosis of solid pancreatic neoplasms: a meta-analysis. Gastrointest Endosc 2012;75:319–31.

18. Hebert-Magee S, Bae S, Varadarajulu S, et al. The presence of a cytopathologist increases the diagnostic accuracy of endoscopic ultrasound-guided fine needle aspiration cytology for pancreatic adenocarcinoma: a meta-analysis. Cytopathology 2013;24:159–71.

19. Eloubeidi MA, Chen VK, Eltoum IA, et al. Endoscopic ultrasound-guided fine needle aspiration biopsy of patients with suspected pancreatic cancer: diagnostic accuracy and acute and 30-day complications. Am J Gastroenterol 2003;98:2663–8.

20. Fritscher-Ravens A, Brand L, Knofel WT, et al. Comparison of endoscopic ultrasound-guided fine needle aspiration for focal pancreatic lesions in patients with normal parenchyma and chronic pancreatitis. Am J Gastroenterol 2002;97:2768–75.

21. Bang JY, Magee SH, Ramesh J, et al. Randomized trial comparing fanning with standard technique for endoscopic ultrasound-guided fine-needle aspiration of solid pancreatic mass lesions. Endoscopy 2013;45:445–50.

22. Madhoun MF, Wani SB, Rastogi A, et al. The diagnostic accuracy of 22-gauge and 25-gauge needles in endoscopic ultrasound-guided fine needle aspiration of solid pancreatic lesions: a meta-analysis. Endoscopy 2013;45:86–92.

23. Wang KX, Ben QW, Jin ZD, et al. Assessment of morbidity and mortality associated with EUS-guided FNA: a systematic review. Gastrointest Endosc 2011;73:283–90.

24. Gouya H, Vignaux O, Augui J, et al. CT, endoscopic sonography, and a combined protocol for preoperative evaluation of pancreatic insulinomas. AJR Am J Roentgenol 2003;181:987–92.

25. Khashab MA, Yong E, Lennon AM, et al. EUS is still superior to multidetector computerized tomography for detection of pancreatic neuroendocrine tumors. Gastrointest Endosc 2011;73:691–6.

26. Semelka RC, Custodio CM, Cem Balci N, et al. Neuroendocrine tumors of the pancreas: spectrum of appearances on MRI. J Magn Reson Imaging 2000;11:141–8.

27. Van Nieuwenhove Y, Vandaele S, Op de Beeck B, et al. Neuroendocrine tumors of the pancreas. Surg Endosc 2003;17:1658–62.

28. Thoeni RF, Mueller-Lisse UG, Chan R, et al. Detection of small, functional islet cell tumors in the pancreas: selection of MR imaging sequences for optimal sensitivity. Radiology 2000;214:483–90.

29. Proye C, Malvaux P, Pattou F, et al. Noninvasive imaging of insulinomas and gastrinomas with endoscopic ultrasonography and somatostatin receptor scintigraphy. Surgery 1998;124:1134–43.

30. Puli SR, Kalva N, Bechtold ML, et al. Diagnostic accuracy of endoscopic ultrasound in pancreatic neuroendocrine tumors: a systematic review and meta analysis. World J Gastroenterol 2013;19:3678–84.
31. Brandwein SL, Farrell JJ, Centeno BA, et al. Detection and tumor staging of malignancy in cystic, intraductal, and solid tumors of the pancreas by EUS. Gastrointest Endosc 2001;53:722–7.
32. Brugge WR, Lewandrowski K, Lee-Lewandrowski E, et al. Diagnosis of pancreatic cystic neoplasms: a report of the cooperative pancreatic cyst study. Gastroenterology 2004;126:1330–6.
33. Yee NS. Immunotherapeutic approaches in pancreatic adenocarcinoma: current status and future perspectives. Curr Mol Pharmacol 2015. [Epub ahead of print].
34. Kaufman M, Singh G, Das S, et al. Efficacy of endoscopic ultrasound-guided celiac plexus block and celiac plexus neurolysis for managing abdominal pain associated with chronic pancreatitis and pancreatic cancer. J Clin Gastroenterol 2010;44:127–34.
35. Wyse JM, Carone M, Paquin SC, et al. Randomized, double-blind, controlled trial of early endoscopic ultrasound-guided celiac plexus neurolysis to prevent pain progression in patients with newly diagnosed, painful, inoperable pancreatic cancer. J Clin Oncol 2011;29:3541–6.
36. Ramesh J, Porterfield J, Varadarajulu S. Endoscopic ultrasound-guided gold fiducial marker placement for intraoperative identification of insulinoma. Endoscopy 2012;44(Suppl 2 UCTN):E327–8.
37. Varadarajulu S, Trevino JM, Shen S, et al. The use of endoscopic ultrasound-guided gold markers in image-guided radiation therapy of pancreatic cancers: a case series. Endoscopy 2010;42:423–5.
38. Kandula M, Moole H, Cashman M, et al. Success of endoscopic ultrasound-guided ethanol ablation of pancreatic cysts: A meta-analysis and systematic review. Indian J Gastroenterol 2015;34:193–9.
39. Varadarajulu S, Trevino JM, Christein JD. EUS for the management of peripancreatic fluid collections after distal pancreatectomy. Gastrointest Endosc 2009;70:1260–5.
40. Varadarajulu S, Wilcox CM, Christein JD. EUS-guided therapy for management of peripancreatic fluid collections after distal pancreatectomy in 20 consecutive patients. Gastrointest Endosc 2011;74:418–23.
41. Stewart CJR, Mills PR, Carter R, et al. Prospective evaluation of brush cytology of biliary strictures during endoscopic strictures: A review of 406 cases. J Clin Pathol 2001;54:449–55.
42. Jailwala J, Fogel EL, Sherman S, et al. Triple-tissue sampling at ERCP in malignant biliary obstruction. Gastrointest Endosc 2000;51:383–90.
43. Macken E, Drijkoningen M, Van Aken E, et al. Brush cytology of ductal strictures during ERCP. Acta Gastroenterol Belg 2000;63:254–9.
44. Howell DA, Beveridge RP, Bosco J, et al. Endoscopic needle aspiration biopsy at ERCP in the diagnosis of biliary strictures. Gastrointest Endosc 1992;38:531–5.
45. de Bellis M, Sherman S, Fogel EL, et al. Tissue sampling at ERCP in suspected malignant biliary strictures (part 2). Gastrointest Endosc 2002;56:720–30.
46. Ponchon T, Gagnon P, Berger F, et al. Value of endobiliary brush cytology and biopsies for the diagnosis of malignant bile duct stenosis: Results of a prospective study. Gastrointest Endosc 1995;42:565–72.
47. Nguyen NQ, Schoeman MN, Ruszkiewicz A. Clinical utility of EUS before cholangioscopy in the evaluation of difficult biliary strictures. Gastrointest Endosc 2013;78:868–74.

48. Andersen JR, Sorensen SM, Kruse A, et al. Randomised trial of endoscopic endoprosthesis versus operative bypass in malignant obstructive jaundice. Gut 1989;30:1132–5.
49. Smith AC, Dowsett JF, Russell RC, et al. Randomised trial of endoscopic stenting versus surgical bypass in malignant low bile duct obstruction. Lancet 1994;344: 1655–60.
50. van der Gaag NA, Rauws EA, van Eijck CH, et al. Preoperative biliary drainage for cancer of the head of the pancreas. N Engl J Med 2010;362:129–37.
51. Isayama H, Komatsu Y, Tsujino T, et al. A prospective randomised study of "covered" versus "uncovered" diamond stents for the management of distal malignant biliary obstruction. Gut 2004;53:729–34.
52. Kullman E, Frozanpor F, Söderlund C, et al. Covered versus uncovered self-expandable nitinol stents in the palliative treatment of malignant distal biliary obstruction: results from a randomized, multicenter study. Gastrointest Endosc 2010;72:915–23.
53. Walter D, van Boeckel PGA, Groenen MJ, et al. Cost efficacy of metal stents for palliation of extrahepatic bile duct obstruction in a randomized controlled trial. Gastroenterology 2015;149:130–8.
54. Decker C, Christein JD, Phadnis MA, et al. Biliary metal stents are superior to plastic stents for preoperative biliary decompression in pancreatic cancer. Surg Endosc 2011;25:2364–7.
55. Holt BA, Hawes R, Hasan M, et al. Biliary drainage: role of EUS guidance. Gastrointest Endosc 2015. [Epub ahead of print].
56. Chen JJ, Wang XM, Liu XQ, et al. Risk factors for post-ERCP pancreatitis: a systematic review of clinical trials with a large sample size in the past 10 years. Eur J Med Res 2014;19:26.
57. Glomsaker T, Hoff G, Kvaløy JT, et al. Patterns and predictive factors of complications after endoscopic retrograde cholangiopancreatography. Br J Surg 2013; 100:373–80.
58. Choudari CP, Sherman S, Fogel EL, et al. Success of ERCP at a referral center after a previously unsuccessful attempt. Gastrointest Endosc 2000;52:478–83.
59. Poincloux L, Rouquette O, Buc E, et al. Endoscopic ultrasound-guided biliary drainage after failed ERCP: cumulative experience of 101 procedures at a single center. Endoscopy 2015;47(9):794–801.

Minimally Invasive Approaches to Pancreatic Surgery

Deepa Magge, MD[a],*, Amer Zureikat, MD[a], Melissa Hogg, MD[a],
Herbert J. Zeh III, MD[b]

KEYWORDS

- Pancreatic adenocarcinoma • Whipple • Distal pancreatectomy • Minimally invasive
- Open

KEY POINTS

- Open and minimally invasive approaches to pancreatic surgery for benign and malignant lesions have been shown to be equivalent in regards to their safety profiles in multiple large single institution series.
- Emerging multicenter data indicate that outcomes including morbidity/mortality, fistula occurrence, and overall survival are equivalent between the two distinct operative techniques.
- Laparoscopic and robotic surgical techniques have gained increasing acceptance over the last few years especially in the setting of pancreatic malignancy and may be associated with decreased patient hospital stays and comparable oncologic outcomes.

INTRODUCTION

Minimally invasive techniques have the potential to revolutionize the surgical management of pancreatic disease in the setting of benign and malignant processes. Both laparoscopic and robot-assisted approaches to pancreatic surgery have made open procedures, traditionally wrought with high morbidity, safer and more feasible.[1] There still remains no consensus regarding the oncologic efficacy of minimally invasive surgery for pancreatic cancer even though median survival after open resection remains 16 to 19 months with 5-year overall survival averaging 22% to 25%.[2] Recent advances in minimally invasive surgery seem to reduce the perioperative morbidity of

The authors have nothing to disclose.
[a] Division of GI Surgical Oncology, University of Pittsburgh Medical Center, 200 Lothrop Street, Pittsburgh, PA 15213, USA; [b] Division of GI Surgical Oncology, University of Pittsburgh Medical Center, 5150 Centre Avenue, Suite 417, Pittsburgh 15232, PA, USA
* Corresponding author.
E-mail address: maggedr@upmc.edu

Surg Oncol Clin N Am 25 (2016) 273–286
http://dx.doi.org/10.1016/j.soc.2015.11.001
1055-3207/16/$ – see front matter © 2016 Elsevier Inc. All rights reserved.

surgonc.theclinics.com

pancreaticoduodenectomy for benign tumors while maintaining a perioperative safety profile equivalent to open approaches. The laparoscopic pancreaticoduodenectomy (LPD) was initially met with skepticism because of long operative times, but has now been established as safe and feasible when performed by select high-volume surgeons at experienced centers.[3] The robotic pancreaticoduodenectomy (RPD), first performed in 2007, is now being increasingly used because of the perceived benefits of stereotactic vision, magnification, platform stability, and favorable ergonomics.[4] Our institution is a strong advocate for minimally invasive approaches to pancreatic surgery and has demonstrated equivalent outcomes between open, laparoscopic, and robotic approaches and favors the robotic technique for benign and malignant processes of the pancreas. The urgency and potential benefits of minimally invasive surgery for patients with pancreatic cancer are highlighted by two recent observations: findings from the National Cancer Database show that 71.4% of patients with clinical stage 1 pancreatic adenocarcinoma currently choose no therapy for their disease and experience shorter survival compared with patients treated with pancreatectomy ($P<.001$) suggesting a nihilism and fear about pancreatic surgery; and nearly half of patients undergoing open pancreaticoduodenectomy (OPD) have complications preventing administration of proven adjuvant chemotherapy.[5] Wu and colleagues[6] have demonstrated the impact of postoperative complications on the administration of adjuvant therapy following pancreaticoduodenectomy for adenocarcinoma. In their retrospective review of 1144 patients who underwent pancreaticoduodenectomy between 1995 and 2011, they noted an overall complication rate of 49.1%, and overall, 54% of the patients received adjuvant chemotherapy. Presence of a postoperative complication led to a definite delay in time to adjuvant therapy and reduced the likelihood of receiving multimodality therapy.

This article presents a review of two minimally invasive techniques for distal pancreatectomy (DP) and pancreaticoduodenectomy, focusing on metrics of technique, safety, morbidity, and oncologic outcomes and potential benefits.

LAPAROSCOPIC DISTAL PANCREATECTOMY
Indications for Minimally Invasive Distal Pancreatectomy

The minimally invasive approach to the DP (MIDP) is now considered by many to be the preferred method of resection for benign and malignant tumors of the distal pancreas. Several studies have been performed, collectively supporting that LDP and RDP can be performed with superior results to the open approach in patients with benign and malignant disease.[1,3,4] Specifically, the minimally invasive approach results in shorter hospital stay, reduced blood loss (EBL), and decreased complication rates.[4,7,8] Similar oncologic resections can be accomplished in terms of lymph node dissection and resection margins, although larger reports of long-term survival are still lacking. Current absolute contraindications to LDP or RDP include prohibitive medical comorbidities and poor patient functional status. Relative contraindications include locally advanced malignancies, vascular invasion, and prior major abdominal operations.[8] Involvement of the celiac trunk is not an absolute contraindication to minimally invasive approach.

Technique of Laparoscopic Distal Pancreatectomy

The patient is placed in supine position, and the peritoneum is accessed either via a Veress needle approach or optical separator technique, which are both inserted in the left subcostal area to induce pneumoperitoneum. The second trocar is then inserted in the right supraumbilical region (12 mm). The remaining trocars are then placed in the left paraxiphoid region (5 mm), right subcostal area (5 mm), and left supraumbilical region (12 mm). Dissection begins with division of the gastrocolic ligament to enter the lesser sac. The splenic flexure of the colon is then mobilized inferiorly, and the anterior surface of the pancreas is inspected. The transverse mesocolon is then dissected off the inferior border of the pancreas, and the pancreas is dissected out of the retroperitoneum at the site of transection, creating a subpancreatic tunnel. Early identification of the splenic vessels and dissection of the vein and artery off the superoposterior aspect of the pancreas allows safer pancreatic transection. Once the vessels have been mobilized, the pancreatic parenchyma is divided using a linear stapler or harmonic scalpel, which is followed by division of the splenic vessels using a stapling device or clips. The spleen is then mobilized by sectioning the suspending ligaments, and the specimen is then placed in a large bag and brought through an access incision.[9]

Outcomes of Laparoscopic Distal Pancreatectomy

Two methodologic problems complicate prospective studies of surgical technique for distal pancreatic cancer: only 20.8% of pancreatic ductal adenocarcinomas (PDA) arise in the distal pancreas; and the 1640 distal pancreatic resections performed annually in the United States are distributed among 1743 hospitals according to 1998 to 2003 data in the Nationwide Inpatient Sample, an average annual case volume of one per hospital. As a result, most comparative effectiveness research has been retrospective and confined to single institution data.[10] Published outcomes after minimally invasive pancreatic resection demonstrate technical equivalence to open DP with reduced intraoperative blood loss and shortened hospital stay. There are only three published studies comparing open and laparoscopic DP (ODP and LDP) in patients with PDA. A single study of 23 patients undergoing LDP for PDC at nine centers has demonstrated median survival identical to open at 16 months by means of a 3:1 matched comparison with historical open DP control subjects.[11]

Our institution performed a retrospective case series comparing clinicopathologic and long-term oncologic outcomes after MIDP and ODP for pancreatic ductal carcinoma in 62 consecutive patients at a single institution. Intention-to-treat analysis demonstrated no evidence for inferiority of MIDP compared with ODP in terms of postoperative outcomes or long-term survival.[12] Another recent study by Nakamura and colleagues[13] comparing LDP and ODP using propensity score-matching indicated the superiority of the laparoscopic approach over the open technique in regards to perioperative outcomes, including higher rate of preservation of spleen and splenic vessels ($P<.001$), lower rates of intraoperative transfusion ($P = .020$), clinical-grade pancreatic fistula ($P<.001$), and morbidity ($P<.001$). The laparoscopic cohort also had a shorter hospital stay ($P = .001$), but a longer operative time ($P<.001$).

ROBOT-ASSISTED DISTAL PANCREATECTOMY
Technique of Robot-Assisted Distal Pancreatectomy

MIDP has several advantages to its open counterpart with regards to blood loss, operative time, hospital length of stay, and complications particularly for benign disease. Furthermore, emerging data suggest that the robotic technique is a superior minimally invasive platform. Since 2009, our institution has performed hundreds of RDPs and has been able to demonstrate specific technical advantages provided by the robot-assisted approach, which are particularly important in the setting of pancreatic adenocarcinoma where adherence to oncologic principles are key to successful resections.[14]

After the peritoneum is accessed in a similar fashion to that obtained in the laparoscopic approach, additional trocars are placed, and the robot is docked. Again, the lesser sac is entered by division of the gastrocolic ligament and the colonic splenic flexure is mobilized inferiorly. Focus is then paid on division of the pancreatic neck. Stereotactic vision and the robotic camera angle allow safe and quick isolation of the pancreatic neck over the superior mesenteric vein (SMV)–splenic vein confluence.[14] The splenic artery is isolated at its takeoff from the celiac trunk, and divided with a vascular stapler (**Figs. 1** and **2**).[14]

A lymphadenectomy is then carried out starting from the left side of the superior mesenteric artery (SMA) laterally, taking the posterior pancreatic fascia en bloc, and a comprehensive celiac lymphadenectomy is completed. With large tumors involving the fourth portion of the duodenum or colon, the robot allows meticulous en bloc resections with reconstructions performed in a similar fashion to the open technique.[14]

Outcomes of Robot-Assisted Distal Pancreatectomy

At the University of Pittsburgh, we compared our prospectively gathered data from the first 30 cases of RDP (performed between 2008 and 2011) with a historical control group of 94 laparoscopic cases (2004–2007, before the robot became available, and well after the group had established maturity with LDP).[15] Patients undergoing RDP and LDP demonstrated equivalent age, gender, ethnicity, ASA (American Society of Anesthesiologists) score, and tumor size. No conversions to open surgery occurred in the RDP group compared with 16% in the LDP group ($P<.05$). This was despite that more PDA were approached robotically than laparoscopically (43% vs 15%; $P<.05$).[15] A more recent updated series of 100 RDPs by our institution demonstrated a persistently low conversion rate of (2%). This may be secondary to the ability of the surgeon at the console to control large vessels and manage unexpected bleeding via intracorporeal suturing more readily with the robot than using laparoscopy. In this experience, RDP outcomes were optimized after 40 cases.[16]

Additionally, the robot platform has been shown to allow improved ability over laparoscopy to perform splenic preservation. In our institutional experience, we have demonstrated enhanced ability to preserve the spleen given increased maneuverability of the robotic arms to carefully dissect out the splenic vessels.[17] In the difficult scenario where the splenic artery is embedded within the superior pancreatic parenchyma, robotic visualization, magnification, and improved dexterity of the instruments allow for rapid and efficient isolation and division of this vessel thereby avoiding a conversion.[15]

The oncologic outcomes between the minimally invasive approach and the open technique for DP have been shown to be equivalent. Use of the robot seems to offer

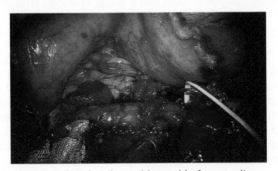

Fig. 1. The splenic artery is isolated and vessel looped before stapling.

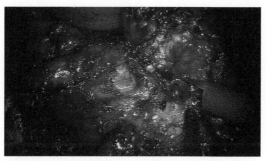

Fig. 2. Completed medial to lateral pancreatic body/tail mobilization.

an increased advantage over laparoscopy, based on the authors' experience. Our institutional experience demonstrated that despite a higher percentage of adenocarcinoma in the robotic group (43% vs 15%; P<.05) and a similar median tumor size of approximately 3 cm, RDP was associated with improved R0 resection rates (100% vs 64%; P<.05), and median lymph node count (19 vs 9; P<.01) when compared with laparoscopy.[15] Although single institution outcomes may not be generalizable, we believe this observation reflects the ability to better recapitulate open oncologic principles with the robotic approach. A more comprehensive lymphadenectomy is completed given enhanced magnification and maneuverability of the robot.

Lastly, it has been shown that patients having undergone RDP as opposed to LDP or ODP have shorter hospital stays given decreased wound complications and increased rates of splenic preservation.[15] As further experience with the robot-assisted approach is gained, additional advantages may be realized (**Table 1**).

LAPAROSCOPIC PANCREATICODUODENECTOMY
Anatomic Considerations When Considering Approach/Indications for Minimally Invasive Approach

Determining the resectability of pancreatic adenocarcinoma of the head of the pancreas depends primarily on the involvement of the mesenteric vessels. Preoperative assessment of the presence of metastatic disease or superior mesenteric arterial or venous involvement in the tumor process is critical in determining whether a patient is a candidate for an open versus minimally invasive approach to the pancreaticoduodenectomy, or whether they are a candidate for surgical resection at all. Based on consensus guidelines, resectable tumors are those that have no distant metastasis; have no radiographic evidence of abutment or distortion of the SMV and portal vein (PV); and have clear fat planes surrounding the celiac axis, hepatic artery, and SMA.[18] Patients with tumor abutment of the SMV/PV, gastroduodenal artery abutment or encasement up to the hepatic artery, or abutment of the SMA less than 180° are considered to be borderline resectable and benefit from neoadjuvant treatment.[18]

Minimally invasive approaches, including laparoscopic and robotic techniques, do not allow for palpation of the tumor intraoperatively, which often precludes determination of resectability. Therefore, the use of the triple-phase computed tomography to determine operative resectability is key before proceeding with surgical resection. The close relationship of these large vessels to tumors in the head of the pancreas frequently results in abutment or invasion often requiring vascular resection, which has not been often performed using a minimally invasive approach, but has been described.

Table 1
Select series of minimally invasive surgery distal pancreatectomy

Author, Year	Technique	N (Total)/N (Malignant)	EBL (mL)	Operative Time (min)	Fistula Rate (Grade C)	Mortality Rate	Oncologic Outcomes (R0 Rate, LN)
Fernandez Cruz et al,[34–41] 2007	Laparoscopic	82/13	370	222	7%	0%	77%, 14.5
Kooby et al,[11] 2008	Laparoscopic	142/54	357	230	26%	0%	93%, NR
Jayarman,[9] 2010	Laparoscopic	107/16	150	193	16%	NR	97%, 6
Kang et al,[42] 2011	Robot	20/18	372	348	NR	0%	NR, NR
Zureikat et al,[18] 2013	Robot	83/60	150	256	36%	0%	97%, 16

Abbreviations: LN, lymph node; NR, not reported.

Recent literature has revealed oncologic equivalency between open and minimally invasive pancreaticoduodenectomy.[18,19] Most high-volume pancreatic centers are now performing laparoscopic and/or robotic surgery for benign and malignant processes. Song and colleagues[20] demonstrated in a case-control fashion comparable oncologic outcomes between patients undergoing open and laparoscopic pylorus-preserving pancreaticoduodenectomy. Similarly, Croome and colleagues[21] demonstrated better operative outcomes and improved oncologic efficacy using the laparoscopic approach compared with the traditional open technique to the Whipple for PDA. An increasing number of pancreatic resections are being performed using minimally invasive approaches, but it remains to be determined if the benefits of this technique outweigh its longer operative times and higher costs. Minimally invasive pancreaticoduodenectomy is a feasible procedure in selected patients who are cared for in select centers by experts in pancreatic surgery.[22] Patients who are candidates for an OPD are not precluded from a minimally invasive approach based on age, body mass index, or comorbidities. However, prior major abdominal surgery or evidence of vascular involvement most likely requiring vascular reconstruction were previously considered relative contraindications to using a minimally invasive approach to pancreatic resection.

Technique of Laparoscopic Pancreaticoduodenectomy

LPD has been described by Zureikat and colleagues[23] and involves complete laparoscopic mobilization of the pancreas and duodenum. The patient is placed supine on a standard operating room table. After gaining access to the abdomen using an optical-separator device in the left upper quadrant, a total of seven ports are placed in a crescent shape around the xiphoid process. A right lower quadrant incision with muscle-sparing technique is used to extract the specimen. On access to the abdomen, the peritoneal cavity is systematically explored to evaluate for metastatic disease. The laparoscopic procedure mirrors that of the open with a few minor modifications. The authors prefer to dissect the inferior border of the pancreas and SMV before the Kocher maneuver. The hepatic flexure is then mobilized and the duodenum fully kocherized. The porta hepatitis is dissected in a similar fashion used for open surgery. A tunnel is created between the PV and pancreatic neck and the pancreas is divided using bipolar electrocautery.[23] An antrectomy is typically performed rather than pylorus preservation procedure based on surgeon preference.

Reconstruction begins with an end-to-side duct to mucosa pancreaticojejunostomy using two-layered running absorbable monofilament. A running 4–0 absorbable monofilament suture is used for the hepaticojejunostomy. A stapled technique is used for the gastrojejunostomy. Two drains are left around the pancreaticojejunostomy before closure.[23]

Outcomes of Laparoscopic Pancreaticoduodenectomy

The LPD is a technically challenging operation. The initial report of Gagner and Pomp[24] of 10 LPDs in 1997 did not favor use of the laparoscopic technique over the open approach because of the high conversion rate (40%) and lack of any perceived benefits. Subsequently, several reports have emerged attempting to further characterize the safety and oncologic efficacy of the LPD, and some have directly compared it with the OPD. Senthilnathan and colleagues[25] described one of the largest initial series of 150 LPDs (130 of which were for adenocarcinomas). This report demonstrated the advantages and feasibility of the minimally invasive approach when performed by highly skilled surgeons. Mean operative time for the entire cohort was 310 minutes (range, 276–344) with a mean EBL of 110 mL (range, 88–132), and one conversion to OPD.

Average hospital stay was 8 days (range, 5.4–10.6) and overall postoperative morbidity was 29.7%. Reoperation was required in five cases (3.84%; two with hemorrhage, one with jejunal loop obstruction, and two with grade C pancreatic fistula). Grade B and C postoperative pancreatic fistula rate was 8.46%. Resected margins were positive in 9.23% of cases, and the mean number of retrieved lymph nodes was 18. The overall 5-year actuarial survival was 29.42%, and the median survival was 33 months.[25]

Kim and colleagues[26] describe another large series of laparoscopic pylorus preserving PD with 100 cases performed between 2007 and 2011 for patients with benign and malignant periampullary lesions. A median operative time of 7.9 hours with mean hospital stay of 14 days was reported for the entire cohort. Overall morbidity rate was 25%, with a 6% pancreatic fistula rate (International Study Group for Pancreatic Fistula grade B or C), all of which were treated conservatively. Postoperative hemorrhage occurred in five patients, only one of whom required reoperation, and DGE (Delayed gastric emptying) occurred in two patients.[26]

In another series of 62 LPDs (45 patients with malignant disease) by Kendrick and Cusati,[27] operative metrics were impressive with a median operative time of 368 minutes and median EBL of 240 mL. Outcomes for the patients with cancer were not detailed separately. Mean length of hospital stay was 7 days and overall morbidity rate was 42%, which included DGE in nine patients and pancreatic fistula in 18% of the patients. Reoperation was required in three (5%) patients for control of sepsis secondary to a pancreatic leak (one), control of hemorrhage following percutaneous drain placement (one), and revision of a biliary leak (one). The reported 30-day operative mortality was 1.6%.[27]

Another comparative review performed by Kendrick and colleagues[28] compared 31 patients undergoing LPD with major vascular resection with 58 patients undergoing the open approach. Mean operative blood loss was significantly less in the laparoscopic (842 mL) compared with the open group (1452 mL) ($P<.001$), as was median hospital stay, 6 (4–118) versus 9 (6–73) days, respectively ($P = .006$). There was no significant difference in the total number of complications (laparoscopic, 35%; open, 48%) or severe complications (laparoscopic, 6.4%; open, 3.4%) in the two groups. In-hospital mortality and 30-day mortality were also not statistically different between the laparoscopic and open groups, 3.2% and 3.4%, respectively. This review demonstrated that the minimally invasive approach to pancreatic resection with major vascular resection is not only feasible and safe but can also result in equivalent oncologic and operative outcomes to the traditional open technique, and although vascular reconstruction used to be considered a contraindication to the minimally invasive approach, it no longer is considered as such.[28]

Kendrick and colleagues[21] focused on the oncologic effectiveness of the MIDP in another review directly comparing 108 patients who underwent LPD with 214 patients who underwent OPD for PDA. They found a significantly higher proportion of patients in the OPD group (12%) who had a delay of greater than 90 days or who did not receive adjuvant chemotherapy at all compared with that in the TLPD (total laparoscopic pancreaticoduodenectomy) group (5%; $P = .04$). There was no significant difference in overall survival between the two groups, but a significantly longer progression-free survival was seen in the TLPD group than in the OPD group ($P = .03$). This study reveals a possible oncologic advantage to the laparoscopic approach over the open technique.[21]

The previously mentioned studies clearly indicate that these initial LPD outcomes are comparable with historic open control subjects, with equivalent operative time, morbidity, and mortality. Blood loss is consistently better than open series, and oncologic outcomes have also been shown to equivalent between the two approaches (**Table 2**).

ROBOT-ASSISTED PANCREATICODUODENECTOMY
Technique

The reported advantages of minimally invasive pancreaticoduodenectomy include better visualization, faster recovery time, and decreased length of hospital stay. In cases of robotic approaches, some of the proposed advantages include increased dexterity and a superior ergonomic position for the operating surgeon.

As described by Zeh and coworkers[29] and Zureikat and colleagues, the robot is now docked very early in the robot-assisted approached to the pancreaticoduodenectomy. The first step is achieved robotically and includes mobilization of the right colon and kocherization of the duodenum along with mobilization of its third and fourth portions. A near total Cattell-Brasch maneuver is performed to expose the SMV at the root of the small bowel mesentery. An extended Kocher maneuver is completed to pull the jejunum into the right upper quadrant via division of the ligament of Treitz. The jejunum is transected around 10 cm distal to the ligament of Treitz using a linear stapler then marked with a suture around 50 cm distally and tacked to the stomach. The second step involves division of the gastrocolic omentum and entrance into the lesser sac, followed by dissection of the posterior stomach from the anterior surface of the pancreas. The right gastric artery is ligated close to the stomach and the right gastroepiploic artery is then ligated at the corresponding greater curvature side. The stomach is divided with a linear stapler at this time and an automated liver retractor is inserted to facilitate exposure.

Dissection is then carried out at the level of the superior border of the pancreas using the robotic hook to identify the common hepatic artery. The right gastric artery is again divided, now at its origin, and the gastroduodenal artery is transected. Cholecystectomy is performed and the lymph nodes are dissected along the lateral border of the common bile duct taking care to identify any aberrant right hepatic artery. The common bile duct is identified and divided followed by thorough portal dissection. The right gastroepiploic vein is identified and followed to its origin to locate the SMV and middle colic vein. The gastroepiploic vein is doubly clipped or tied and divided. The SMV is dissected off the inferior border of the pancreas and a tunnel is created over the PV. The angle afforded by the robotic camera ensures safe visualization of the tunnel. After completion of the tunnel, the neck of the pancreas is divided with electrocautery, reserving sharp robotic scissor transection for the PD. The pancreas is then mobilized from the lateral border of the SMV-PV working caudad to cephalad. The first jejunal branch is divided with a vascular stapler. The SMV-PV is reflected medially and the SMA is identified. Dissection proceeds along the SMA by clearing all the tissue around the anterior, right side, and posterior surface of the SMA.[29,30]

Reconstruction is started with a two-layered end-to-side duct to mucosa pancreaticojejunostomy in a modified Blumgart fashion. The choledochojejunostomy is then performed in a running fashion. An antecolic Hoffmeister end-to-side gastrojejunostomy is hand-sewn in two layers.[29,30]

Outcomes of Robot-Assisted Pancreaticoduodenectomy

Despite substantial literature supporting advantages to the minimally invasive approach for the DP, evidence supporting similar benefits for the minimally invasive pancreaticoduodenectomy is still lacking. Both LPD and RPD outcomes are similar, and are not inferior to OPD in carefully selected patients. Additionally, both minimally

Table 2
Select series of minimally invasive surgery pancreaticoduodenectomy

Author, Year	Technique	N (Total)/N (Malignant)	EBL (mL)	Operative Time (min)	Fistula Rate (Grade C)	Mortality Rate	Oncologic Outcomes (R0 Rate, LN)
Guilianotti et al,[4] 2010	Robot	60/45	394	421	31.6%	3%	90%, 18
Kim et al,[26] 2013	Laparoscopic	100/12	—	474	6%	—	100%, 13
Kendrick,[21] 2014	Laparoscopic	108/108	492.4	379.4	11%	1%	77.8%, 21.4
Palanivelu,[25] 2015	Laparoscopic	150/130	110	310	8.5%	0%	90.8%, 18
Zureikat,[31] (last 120 cases) 2015	Robot	200/166	250	417	6.9%	3.3%	91.4%, 26

Abbreviation: LN, lymph node.

invasive platforms seem to be advantageous to OPD with respect to blood loss. Other potential advantages need to be explored in larger control matched series.

Several case control studies evaluating outcomes of RPDs have been performed and have shown that estimated blood loss and length of stay is significantly better in the RPD with no increase in operative mortality compared with the open cohort. None of the studies to date have demonstrated an improvement in overall morbidity, fistula rate, or operative times. However, it should be noted that the largest of these case control studies is 44 robotic cases; thus, all published comparisons between open and robotic PDs suffer from low numbers that compare early robotic experiences with mature open ones. The learning curve for OPD is estimated to be around 60 to 70 cases and according to Boone and colleagues[31] it is likely that the RAPD learning curve is similar.

Our institution has now performed more than 300 RPDs to date. In an analysis of the first 132 RPD, improvements in operative times, open conversion and EBL, morbidity, and pancreatic fistula rates have been observed. Although the operative time is often the main criticism of RPD, there has been a decline in this key point. The last 100 RPD at our institution have been performed with median time 340 minutes. A recent RPD analysis from the University of Pittsburgh confirmed that outcomes are optimized after an initial steep learning curve of approximately 80 cases. In-depth analysis of this learning curve revealed that blood loss and conversions were optimized after 20 cases (600 vs 250, $P<.05$, and 35% vs 3%, $P<.05$ respectively), incidence of pancreatic fistula after 40 cases (27% vs 14%; $P<.05$), and operative time after 80 cases (582 minutes vs 417 minutes; $P<.05$).[31] Complication rates, length of stay, and readmissions also improved but the sample size was underpowered to detect a significant difference. In the last 100 cases, we found a fistula rate of 6%, a 90-day mortality rate of 3%, and a median length of stay of 8 days. Importantly, a two-attending approach was used throughout the learning curve period to ensure patient safety and procedural efficacy.[31] These data suggest that meaningful comparative effectiveness studies of minimally invasive and open PD should take into consideration the impact of the learning curve before any outcomes are assessed.

Clavien grade 3 and 4 complications (requiring radiologic, endoscopic, or anesthetic intervention and/or causing end organ damage) have decreased from 30.7% in the first 80% to 13.7 % ($P = .035$). This compares favorably with published reports of OPD that estimate major morbidity using the Clavien system to be between 30% and 40%. This improved morbidity profile has not translated into shorter length of stay (median RPD hospital stay in the authors series = 10 days), but this may be largely a reflection of a cautious approach in our assessment of this early technology. Overall International Study Group on Pancreatic Fistula leak rate was 17% (grade C = 3.7%), comparing favorably with the most recent large analysis by Denbo and colleagues[32,33] of more than 2700 OPDs (18% overall leak rate, grade C ≤5%).

The conversion rate and blood loss metrics have also improved with increased experience. The conversion rate and EBL have decreased from 35% and 600 mL in the first 20 cases to 3% and 250 mL in the subsequent cohort ($P = .0001$ and 0.002, respectively). The conversion rate compares favorably with most LPD series, and the EBL is well below most OPD reports.[31]

Our institution's early optimization of the RPD was performed without the assistance of simulators and bioartificial organs. Over the past year, University of Pittsburgh Medical Center has implemented a robotic curriculum in the training of its surgical oncology fellows using a step-wise approach to advanced robot training. The past six fellows all completed RPDs on the pancreaticobiliary service, with no decrease to the attending team's median operative time. This illustrates the benefit of an established robotic curriculum in surgical training.

Minimally invasive approaches to major gastrointestinal surgery have been shown to be as effective as the traditional open approach. Laparoscopic surgery offers patients distinct benefits but is not without its disadvantages to surgeons in terms of maneuverability and visualization. Robotic telemanipulation systems were introduced with the objective of providing a solution to the problems in this field of surgery. Pancreatic surgery, in particular, may be aided significantly by minimal access surgery given the high morbidity associated with traditional open pancreatic procedures. Our institutional experience demonstrates that minimally invasive pancreas resections are safe, feasible, and associated with equivalent outcomes to historical series of OPD. Moreover, our experience suggests that the robot-assisted approach may offer benefit over open and laparoscopic approaches. Currently, multicenter comparative effectiveness trials are hindered by the low number of centers with enough experience with these approaches to allow for either randomization or propensity scoring. However, as the minimally invasive approach continues to be widely adopted by specialized centers, these further investigations will be possible.

REFERENCES

1. Mack MJ. Minimally invasive and robotic surgery. JAMA 2001;285:568–72.
2. Shoup M, Conlon KC, Klimstra D, et al. Is extended resection for adenocarcinoma of the body or tail of the pancreas justified? J Gastrointest Surg 2003;7(8):946–52.
3. Cadiere GB, Himpens J, Germay O, et al. Feasibility of robotic laparoscopic surgery: 146 cases. World J Surg 2001;25:1467–77.
4. Giulianotti PC, Sbrana F, Bianco FM, et al. Robot-assisted laparoscopic pancreatic surgery: single-surgeon experience. Surg Endosc 2010;24(7):1646–57.
5. Bilimoria KY, Bentrem DJ, Ko CY, et al. National failure to operate on early stage pancreatic cancer. Ann Surg 2007;246(2):173–80.
6. Wu W, He J, Cameron JL, et al. The impact of postoperative complications on the administration of adjuvant therapy following pancreaticoduodenectomy for adenocarcinoma. Ann Surg Oncol 2014;21(9):2873–81.
7. Asbun HJ, Stauffer JA. Laparoscopic vs open pancreaticoduodenectomy: overall outcomes and severity of complications using the Accordion Severity Grading System. J Am Coll Surg 2012;215(6):810–9.
8. Kooby DA, Hawkins WG, Schmidt CM, et al. A multicenter analysis of distal pancreatectomy for adenocarcinoma: is laparoscopic resection appropriate? J Am Coll Surg 2010;210(5):779–85, 786–7.
9. Jayaraman S, Gonen M, Brennan M, et al. Laparoscopic distal pancreatectomy: evolution of a technique at a single institution. J Am Coll Surg 2010;211:503–9.
10. McPhee JT, Hill JS, Whalen GF, et al. Perioperative mortality for pancreatectomy: a national perspective. Ann Surg 2007;246:246–53.
11. Kooby DA, Gillespie T, Bentrem D, et al. Left-sided pancreatectomy: a multicenter comparison of laparoscopic and open approaches. Ann Surg 2008;248(3):438–46.
12. Magge D, Zeh HJ 3rd, Moser AJ, et al. Comparative effectiveness of minimally invasive and open distal pancreatectomy for ductal adenocarcinoma. JAMA Surg 2013;148(6):525–31.
13. Nakamura M, Wakabayashi G, Miyasaka Y, et al. Multicenter comparative study of laparoscopic and open distal pancreatectomy using propensity score-matching. J Hepatobiliary Pancreat Sci 2015;22(10):731–6.

14. Winer J, Can MF, Bartlett DL, et al. The current state of robotic-assisted pancreatic surgery. Nat Rev Gastroenterol Hepatol 2012;9(8):468–76.
15. Daouadi M, Zureikat AH, Zenati MS, et al. Robot-assisted minimally invasive distal pancreatectomy is superior to the laparoscopic technique. Ann Surg 2013;257(1):128–32.
16. Shakir M, Boone BA, Zeh HJ, et al. The learning curve for robotic distal pancreatectomy: an analysis of outcomes of the first 100 consecutive cases at a high-volume pancreatic centre. HPB (Oxford) 2015;17(7):580–6.
17. Chong C, Lee KF, Fong AK, et al. Robot-assisted laparoscopic spleen-preserving distal pancreatectomy. Surg Pract 2015;19(1):40–1.
18. Zureikat AH, Moser AJ, Boone BA, et al. 250 robotic pancreatic resections: safety and feasibility. Ann Surg 2013;258(4):554–9.
19. Callery MP, Chang KJ, Fishman EK, et al. Pretreatment assessment of resectable and borderline resectable pancreatic cancer: expert consensus statement. Ann Surg Oncol 2009;16(7):1727–33.
20. Song KB, Kim SC, Hwang DW, et al. Matched case-control analysis comparing laparoscopic and open pylorus-preserving pancreaticoduodenectomy in patients with periampullary tumors. Ann Surg 2015;262(1):146–55.
21. Croome KP, Farnell MB, Kendrick ML, et al. Total laparoscopic pancreaticoduodenectomy for pancreatic ductal adenocarcinoma: oncologic advantages over open approaches. Ann Surg 2014;260(4):633–8.
22. Cho A, Yamamoto H, Nagata M, et al. Comparison of laparoscopy-assisted and open pylorus–preserving pancreaticoduodenectomy for periampullary disease. Am J Surg 2009;198:445–9.
23. Zureikat AH, Breaux JA, Steel JL, et al. Can laparoscopic pancreaticoduodenectomy be safely implemented? J Gastrointest Surg 2011;15(7):1151–7.
24. Gagner M, Pomp A. Laparoscopic pylorus-preserving pancreatoduodenectomy. Surg Endosc 1994;8(5):408–10.
25. Senthilnathan P, Gurumurthy SS, Palanivelu C, et al. Long-term results of laparoscopic pancreaticoduodenectomy for pancreatic and periampullary cancer—experience of 130 cases from a tertiary-care center in South India. J Laparoendosc Adv Surg Tech A 2015;25(4):295–300.
26. Kim SC, Song KB, Jung YS, et al. Short-term clinical outcomes for 100 consecutive cases of laparoscopic pylorus-preserving pancreatoduodenectomy: improvement with surgical experience. Surg Endosc 2013;27(1):95–103.
27. Kendrick ML, Cusati D. Total laparoscopic pancreaticoduodenectomy: feasibility and outcome in an early experience. Arch Surg 2010;145(1):19–23.
28. Croome KP, Farnell MB, Kendrick ML, et al. Pancreaticoduodenectomy with major vascular resection: a comparison of laparoscopic versus open approaches. J Gastrointest Surg 2015;19(1):189–94.
29. Zeh HJ, Bartlett DL, Moser AJ. Robotic-assisted major pancreatic resection. Adv Surg 2011;45(1):323–40.
30. Nguyen KT, Zureikat AH, Chalikonda S, et al. Technical aspects of robotic-assisted pancreaticoduodenectomy (RAPD). J Gastrointest Surg 2011;15(5):870–5.
31. Boone BA, Zenati M, Zureikat AH, et al. Assessment of quality outcomes for robotic pancreaticoduodenectomy: identification of the learning curve. JAMA Surg 2015;150(5):416–22.
32. Denbo JW, Orr WS, Zarzaur BL, et al. Toward defining grade C pancreatic fistula following pancreaticoduodenectomy: incidence, risk factors, management and outcome. HPB (Oxford) 2012;14(9):589–93.

33. Lai EC, Yang GP, Tang CN. Robot-assisted laparoscopic pancreaticoduodenectomy versus open pancreaticoduodenectomy–a comparative study. Int J Surg 2012;10(9):475–9.

34. Fernandez-Cruz L, Cosa R, Blanco L, et al. Curative laparoscopic resection for pancreatic neoplasms: a critical analysis from a single institution. J Gastrointest Surg 2007;11(12):1607–21 [discussion: 1621–2].

35. Kang CM, Kim DH, Lee WJ, et al. Initial experiences using robot-assisted central pancreatectomy with pancreaticogastrostomy: a potential way to advanced laparoscopic pancreatectomy. Surg Endosc 2011;25(4):1101–6.

36. Giulianotti PC, Sbrana F, Bianco FM, et al. Robotic-assisted laparoscopic middle pancreatectomy. J Laparoendosc Adv Surg Tech A 2010;20(2):135–9.

37. Corcione F, Pirozzi F, Cuccurullo D, et al. Laparoscopic pancreaticoduodenectomy: experience of 22 cases. Surg Endosc 2013;27(6):2131–6.

38. Kuroki T, Adachi T, Okamoto T, et al. A non-randomized comparative study of laparoscopy-assisted pancreaticoduodenectomy and open pancreaticoduodenectomy. Hepatogastroenterology 2012;59(114):570–3.

39. Gumbs AA, Rodriguez Rivera AM, Milone L, et al. Laparoscopic pancreatoduodenectomy: a review of 285 published cases. Ann Surg Oncol 2011;18(5):1335–41.

40. Mesleh MG, Stauffer JA, Bowers SP, et al. Cost analysis of open and laparoscopic pancreaticoduodenectomy: a single institution comparison. Surg Endosc 2013;27(12):4518–23.

41. Hwang HK, Kang CM, Chung YE, et al. Robot-assisted spleen-preserving distal pancreatectomy: a single surgeon's experiences and proposal of clinical application. Surg Endosc 2013;27(3):774–81.

42. Kang CM, Kim DH, Lee WJ, et al. Conventional laparoscopic and robot-assisted spleen-preserving pancreatectomy: does da Vinci have clinical advantages? Surg Endosc 2011;25:2004–9.

Advances in the Surgical Management of Resectable and Borderline Resectable Pancreas Cancer

Beth A. Helmink, MD, PhD[a], Rebecca A. Snyder, MD, MPH[b],
Kamran Idrees, MD[a], Nipun B. Merchant, MD[c],
Alexander A. Parikh, MD, MPH[a],*

KEYWORDS

- Resectability • Borderline resectable • Vascular resection
- Aberrant vascular anatomy • Lymphadenectomy • Pancreatic fistula
- Delayed gastric emptying • Palliation

KEY POINTS

- Despite successful surgical resection, recurrence rates remain high and overall survival is less than 20%.
- Advances in cross-sectional imaging and diagnostic modalities such as endoscopic ultrasound have allowed better characterization and selection of patients that will benefit from upfront surgical resection versus neoadjuvant therapy to improve the probability of achieving microscopically negative margins (R0).
- Margin-negative resection is possible in the setting of vascular involvement in borderline resectable and selected locally advanced patients after neoadjuvant therapy with vascular resection and/or reconstruction.
- Although mortality rates in high-volume centers are low, morbidity rates after resection remain significant, and efforts to minimize these complications are important to allow for the expeditious use of adjuvant therapy.

The authors have nothing to disclose.
[a] Division of Surgical Oncology, Vanderbilt University Medical Center, 597 PRB, 2220 Pierce Avenue, Nashville, TN 37232, USA; [b] Department of Surgical Oncology, University of Texas M.D. Anderson Cancer Center, 1400 Pressler Street, Unit Number: 1484, Houston, TX 77030, USA; [c] Division of Surgical Oncology, Sylvester Comprehensive Cancer Center, University of Miami Medical Center, 1120 Northwest 14th Street, Clinical Research Building, Suite 410, Miami, FL 33136, USA
* Corresponding author. Division of Surgical Oncology, Vanderbilt University Medical Center, 597 PRB, 2220 Pierce Avenue, Nashville, TN 37232.
E-mail address: alexander.parikh@vanderbilt.edu

Surg Oncol Clin N Am 25 (2016) 287–310
http://dx.doi.org/10.1016/j.soc.2015.11.008
1055-3207/16/$ – see front matter © 2016 Elsevier Inc. All rights reserved.

surgonc.theclinics.com

INTRODUCTION

Pancreatic cancer remains one of the most lethal diseases worldwide. Although surgical resection combined with multimodality therapy affords a significant survival advantage in some patients, the vast majority of patients present with locally advanced (LA) or metastatic disease for which palliation is the only option. For those patients who are candidates for resection, surgical options include a pancreaticoduodenectomy (PD), distal or left pancreatectomy (LP), or total pancreatectomy (TP), depending on the location of tumor within the pancreas.

Although surgical resection was initially associated with significant perioperative mortality, advances in surgical technique and perioperative care have reduced the mortality to the low single digits in high-volume centers.[1,2] In addition, improvements in preoperative imaging modalities have enabled better determination of the extent of disease and have thus allowed for better operative planning and patient selection as well as better standardization of treatment regimens. Nevertheless, perioperative morbidity remains a significant problem and can often result in inadequate administration of appropriate adjuvant therapy. However, even in those patients who undergo successful surgical resection and appropriate adjuvant therapy, 5-year survival rates remain low, ranging from 5% to 15%.[3]

In this review, the current state of surgical management of resectable and borderline-resectable (BR) pancreatic cancer is discussed, focusing on both the technical aspects and the common postoperative complications and their management.

DETERMINING RESECTABILITY

Whether a pancreatic tumor is amenable to surgical intervention is defined by the probability of achieving microscopically negative margins (R0) at the time of resection. Numerous studies have demonstrated a strong correlation between R0 resections and decreased recurrence rates and improved overall survival (OS).[4–12] Accordingly, margin status remains one of the most important predictors of long-term survival in pancreatic cancer.[4,6,13] The status of the resection margin is often cited as a significant predictor of patient outcomes following PD, with the median survival of patients with microscopically positive (R1) resection significantly decreased as compared with those undergoing R0 resection.[10,14,15] However, this is not without some controversy, as some studies do not indicate significant differences in survival between these 2 groups when controlled for other prognostic factors.[10,14,15] Overall, in patients undergoing PD for resectable disease, there is wide variance in the reported R1 resection rates with those rates varying from 20 to more than 80%.[10,14,15] These differences represent differences not only in patient selection and operative technique but also in the identification and analysis of the specimen by pathologists.

Although dependent on what type of resection being performed, margins during pancreatic resection typically include the following:

- Transection margins
  - Pancreatic neck margin
  - Common bile duct (CBD)/hepatic duct (CHD) margin
  - Distal stomach/proximal duodenum
- Circumferential margins
  - Anterior pancreatic margin
  - Posterior pancreatic margin

- ○ Superior mesenteric artery (SMA) margin
- ○ Superior mesenteric vein (SMV) margin
- ○ Radial CBD/CHD margin

Importantly, the transection margins can generally be extended if intraoperative analysis (usually by frozen section) suggests disease involvement. Circumferential margins are less clearly defined, and extending these margins is more difficult.

Unfortunately, there are no clear consensus guidelines addressing the pathologic analysis of PD specimens, including the number or types of margins, inking practices, or even diagnostic criteria for positivity. For example, in European studies, tumor found within 1 mm of the resection is defined as R1 resection, whereas in the United States, tumor must be present at the margin.[10,14] Moreover, the inflammation, atrophy, and fibrosis associated with pancreatic cancer, particularly in the setting of prior pancreatitis or neoadjuvant chemoradiation therapy, make the analyses of margins more difficult. Careful multicolor inking of the specimen with extensive sampling and thin axial slices as well as adoption of the European definition of R1 resection has been show to lead to more accurate R1 margin rates.[10,14,16,17] In fact, when careful pathologic analysis is performed, R1 resection rates tend to be higher and the discrepancy between the survival of patients undergoing R0 and R1 resections are more pronounced.[10,14,15] Current College of American Pathologists guidelines are vague and recommend "inking the posterior surface of the pancreas and submission of sections through the tumor at its closest approach to this surface as well as the retroperitoneal (uncinate) margin."[18]

In determining resectability, the main barrier to achieving R0 resection remains the relationship of the tumor to the mesenteric vasculature. The goal of preoperative staging and imaging, therefore, is not only to evaluate for metastatic disease but also to delineate the relationship of the relevant vasculature structures to the tumor, including the common hepatic artery (CHA), gastroduodenal artery (GDA), SMA, celiac axis, SMV, portal vein (PV), and the SMV-PV confluence. Preoperative staging and imaging enable the patient's tumor to be appropriated into 1 of 4 categories: resectable, BR, LA, or metastatic. One of the major obstacles in determining resectability of pancreas cancer has been the lack of a unified definition of these categories. Several institutions and agencies have published definitions; however, significant variation persists.

Resectable Disease

In general, upfront resectable disease is defined as

- Tumor without contact with the celiac artery (CA), hepatic artery (HA), SMA, or SMV, suggesting a high likelihood that margin-negative resection can be achieved without preoperative therapy **(Fig. 1A)**

With improvements in surgical technique and vascular resection, some groups also include tumors with limited involvement of the SMV-PV confluence in which an R0 resection is still possible, albeit with vascular resection and reconstruction in the resectable category **(Fig. 1B)**. For example, the MD Anderson Cancer Center (MDACC) definition deems tumors resectable if there is abutment of the SMV-PV with patent vessels.[19] The National Cancer Center Network (NCCN) also allows for 180° contact or less of the SMV-PV but only in the absence of any vein contour irregularity.[20]

Locally Advanced Disease

The definition of LA disease also varies, although in general, LA characterizes patients in whom the likelihood of attempting to resect the tumor even after treatment with

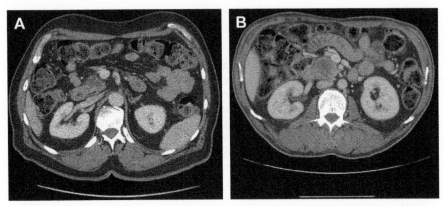

Fig. 1. (*A*) Cross-sectional imaging of a resectable pancreatic adenocarcinoma with preservation of a fat plane between the tumor and the SMV and SMA. (*B*) Resectable pancreatic adenocarcinoma with less than 180° involvement of the SMV but with a preserved fat plane between the tumor and SMA.

systemic or locoregional therapy to allow a margin-negative resection is essentially minimal. Although several varying definitions exist, essentially tumors with extensive vascular involvement especially arterial involvement are deemed LA (**Fig. 2, Table 1**).

Borderline Resectable Disease

The original term marginally resectable was coined to identify patients at high risk of a macroscopically positive (R2) resection with upfront surgery.[21] The term BR pancreas cancer was subsequently adopted by the NCCN in 2006 to describe patients who might benefit from neoadjuvant therapy in order to reduce the likelihood of margin

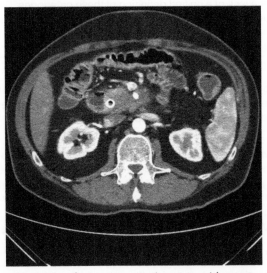

Fig. 2. Cross-sectional imaging of an LA pancreatic cancer with greater than 180° involvement of the SMA.

Table 1
Definitions of locally advanced pancreatic cancer

Vessel Involved	MDACC	AHPBA/SSO/SSAT	NCCN/ISGPS
SMA	Encasement	Encasement	Contact >180° or contact with first jejunal SMA branch
CHA	Encasement—unable to reconstruct	Encasement with extension to CA	Contact with extension to CA or bifurcation
Celiac axis	Encasement	Abutment or encasement	Contact >180°
SMV-PV confluence	Occluded—unable to reconstruct	Occluded—unable to reconstruct	Unable to reconstruct

positivity.[20] Unfortunately, what defines BR disease remains an area of significant controversy.

Over the past decade, several different classification schemes have been published to describe which patients are considered BR pancreatic cancer, including consensus statements and guidelines from the NCCN; the International Study Group of Pancreatic Surgery (ISGPS); MDACC; Americas Hepato-Pancreato-Biliary Association/Society of Surgical Oncology (AHPBA/SSO); the Society for Surgery of the Alimentary Tract (SSAT); and the Moffitt Cancer Center[19,20,22] (**Fig. 3**, **Table 2**).

Despite what would seem to be rather objective criteria, all of these definitions are somewhat subjective and are continually evolving. In the recent Alliance Trial (A021101), a multi-institutional single-armed trial designed to evaluate toxicity and feasibility of neoadjuvant chemotherapy and chemoradiation for BR pancreatic cancer, for example, the investigators advocated for an easily reproducible definition based on more objective data obtained from computed tomographic (CT) imaging, avoiding subjective terms like abutment or encasement. The Alliance definition

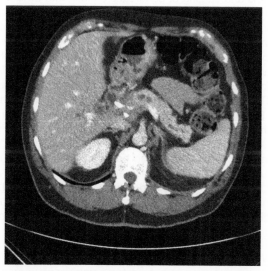

Fig. 3. Cross-sectional imaging of a BR pancreatic adenocarcinoma with encasement of the SMV, but with preservation of a fat plane between the tumor and SMA.

Table 2
Definitions of borderline resectable pancreatic cancer

Vessel Involved	MDACC	AHPBA/SSO/SSAT	NCCN/ISGPS	Moffitt
SMA	Abutment	Abutment	Abutment	Abutment
CHA	Abutment or short segment encasement	Abutment or short segment encasement	Abutment without extension to celiac or HA bifurcation	Abutment or short segment encasement
Celiac axis	Abutment	No abutment or encasement	No contact	Not specified
SMV-PV confluence	Short-segment occlusion amenable to reconstruction	Abutment, encasement, or occlusion amenable to reconstruction	Abutment or encasement amenable to reconstruction	Abutment or encasement amenable to resection

consisted of the following: (1) an interface between the tumor and SMV-PV 180° or greater of the vein wall circumference; (2) short-segment occlusion of the SMV-PV with normal vein above and below the obstruction amenable to resection and reconstruction; (3) short-segment interface of any degree between tumor and HA with normal artery proximal and distal to the interface amenable to arterial resection and reconstruction; and (4) interface between the SMA and CA measuring less than 180° of the circumference of the artery.[23]

DIAGNOSTIC WORKUP
Imaging Modalities

Imaging modalities including CT, MRI, and endoscopic ultrasound (EUS) are the mainstay in the diagnosis and staging of pancreatic cancer, and advances in these techniques have dramatically improved the preoperative determination of resectability for pancreatic cancer. Specifically, the development of multi-detector-row CT allows for high-resolution scan as well as 3-dimensional (3D) reconstructions; this, in addition to a "pancreas protocol CT," which includes 3 phases (arterial phase, pancreatic parenchymal phase, and venous washout phase), has given physicians the ability to analyze the relationship of the pancreatic tumor to important vascular structures discussed above. CT is also effective in detecting lymphadenopathy and peritoneal and liver metastases. Enhanced MRI (with gadolinium or pancreatic tumor, excluding mangafodipir trisodium) is also effective in detecting local extension and vascular involvement. It is often superior to CT in detecting small liver lesions. Magnetic resonance cholangiopancreatography has the added benefit of noninvasively evaluating biliary and pancreatic ducts. Finally, EUS is highly sensitive for the detection of small tumors, surpassing both CT and MRI in this regard, as well as lymph node (LN) metastases and vascular invasion.[24–26] In addition, EUS provides the safest avenue for pathologic confirmation of disease, which is crucial for those patients undergoing neoadjuvant therapy.[26]

The Role for Diagnostic Laparoscopy

Although CT and MRI are highly sensitive for detection of LA as well as distant metastatic disease, small liver metastases and peritoneal disease may be undetectable even with high-quality axial imaging. As a result, many surgeons advocate the use of diagnostic laparoscopy before attempted resection, especially among patients with findings suspicious for advanced disease on imaging, such as ascites, indeterminate liver lesions, or peritoneal or omental thickening. Staging laparoscopy is not as useful for determining resectability of LA disease because tumor involvement of the vasculature, specifically the SMA, which is not easily detected by laparoscopy.[27]

A Cochrane database review of the use of diagnostic laparoscopy demonstrated a decreased laparotomy and aborted resection rate from 40% with CT alone to 17% with CT combined with diagnostic laparoscopy.[28] If metastatic disease is detected, staging laparoscopy not only decreases hospital length of stay but also allows patients to initiate chemotherapy significantly earlier than those undergoing exploratory laparotomy.[29–31]

An adjunct to laparoscopy includes peritoneal washings. Notably, positive peritoneal cytology occurs in 7% to 30% of potentially resectable cases, and those patients have similar outcomes to those with metastatic tumor burden; thus, they are generally not considered candidates for radical resection.[32,33] By NCCN standards, positive washings are considered stage IV disease.[32,34] The use of peritoneal washings for patients with pancreatic cancer, however, is not universally used.

VASCULAR RESECTION DURING PANCREATICODUODENECTOMY

Although historically abandoned due to poor outcomes, vascular resection, particularly venous resection, has now gained widespread acceptance in the resection of pancreatic cancer in selected patients. There is near universal agreement, however, that aggressive vascular resections for patients with BR disease should only be performed in patients with favorable tumor biology who have received neoadjuvant therapy before resection and by surgeons experienced in these procedures.

Ideally, the need for vascular resection is determined preoperatively, although this is not always possible. Signs of vascular involvement on cross-sectional imaging include proximity of tumor, loss of the fat plane or interface between a given vessel and tumor, and narrowing or impingement of venous structures (see **Fig. 1**). Narrowing of vein is highly specific, but not sensitive, for tumor involvement. Arterial involvement is more easily defined by CT preoperatively given the nerve plexus and fat plane normally surrounding an artery[35] (see **Fig. 2**).

However, more than 40% of tumors ultimately requiring vascular resection and reconstruction did not clearly demonstrate findings suggestive of vascular resection on preoperative imaging,[36–39] again underscoring the importance of centralization of pancreatic cancer care to high-volume centers in which surgeons are experienced and facile with vascular reconstruction or to medium volume centers at which a vascular surgeon is available to assist with resection and reconstruction.[40,41] Importantly, one study indicated that the cross-sectional imaging before neoadjuvant therapy was more predictive of vascular involvement than imaging performed after completion of preoperative therapy. The investigators found initial imaging to be 98% predictive of vascular involvement compared with only 25% after neoadjuvant therapy.[42]

Venous Resections

Resection of the SMV, PV, or SMV-PV confluence is not uncommon at high-volume centers. Reports indicate that an average of 30% (7%–80%) of PDs performed at major medical centers now include venous resection and reconstruction.[36,43–45] Perioperative morbidity and mortality associated with venous resection and reconstruction are similar to PDs performed without any venous construction, with short-term mortality ranging from 4% to 12% and complications ranging from 17% to 100%.[46–48]

Venous resection and reconstruction can vary in extent, including the following:

- Partial lateral venorrhaphy with transverse closure
- Resection with vein patch
- Interposition graft with either autologous or prosthetic vein graft

Patch reconstruction with autologous vein is standard practice; however, both cadaveric allografts and xenografts (porcine peritoneum, bovine pericardium) have also been used.[49] The autologous vein of choice for interposition grafts is the internal jugular vein or greater saphenous vein, but other conduits, including the superficial femoral, left renal, and inferior mesenteric veins (IMVs), have also been used.[50,51] The risk of prosthetic graft in a potentially contaminated operative field with risk of pancreatic fistula is significant; thus, prosthetic grafts are not recommended but are sometimes required if suitable autologous vein is not available.[49,52] Notably, up to 5- to 7-cm gaps can be primarily anastomosed with division of splenic vein (SV), mobilization of the right colon, hepatic flexure, and root of the mesentery and full mobilization of the liver, often obviating interposition graft.[52–54]

Splenic Vein Ligation and Sinistral Hypertension

As noted, division of the SV to allow for additional mobilization enabling an end-to-end anastomosis and eliminating need for interposition graft is commonly practiced. In addition, when tumor involvement includes the area of confluence of SV and SMV, the SV is often ligated and divided. However, division of the SV has the theoretic risk of sinistral or left-sided portal hypertension. Some studies have demonstrated increased frequency of sinistral hypertension as defined by an increase in spleen volume or decrease in platelet count. In addition, there are case reports of hypertensive gastropathy with gastric varices and gastrointestinal (GI) bleed following SV ligation during PD.[55,56] Any theoretic risk of SV thrombosis and sinistral hypertension can be avoided by preservation of not only the short gastric vessels but also the SV-IMV confluence, both of which would allow for decompression of the SV to the systemic circulation. In addition, reanastomosis in an end-to-end fashion of SV to IMV, use of an interposition graft, or even a distal splenorenal shunt, mesocaval shunt, or IMV to right gastroepiploic vein anastomosis may be performed.[55]

The incidence and clinical significance of this theoretic complication have been called into question by several studies. In one study, only a very limited number of patients in whom the SV had been ligated actually developed clinically significant splenomegaly.[57] The reasons for this are likely many. For one, survival following PD may not be long enough for this process to manifest itself. In addition, following ligation of the SV, venous blood can re-enter the systemic circulation via the esophageal veins or right colic tributaries.[55] Finally, tumor involvement of the SV or confluence can cause relative stenosis, and collateral vessels may already be well developed at the time of PD.[55]

Arterial Resections

Although venous resection is not uncommon, consensus guidelines still consider extensive tumor involvement of major arteries (SMA, celiac, and common hepatic arteries) to be unresectable. In a recent meta-analysis, patients undergoing arterial reconstruction were associated with increased operative times, higher morbidity rate, including vascular and nonvascular complications, and a higher rate of reoperation, as well as an increased mortality rate.[36] Patients who underwent combined venous and arterial resection had worse outcomes when compared with patients undergoing venous reconstruction alone. In addition, the 1-, 3-, and 5-year survival rates of PD with arterial resection were worse than PD alone and to PD with venous reconstruction.[46] It should be noted, however, that this meta-analysis included a heterogeneous patient population over an extended time period (1977–2010), during which significant improvements in patient outcomes as well as advancements in neoadjuvant therapy regimens took place.[35,46,58]

At the current time, greater than 180° abutment, or encasement of the SMA, is considered a contraindication to resection. There has, however, been limited experience but acceptable outcomes achieved in young, otherwise healthy individuals who underwent extended resection for LA disease involving the CHA or celiac axes after completion of neoadjuvant chemotherapy at high-volume centers.[58,59] In nearly all patients who require arterial resections, venous resections are also required, further increasing the complexity and potential morbidity of the resection.

Postoperative Anticoagulation

Although the risk of mesenteric or PV thrombosis may be increased in patients undergoing resection for malignancy, it appears to be particularly increased when vascular reconstruction is performed.[60] It is important that the anastomoses or graft is not twisted or kinked in any way, and all venous anastomoses should allow for dilation and avoid a "waist" at the suture line once normal venous flow is re-established.[52]

A recent review article in 2014 found a rate of thrombosis of 25% with reconstruction.[52] Thrombosis can range from partial occlusion of the SMV or a lesser tributary to the more feared complication of early or late PV thrombosis. The area and extent of resection and reconstruction almost certainly influence venous thrombosis rates.[61] Rates of thrombosis with polytetrafluoroethylene grafts are consistently higher than interposition grafts using autologous vein; most studies report patency rates of approximately 90% for autologous vein conduit.[49,52,62]

Patients may be asymptomatic or, rarely, may develop severe peritonitis secondary to acute mesenteric ischemia. Early PV thrombosis is associated with a 30% to 40% mortality rate. Although early thrombosis is deadly, patients with delayed PV thrombosis following PD with vascular reconstruction have survival rates greater than those without thrombosis presumably because of interval development of collateral flow.[63]

Intraoperative systemic anticoagulation during reconstruction is not routinely used. Some surgeons advocate its routine use, whereas others advocate its use when the SMA is formally clamped for an extended period; there are no data to support or refute its use. Data supporting the use of postoperative anticoagulation for patients undergoing vascular reconstruction during PD likewise are sparse. Most protocols are based on surgeon preference. A recent review article in 2014 summarized the available data; however, given the wide variation in practice in the primary articles (heparin and warfarin vs aspirin), no firm conclusions could be drawn.[52] A more guided prospective multi-institutional research trial would be necessary to define best practice standards with regards to anticoagulation for venous reconstruction.[49] Current practice at the authors' institution involves the use of low-dose aspirin postoperatively for all PDs requiring vascular reconstruction.

ABERRANT VASCULAR ANATOMY AND CELIAC STENOSIS

As many as 20% to 50% of patients exhibit aberrant vascular anatomy. The variants most critical for the surgeon during PD include an accessory or replaced right hepatic artery (RRHA) and replaced common hepatic artery (RCHA) because they typically course through an area predisposed to tumor involvement. Although these aberrancies may add to the complexity of the operation, it is not clear whether these variants affect resectability. Although traditionally these abnormalities may have been discovered in the operating room, modern multiphase imaging techniques nearly always identify these abnormalities preoperatively and allow for proper operative planning.

Replaced Right and Common Hepatic Arteries

The most common variant overall is an RRHA, which branches from the SMA, and is seen in 11% to 20% of individuals. It typically courses behind or through the pancreatic head, predisposing it to tumor involvement especially with posteriorly located malignancies.[64] Fortunately, an RRHA can often be preserved with careful dissection even with tumor nearby. If division is required, the primary concern is preservation of blood flow to the CBD, which could lead to failure of the bilioenteric anastomosis or delayed anastomotic stenosis.[64,65] Given this, some argue that it is important to attempt to reconstruct if the replaced RHA must be sacrificed (either primarily or using an autologous vein graft), although this may be technically difficult given its small diameter.[66,67] A second anatomic variant of concern to the surgeon performing PD is the rarer RCHA, in which the CHA originates from the SMA. Fortunately, this variant occurs only in 0.4% to 4.5% of population.[64] If the replaced CHA has an intrapancreatic course, reconstruction is usually necessary.[64]

Celiac Artery Stenosis

Celiac artery stenosis is most often secondary to intrinsic disease (plaque) or extrinsic forces secondary to either nodal disease burden, median arcuate ligament syndrome, or a tumor-associated fibroinflammatory process. Celiac stenosis is encountered in up to 5% of all pancreaticoduodenectomies.[68,69] Most patients are asymptomatic due to the propensity for extensive collateralization; the CHA receives retrograde flow via the GDA or dorsal pancreatic artery coming off the SMA, or via the Arc of Buhler, which is a direct connection between SMA and CHA. Elimination of collateral flow by division of the GDA during PD in the setting of celiac stenosis has theoretic and observed implications for compromised flow to liver, stomach, and spleen.[68,69]

Preoperatively, CT imaging has low sensitivity for detecting clinically significant celiac stenosis but significant collateralization or an unusually large GDA raises suspicion.[68] Given this low sensitivity, it should be routine practice during PD to assess flow within the HA by temporarily occluding flow from the GDA before division.[70] Significant stenosis from atherosclerosis that is identified preoperatively can be managed with angioplasty and stent, but the long-term outcome is not clear.[70,71] Intraoperatively, if blood flow in the proper HA becomes significantly reduced following ligation of the GDA, it is recommended that restoration of flow be performed. In cases with eccentric compression, division of the median arcuate ligament is successful in up to 70% of cases.[72–74] If that is not successful or if reduced blood flow is due to other reasons, an autologous graft from the aorta to the proper HA is recommended.

LYMPHADENECTOMY IN PANCREATIC CANCER

A large proportion of pancreatectomy specimens contain positive nodes, ranging from 50% to 80%.[75–77] Lymphatic spread is thought to begin with peripancreatic nodes either by direct invasion or via lymphatic channels, then spreading to SMA and CHA nodes, and finally, to para-aortic nodes.

LN involvement is a significant negative prognostic factor. The 5-year actuarial survival of patients with node positive disease is 5%, as compared with 10% survival among patients with node-negative disease.[75–77] Local recurrence rates are also significantly higher in those with LN-positive disease. Survival is increased dramatically with N0 resection, and, within N0 resections, there is increased survival with increased nodal sampling. In addition, for N1 disease, the LN ratio (positive LN/resected LN) is critical, with ratios of 0 to 0.2 having more favorable outcomes than 0.2 to 0.4,[76,78,79] underscoring the responsibility of both surgeon and pathologist to provide an adequate nodal assessment at the time of PD. At least 12 to 15 nodes are recommended for adequate analysis.[75] Similar to pathologic analysis of specimen margins, however, the quality of LN evaluation within a given surgical specimen varies significantly.[80]

It is not known which groups of nodes offer the most prognostic impact, or whether nodal invasion of peripancreatic LNs, likely by direct invasion, has the same prognostic implication as true lymphatic dissemination into nodal groups further from the primary mass.[81,82] In one study, peripancreatic nodal invasion only had survival rates similar to those without nodal invasion, whereas, in others, direct invasion had similar prognostic implications as true lymphatic spread.[81,82] In general, however, patients with involvement of a single nodal group have better outcomes than involvement of multiple nodal groups.[83]

Extended Lymphadenectomy

Although the prognostic impact of overt nodal spread is rarely disputed, there was, for some time, significant debate as to whether aggressive nodal dissection at the time of PD to attain locoregional control of disease truly affected outcomes.[84]

The need for definition of a standard nodal dissection was addressed at the 2013 ISGPS consensus meeting. The standard lymphadenectomy for PD should include the following:

- The peripancreatic tissue to the right of SMA and proper HA—specifically nodal stations 5, 6, 8a (proper HA), 12b, 12c, 13a, 13b (posterior surface), 14a (right lateral SMA), 14b (right lateral SMA), 17a, 17b (anterior surface) as defined by the Japanese Pancreas Society[75]

Anything beyond this is considered an extended lymphadenectomy.[75]

Several meta-analyses have revealed no improvement in survival with extended lymphadenectomy, as extraregional LN involvement should be considered metastatic disease. In addition, more extensive dissections are associated with higher rates of postoperative complications, including delayed gastric emptying (DGE), increased weight loss, and diarrhea thought to be secondary to autonomic disruption.[85–87]

PYLORUS-SPARING VERSUS STANDARD PANCREATICODUODENECTOMY

The pylorus-preserving PD (PPPD) was first introduced in 1944 by Watson,[88] and interest was reignited in 1980 by Traverso and Longmire.[89] This procedure differs from the standard PD by sparing the pylorus and the proximal 1 to 3 cm of duodenum in an effort to prevent the dumping, bile reflux gastritis, and marginal ulceration associated with the traditional standard PD reconstruction that includes an antrectomy. A 2014 meta-analysis showed no difference in disease outcomes, morbidity, mortality, or OS with pylorus-preserving as compared with standard PD.[90,91] Furthermore, a randomized controlled trial showed a significant increase in DGE with PPPD as compared with standard PD.[92] The decision as to the type of reconstruction is therefore largely based on surgeon preference.

THE ROLE FOR MINIMALLY INVASIVE SURGERY

PD requires intricate dissection deep within the retroperitoneum of tumor that is often adherent to major vessels. Once the specimen is resected, a series of complex anastomoses must be completed. The complexity inherent to this procedure resulted in the late acceptance of minimally invasive approaches as compared with other major abdominal operations. The minimally invasive approach to PD was first introduced by Gagner and Pomp[93] in 1994 for a patient with chronic pancreatitis. Since that time, laparoscopic, laparoscopic hand-assisted, and laparoscopic robot-assisted pancreaticoduodenectomies have all been completed with success, even including vascular resection.[94,95] Robot-assisted minimally invasive surgery has several distinct advantages over pure laparoscopic techniques because it gives the surgeon improved dexterity and better visualization given stereoscopic 3D optic capabilities.[96] Laparoscopic PD is rarely performed outside of specialized institutions now, but laparoscopic robot-assisted PD remains a viable alternative to the conventional open approach.

Available data demonstrate that there is no difference in morbidity, mortality, or major complications of pancreatic fistula and DGE in minimally invasive as compared with open PD. The rate of conversion to an open procedure is approximately 10% to 15%, and there is a steep learning curve.[96] In addition, there is associated increased cost, longer operating room (OR) time, and higher reoperation rates.[96] Benefits may include decreased estimated blood loss (EBL), lower hospital length of stay, and a trend toward starting adjuvant therapy earlier.[97] Little has been written about the overall cost-effectiveness of robot-assisted or laparoscopic-only PD, but one study proposes that the higher upfront cost of equipment, training, and personnel may be balanced by reduced hospital length of stay.[98]

Regarding oncologic outcomes, in theory, the use of high-resolution cameras might enable better visualization and finer dissection and may lead to higher R0 resection rates, especially in borderline tumors following neoadjuvant therapy. This theory has not yet been demonstrated in the literature.[96] In addition, there is no significant improvement in LN dissection; the number of nodes obtained during minimally invasive procedures as compared with open PD is similar.[96,99] It should be noted that the interpretation of any data regarding oncologic outcomes in minimally invasive PD is potentially biased, because those patients with low American Society of Anesthesiologists performance status, with large tumors, or at high risk for R1/R2 resection are generally not offered a minimally invasive procedure.[100] In addition, no data on long-term oncologic outcomes are available. Prospective randomized controlled trials with patients with comparable disease states with long-term follow-up are needed before these minimally invasive techniques are universally recommended; however, because of the low numbers of truly surgically resectable patients, this is likely not feasible. (See Deepa Magge, Amer Zureikat, Melissa Hogg, et al: Minimally Invasive Approaches to Pancreatic Surgery, in this issue.)

COMPLICATIONS FOLLOWING PANCREATICODUODENECTOMY

Although mortality rates after PD remain low (1%–2%) in experienced centers, morbidity rates remain high (40%–50%), even among high-volume centers.[3] Postoperative complications increase hospital length of stay and cost, worsen patient outcomes, and often delay adjuvant therapy plans. Specifically, postoperative complications significantly delay the initiation of adjuvant chemotherapy, decrease the percentage of patients undergoing adjuvant multimodality therapy, and decrease the intensity of the adjuvant therapy tolerated.[101–103]

Delayed Gastric Emptying

The most common complication following PD is DGE with prevalence ranging from 20% to 40%. Although DGE is a transient phenomenon generally resolving in a few days to weeks following the operation, the impact of DGE should not be underestimated. It greatly increases length of hospital stay and readmission rates following PD as well as patient satisfaction and quality of life.

The cause remains unclear, but is generally thought to be a result of the major perturbations in the normal anatomy and physiology of the upper GI tract inherent to PD. Relative gastric antropyloric ischemia, vagal dysfunction, motilin deficiency resulting from duodenal resection, and peripancreatic inflammation have all been implicated.[67,104–106]

The diagnosis of DGE is largely clinical. In 2007, the ISGPS compiled a classification system for DGE based on nasogastric tube output and time to regular diet[107] (**Table 3**). Several risk factors for DGE have been identified and include the following[108–114]:

- Pylorus-preserving PD
- Retrocolic gastrojejunostomy
- Diabetes
- Presence of pancreatic fistula
- Increased OR times
- Increased body mass index
- Other postoperative complications

The use of octreotide in the perioperative period was also found to be an independent risk factor for DGE.[112] If these risk factors are identified preoperatively or intraoperatively, consideration should be given to enteral access; high-risk patients should undergo nasojejunal postanastomotic feeding tube or surgical jejunostomy placement at the time of the resection.

Treatment of DGE is largely based on dietary modification and the use of promotility agents, such as erythromycin, metoclopramide, and domperidone.[105,115] Erythromycin is generally seen as safe, inexpensive, and more effective than either domperidone or metoclopramide but has some important side effects and drug interactions.[116] Gastric stimulators are often used to treat idiopathic or diabetic

Table 3
International Study Group of Pancreatic Surgery classification scheme for delayed gastric emptying

Characteristic	Grade A	Grade B	Grade C
Nasogastric tube required	4–7 d or reinsertion after postoperative day (POD) 3	8–14 d or reinsertion after POD 7	>14 d or reinsertion after POD 14
Unable to tolerate food at:	POD 7	POD 14	POD 21
Gastric distention/ vomiting	Yes	Yes	Yes
Use of prokinetics	Yes	Yes	Yes

gastroparesis but are of no significant utility in the treatment of DGE following PD. Symptoms are managed with antiemetics, generally in combination with promotility agents.

Pancreatic Fistula

Postoperative pancreatic fistula is also a common complication following PD, affecting 25% to 40% of patients and often leading to abscess formation, hemorrhage, or DGE. It is also the most common cause of mortality. Unfortunately, all attempts thus far to prevent pancreatic fistula have largely been unsuccessful.[117] A classification scheme for pancreatic fistulas has been formulated by the ISGPS/International Study Group of Pancreatic Fistula based on severity and need for intervention (**Table 4**).

Major risk factors include a "soft pancreas," which generally indicates that the gland has preserved exocrine function, which would lead to more effluent from ducts. It is also technically more difficult to place sutures in a soft gland. Ducts smaller than 3 mm in diameter are also associated with higher leak rates. Not surprisingly, pancreatic fistula is more commonly seen following resection of ampullary, duodenal, or islet cell tumors in which pancreatic gland function is normal and ductal dilatation is absent, as compared with adenocarcinoma or chronic pancreatitis, which are associated with more atrophic, "harder" glands and chronically dilated ducts. Increased intraoperative blood loss has also been shown to augment the risk of developing a fistula.[117]

The pancreaticojejunostomy can be performed in an end-to-end or end-to-side manner with duct-to-mucosal anastomosis versus an invagination technique. In some studies, direct anastomosis of duct-to-mucosa as compared with invagination technique is associated with lower leak rate, but this has not been recapitulated.[118] There are some scant data suggesting that pancreaticogastrostomy may have a more favorable leak rate than pancreaticojejunostomy, but this has not been confirmed in randomized controlled trials.[119]

The use of fibrin glue at the anastomosis was evaluated in both randomized controlled trials and in systematic reviews and was found to result in no significant change in postoperative pancreatic fistula.[120] Thus, no intraoperative modifications have resulted in clearly demonstrable improvements in pancreatic fistula rates.

In theory, decreasing pancreatic secretion/effluent should decrease fistula severity and/or duration. Various somatostatin analogues have been trialed, including octreotide, which in European centers was effective in reducing fistula rates. A *Cochrane*

Table 4 International Study Group of Pancreatic Surgery classification scheme for pancreatic fistula			
Characteristic	Grade A	Grade B	Grade C
Signs of systemic illness	No	Yes	Yes
Treatment required?	No	Yes	Yes
CT or ultrasound evidence	No	Yes	Yes
Persistent drainage (>3 wk)	No	Yes	Yes
Signs of infection	No	Yes	Yes
Readmission	No	Yes	Yes
Sepsis	No	No	Yes
Reoperation	No	No	Yes
Death	No	No	Yes

Review in 2012 confirmed a decrease in overall pancreatic fistula rate with postoperative somatostatin therapy; however, there were no differences in rates of clinically significant fistulas, no change in reoperation rates, no increased rate of fistula closure, and most importantly, no change in mortality.[121] Other somatostatin analogues with longer half-lives and broader and stronger binding profiles are in various stages of development and have shown promise.[122] Specifically, pasireotide has recently been shown in randomized controlled trials to decrease clinically significant pancreatic fistula rates (ISGPS grade 2 or higher) by almost 50% for pancreatectomies, including those with dilated or normal pancreatic ducts.[122] Although these data are very convincing, its generalized use, however, is still lacking—perhaps due to cost.

Hemorrhage

Postoperative hemorrhage is the third most common severe complication following PD. The most common sites of hemorrhage include the GDA stump, tributaries of the PV or SMV, branches of HA or SMA, the cut surface of the pancreas, suture lines, and the gallbladder fossa.[123] The ISGPS has devised a classification scheme for postoperative hemorrhage based on time of onset in addition to location and severity of bleed (**Table 5**). Early-onset hemorrhage (postoperative days 1–5) is most likely secondary to technical failure or postoperative coagulopathy, whereas late-onset (after postoperative day 5) bleeds most often result from the erosion of peripancreatic vessels or pseudoaneurysm formation due to pancreatic leak or intra-abdominal abscess.[123] Severity can be mild or severe with transfusion requirement or need for reoperation or an interventional radiologic procedure. Overall, treatment algorithms differ for early versus delayed postpancreatectomy hemorrhage. Severe early bleeding into the peritoneal cavity warrants relaparotomy for ligation of the bleeding vessel, whereas bleeding into the GI tract (likely from gastrojejunal or enteroenteroanastomosis) may be amenable to endoscopic intervention. Late-onset hemorrhage can be addressed with angiography with coiling/embolization/stenting if technically feasible provided that the patient is hemodynamically stable with appropriate resuscitation and lesion is visualized. If these conditions are not met, relaparotomy is again warranted.[124,125]

PALLIATIVE OPTIONS

As mentioned earlier, only 20% of patients present with resectable disease; the remainder of patients unfortunately present with LA (40%) or metastatic disease (40%). Therapy for LA and metastatic disease focuses on palliative systemic therapy,

Table 5 International Study Group of Pancreatic Surgery classification scheme for postoperative hemorrhage following pancreatectomy			
Characteristic	**Grade A**	**Grade B**	**Grade C**
Time of onset	Early	Early/late	Late
Site	Intraluminal or extraluminal	Intraluminal or extraluminal	Intraluminal or extraluminal
Clinical impact	Mild	Severe early/mild late	Severe
Therapeutic consequences	No	Yes	Yes

with median survival of 9 to 11 months.[126] Although these patients have no options for potential cure, there remains a possibility for palliative surgery for the treatment of symptoms caused by their disease, including obstructive jaundice, gastric outlet obstruction, and intractable pain. Patients who are candidates for minimally invasive options available for palliation may benefit from a shorter recovery period, even more important given their expected short life expectancy.[38]

In general, obstructive jaundice is best addressed with endoscopic stent placement. Expandable metal stents offer the best long-term patency and lowest complication rate. Surgical approaches for biliary obstruction not amenable to endoscopic therapy include biliary bypass procedures such as hepaticojejunostomies or choledochojejunostomies. Although a cholecystojejunostomy is less frequently used, it is an attractive option in patients with tumors at least 1 cm away from the cystic duct/hepatic duct junction because it can often be performed using minimally invasive techniques.[127,128]

In contrast to obstructive jaundice, endoscopic approaches to the treatment of gastric outlet obstruction have been largely unsuccessful. Duodenal stents are associated with significant risk of migration, perforation, or biliary obstruction and require significant changes in diet that impact quality of life.[129] Although often used in patients with a life expectancy of only a few months, surgical gastrojejunostomy, either open or minimally invasive, is preferred in those expected to live more than 2 months.[129,130] Studies have shown that gastrojejunostomy for palliation is best performed in a retrocolic position in an isoperistaltic configuration with the anastomosis below the mesocolon to prevent stricture.[131] Prophylactic gastrojejunostomy performed in the setting of exploratory laparoscopy/laparotomy and discovery of unresectable disease with high risk of obstruction generally does not lead to increased morbidity and mortality.[131] (See Christopher Wolfgang, Katherine E. Poruk: Palliative Management of Unresectable Pancreatic Cancer, in this issue, for further details of palliative management of pancreatic diseases.)

Pancreatic cancer, particularly LA disease, is particularly painful because of involvement of the celiac nerve plexus. In the treatment of intractable abdominal/back pain, all standard pharmacologic options should be exhausted before any attempts at additional intervention are made. Potential invasive therapies include ethanol injection or ablation of the celiac plexus. These procedures can be performed percutaneously, endoscopically, laparoscopically, or in an open fashion at the time of exploration. There are no significant benefits of neurolysis over pharmacologic agents, however, and any manipulation of the nerve plexus can result in significant morbidity, including debilitating diarrhea, significant orthostasis, and even spinal cord hematomas.[132–134]

Notably, there is no role for palliative resection of the primary mass. There has, however, been some interest recently in tumor ablation either through thermal damage (radiofrequency ablation, high-intensity focused ultrasound, cryoablation, and microwave ablation), or nonthermal techniques (irreversible electroporation, stereotactic body radiation therapy, photodynamic therapy, and ^{125}I seeding).[126] Nonthermal techniques have garnered significant attention as the "heat sink" associated with thermal techniques is especially problematic given nearby structures, such as the duodenum, biliary tree, and mesenteric vasculature.[135] Importantly, all have been associated with some relief of pain.[126,135] To date, however, there are no prospective data comparing ablative therapies with standard of care in terms of safety or even efficacy; most of the analyses thus far have been single-institution studies. Most available data, however, suggest that these strategies may be more efficacious in combination with other therapies (chemoradiation and others).[135]

SUMMARY

For pancreatic cancer, successful surgical resection offers the only chance for cure. It is possible in a small minority of patients, however, even with successful resection; recurrence rates remain high, and OS is less than 25%. Over the past several years, advances in imaging and diagnostic modalities have allowed better characterization and selection of patients that are potentially resectable as well as BR and LA in an attempt to standardize resectional, neoadjuvant, and palliative therapeutic strategies. Response to neoadjuvant therapy has resulted in a higher number of patients eligible for resection. In addition, a better understanding of the biology of disease has allowed us to better define the factors important for improved outcomes.

Although mortality rates in high-volume centers are low, morbidity rates after resection remain significant. A thorough understanding of the factors related to these complications is crucial to minimize these events and allow for the expeditious use of adjuvant therapy. It is hoped that further understanding of the biology of this lethal disease will lead to the development of novel targeted therapies and a subsequent increase in the number of patients eligible for resection as well as improved long-term survival.

REFERENCES

1. Sosa JA, Bowman HM, Gordon TA, et al. Importance of hospital volume in the overall management of pancreatic cancer. Ann Surg 1998;228(3):429–38.
2. Birkmeyer JD, Finlayson SR, Tosteson AN, et al. Effect of hospital volume on in-hospital mortality with pancreaticoduodenectomy. Surgery 1999;125(3):250–6.
3. Hariharan D, Saied A, Kocher HM. Analysis of mortality rates for pancreatic cancer across the world. HPB 2008;10(1):58–62.
4. Winter JM, Cameron JL, Campbell KA, et al. 1423 pancreaticoduodenectomies for pancreatic cancer: a single-institution experience. J Gastrointest Surg 2006; 10(9):1199–210 [discussion: 1210–1].
5. Moon HJ, An JY, Heo JS, et al. Predicting survival after surgical resection for pancreatic ductal adenocarcinoma. Pancreas 2006;32(1):37–43.
6. Kuhlmann KF, de Castro SM, Wesseling JG, et al. Surgical treatment of pancreatic adenocarcinoma; actual survival and prognostic factors in 343 patients. Eur J Cancer 2004;40(4):549–58.
7. Han SS, Jang JY, Kim SW, et al. Analysis of long-term survivors after surgical resection for pancreatic cancer. Pancreas 2006;32(3):271–5.
8. Jarufe NP, Coldham C, Mayer AD, et al. Favourable prognostic factors in a large UK experience of adenocarcinoma of the head of the pancreas and periampullary region. Dig Surg 2004;21(3):202–9.
9. Westgaard A, Tafjord S, Farstad IN, et al. Resectable adenocarcinomas in the pancreatic head: the retroperitoneal resection margin is an independent prognostic factor. BMC Cancer 2008;8:5.
10. Verbeke CS. Resection margins and R1 rates in pancreatic cancer–are we there yet? Histopathology 2008;52(7):787–96.
11. Yeo CJ, Cameron JL, Lillemoe KD, et al. Pancreaticoduodenectomy for cancer of the head of the pancreas. 201 patients. Ann Surg 1995;221(6):721–31 [discussion: 731–3].
12. Fatima J, Schnelldorfer T, Barton J, et al. Pancreatoduodenectomy for ductal adenocarcinoma: implications of positive margin on survival. Arch Surg 2010; 145(2):167–72.

13. Sohn TA, Yeo CJ, Cameron JL, et al. Resected adenocarcinoma of the pancreas—616 patients: results, outcomes, and prognostic indicators. J Gastrointest Surg 2000;4(6):567–79.

14. Verbeke CS. Resection margins in pancreatic cancer: are we entering a new era? HPB 2014;16(1):1–2.

15. Verbeke CS, Menon KV. Redefining resection margin status in pancreatic cancer. HPB 2009;11(4):282–9.

16. Esposito I, Kleeff J, Bergmann F, et al. Most pancreatic cancer resections are R1 resections. Ann Surg Oncol 2008;15(6):1651–60.

17. Campbell F, Smith RA, Whelan P, et al. Classification of R1 resections for pancreatic cancer: the prognostic relevance of tumour involvement within 1 mm of a resection margin. Histopathology 2009;55(3):277–83.

18. Washington K, Berlin J, Branton P, et al. Protocol for the examination of specimens from patients with carcinoma of the exocrine pancreas. Guidelines of the College of American Pathologists. 2015.

19. Varadhachary GR, Tamm EP, Abbruzzese JL, et al. Borderline resectable pancreatic cancer: definitions, management, and role of preoperative therapy. Ann Surg Oncol 2006;13(8):1035–46.

20. TME a. NCCN clinical practice guidelines in oncology: pancreatic adenocarcinoma. 2nd edition. National Comprehensive Cancer Network.

21. Mehta VK, Fisher G, Ford JA, et al. Preoperative chemoradiation for marginally resectable adenocarcinoma of the pancreas. J Gastrointest Surg 2001;5(1):27–35.

22. Abrams RA, Lowy AM, O'Reilly EM, et al. Combined modality treatment of resectable and borderline resectable pancreas cancer: expert consensus statement. Ann Surg Oncol 2009;16(7):1751–6.

23. Katz MH, Marsh R, Herman JM, et al. Borderline resectable pancreatic cancer: need for standardization and methods for optimal clinical trial design. Ann Surg Oncol 2013;20(8):2787–95.

24. Muller MF, Meyenberger C, Bertschinger P, et al. Pancreatic tumors: evaluation with endoscopic US, CT, and MR imaging. Radiology 1994;190(3):745–51.

25. Legmann P, Vignaux O, Dousset B, et al. Pancreatic tumors: comparison of dual-phase helical CT and endoscopic sonography. AJR Am J Roentgenol 1998;170(5):1315–22.

26. Miura F, Takada T, Amano H, et al. Diagnosis of pancreatic cancer. HPB 2006; 8(5):337–42.

27. Hennig R, Tempia-Caliera AA, Hartel M, et al. Staging laparoscopy and its indications in pancreatic cancer patients. Dig Surg 2002;19(6):484–8.

28. Allen VB, Gurusamy KS, Takwoingi Y, et al. Diagnostic accuracy of laparoscopy following computed tomography (CT) scanning for assessing the resectability with curative intent in pancreatic and periampullary cancer. Cochrane Database Syst Rev 2013;(11):CD009323.

29. Beenen E, van Roest MH, Sieders E, et al. Staging laparoscopy in patients scheduled for pancreaticoduodenectomy minimizes hospitalization in the remaining life time when metastatic carcinoma is found. Eur J Surg Oncol 2014; 40(8):989–94.

30. Hashimoto D, Chikamoto A, Sakata K, et al. Staging laparoscopy leads to rapid induction of chemotherapy for unresectable pancreatobiliary cancers. Asian J Endosc Surg 2015;8(1):59–62.

31. Velanovich V, Wollner I, Ajlouni M. Staging laparoscopy promotes increased utilization of postoperative therapy for unresectable intra-abdominal malignancies. J Gastrointest Surg 2000;4(5):542–6.

32. Ferrone CR, Haas B, Tang L, et al. The influence of positive peritoneal cytology on survival in patients with pancreatic adenocarcinoma. J Gastrointest Surg 2006;10(10):1347–53.

33. Clark CJ, Traverso LW. Positive peritoneal lavage cytology is a predictor of worse survival in locally advanced pancreatic cancer. Am J Surg 2010;199(5): 657–62.

34. Tempero MA, Arnoletti JP, Behrman S, et al. Pancreatic adenocarcinoma. J Natl Compr Canc Netw 2010;8(9):972–1017.

35. Christians K, Evans DB. Pancreaticoduodenectomy and vascular resection: persistent controversy and current recommendations. Ann Surg Oncol 2009; 16(4):789–91.

36. Porembka MR, Hawkins WG, Linehan DC, et al. Radiologic and intraoperative detection of need for mesenteric vein resection in patients with adenocarcinoma of the head of the pancreas. HPB 2011;13(9):633–42.

37. Li H, Zeng MS, Zhou KR, et al. Pancreatic adenocarcinoma: the different CT criteria for peripancreatic major arterial and venous invasion. J Comput Assist Tomogr 2005;29(2):170–5.

38. Buchs NC, Chilcott M, Poletti PA, et al. Vascular invasion in pancreatic cancer: imaging modalities, preoperative diagnosis and surgical management. World J Gastroenterol 2010;16(7):818–31.

39. Vollmer CM, Drebin JA, Middleton WD, et al. Utility of staging laparoscopy in subsets of peripancreatic and biliary malignancies. Ann Surg 2002;235(1):1–7.

40. Marangoni G, O'Sullivan A, Faraj W, et al. Pancreatectomy with synchronous vascular resection–an argument in favour. Surgeon 2012;10(2):102–6.

41. Turley RS, Peterson K, Barbas AS, et al. Vascular surgery collaboration during pancreaticoduodenectomy with vascular reconstruction. Ann Vasc Surg 2012; 26(5):685–92.

42. Valls C, Andia E, Sanchez A, et al. Dual-phase helical CT of pancreatic adenocarcinoma: assessment of resectability before surgery. AJR Am J Roentgenol 2002;178(4):821–6.

43. Siriwardana HP, Siriwardena AK. Systematic review of outcome of synchronous portal-superior mesenteric vein resection during pancreatectomy for cancer. Br J Surg 2006;93(6):662–73.

44. Ramacciato G, Mercantini P, Petrucciani N, et al. Does portal-superior mesenteric vein invasion still indicate irresectability for pancreatic carcinoma? Ann Surg Oncol 2009;16(4):817–25.

45. Chua TC, Saxena A. Extended pancreaticoduodenectomy with vascular resection for pancreatic cancer: a systematic review. J Gastrointest Surg 2010;14(9): 1442–52.

46. Mollberg N, Rahbari NN, Koch M, et al. Arterial resection during pancreatectomy for pancreatic cancer: a systematic review and meta-analysis. Ann Surg 2011;254(6):882–93.

47. Zhou Y, Zhang Z, Liu Y, et al. Pancreatectomy combined with superior mesenteric vein-portal vein resection for pancreatic cancer: a meta-analysis. World J Surg 2012;36(4):884–91.

48. Tseng JF, Raut CP, Lee JE, et al. Pancreaticoduodenectomy with vascular resection: margin status and survival duration. J Gastrointest Surg 2004;8(8):935–49 [discussion: 949–50].

49. Krepline AN, Christians KK, Duelge K, et al. Patency rates of portal vein/superior mesenteric vein reconstruction after pancreatectomy for pancreatic cancer. J Gastrointest Surg 2014;18(11):2016–25.

50. Lee DY, Mitchell EL, Jones MA, et al. Techniques and results of portal vein/superior mesenteric vein reconstruction using femoral and saphenous vein during pancreaticoduodenectomy. J Vasc Surg 2010;51(3):662–6.

51. Suzuki T, Yoshidome H, Kimura F, et al. Renal function is well maintained after use of left renal vein graft for vascular reconstruction in hepatobiliary-pancreatic surgery. J Am Coll Surg 2006;202(1):87–92.

52. Chandrasegaram MD, Eslick GD, Lee W, et al. Anticoagulation policy after venous resection with a pancreatectomy: a systematic review. HPB 2014; 16(8):691–8.

53. Wang F, Arianayagam R, Gill A, et al. Grafts for mesenterico-portal vein resections can be avoided during pancreatoduodenectomy. J Am Coll Surg 2012; 215(4):569–79.

54. Fujisaki S, Tomita R, Fukuzawa M. Utility of mobilization of the right colon and the root of the mesentery for avoiding vein grafting during reconstruction of the portal vein. J Am Coll Surg 2001;193(5):576–8.

55. Ferreira N, Oussoultzoglou E, Fuchshuber P, et al. Splenic vein-inferior mesenteric vein anastomosis to lessen left-sided portal hypertension after pancreaticoduodenectomy with concomitant vascular resection. Arch Surg 2011;146(12):1375–81.

56. Ono Y, Matsueda K, Koga R, et al. Sinistral portal hypertension after pancreaticoduodenectomy with splenic vein ligation. Br J Surg 2015;102(3):219–28.

57. Strasberg SM, Bhalla S, Sanchez LA, et al. Pattern of venous collateral development after splenic vein occlusion in an extended Whipple procedure: comparison with collateral vein pattern in cases of sinistral portal hypertension. J Gastrointest Surg 2011;15(11):2070–9.

58. Christians KK, Pilgrim CH, Tsai S, et al. Arterial resection at the time of pancreatectomy for cancer. Surgery 2014;155(5):919–26.

59. Amano R, Kimura K, Nakata B, et al. Pancreatectomy with major arterial resection after neoadjuvant chemoradiotherapy gemcitabine and S-1 and concurrent radiotherapy for locally advanced unresectable pancreatic cancer. Surgery 2015;158(1):191–200.

60. Kang MJ, Jang JY, Chang YR, et al. Portal vein patency after pancreatoduodenectomy for periampullary cancer. Br J Surg 2015;102(1):77–84.

61. Ouaissi M, Sielezneff I, Pirro N, et al. Therapeutic anticoagulant does not modify thromboses rate vein after venous reconstruction following pancreaticoduodenectomy. Gastroenterol Res Pract 2008;2008:896320.

62. Chu CK, Farnell MB, Nguyen JH, et al. Prosthetic graft reconstruction after portal vein resection in pancreaticoduodenectomy: a multicenter analysis. J Am Coll Surg 2010;211(3):316–24.

63. Sgroi MD, Narayan RR, Lane JS, et al. Vascular reconstruction plays an important role in the treatment of pancreatic adenocarcinoma. J Vasc Surg 2015; 61(2):475–80.

64. Shukla PJ, Barreto SG, Kulkarni A, et al. Vascular anomalies encountered during pancreatoduodenectomy: do they influence outcomes? Ann Surg Oncol 2010; 17(1):186–93.

65. Traverso LW, Freeny PC. Pancreaticoduodenectomy. The importance of preserving hepatic blood flow to prevent biliary fistula. Am Surg 1989;55(7):421–6.

66. Allendorf JD, Bellemare S. Reconstruction of the replaced right hepatic artery at the time of pancreaticoduodenectomy. J Gastrointest Surg 2009;13(3):555–7.

67. Kim DK, Hindenburg AA, Sharma SK, et al. Is pylorospasm a cause of delayed gastric emptying after pylorus-preserving pancreaticoduodenectomy? Ann Surg Oncol 2005;12(3):222–7.

68. Sakorafas GH, Sarr MG, Peros G. Celiac artery stenosis: an underappreciated and unpleasant surprise in patients undergoing pancreaticoduodenectomy. J Am Coll Surg 2008;206(2):349–56.
69. Bong JJ, Karanjia ND, Menezes N, et al. Total gastric necrosis due to aberrant arterial anatomy and retrograde blood flow in the gastroduodenal artery: a complication following pancreaticoduodenectomy. HPB 2007;9(6):466–9.
70. Lai EC. Vascular resection and reconstruction at pancreatico-duodenectomy: technical issues. Hepatobiliary Pancreat Dis Int 2012;11(3):234–42.
71. Pallisera A, Morales R, Ramia JM. Tricks and tips in pancreatoduodenectomy. World J Gastrointest Oncol 2014;6(9):344–50.
72. Nara S, Sakamoto Y, Shimada K, et al. Arterial reconstruction during pancreato-duodenectomy in patients with celiac axis stenosis–utility of Doppler ultrasonography. World J Surg 2005;29(7):885–9.
73. Farma JM, Hoffman JP. Nonneoplastic celiac axis occlusion in patients undergoing pancreaticoduodenectomy. Am J Surg 2007;193(3):341–4 [discussion: 344].
74. Kurosaki I, Hatakeyama K, Nihei KE, et al. Celiac axis stenosis in pancreaticoduodenectomy. J Hepatobiliary Pancreat Surg 2004;11(2):119–24.
75. Tol JA, Gouma DJ, Bassi C, et al. Definition of a standard lymphadenectomy in surgery for pancreatic ductal adenocarcinoma: a consensus statement by the International Study Group on Pancreatic Surgery (ISGPS). Surgery 2014; 156(3):591–600.
76. Slidell MB, Chang DC, Cameron JL, et al. Impact of total lymph node count and lymph node ratio on staging and survival after pancreatectomy for pancreatic adenocarcinoma: a large, population-based analysis. Ann Surg Oncol 2008; 15(1):165–74.
77. Riediger H, Keck T, Wellner U, et al. The lymph node ratio is the strongest prognostic factor after resection of pancreatic cancer. J Gastrointest Surg 2009; 13(7):1337–44.
78. Sierzega M, Popiela T, Kulig J, et al. The ratio of metastatic/resected lymph nodes is an independent prognostic factor in patients with node-positive pancreatic head cancer. Pancreas 2006;33(3):240–5.
79. Zhan HX, Xu JW, Wang L, et al. Lymph node ratio is an independent prognostic factor for patients after resection of pancreatic cancer. World J Surg Oncol 2015;13:105.
80. Adsay NV, Basturk O, Altinel D, et al. The number of lymph nodes identified in a simple pancreatoduodenectomy specimen: comparison of conventional vs orange-peeling approach in pathologic assessment. Mod Pathol 2009;22(1): 107–12.
81. Pai RK, Beck AH, Mitchem J, et al. Pattern of lymph node involvement and prognosis in pancreatic adenocarcinoma: direct lymph node invasion has similar survival to node-negative disease. Am J Surg Pathol 2011;35(2):228–34.
82. Konstantinidis IT, Deshpande V, Zheng H, et al. Does the mechanism of lymph node invasion affect survival in patients with pancreatic ductal adenocarcinoma? J Gastrointest Surg 2010;14(2):261–7.
83. Gnerlich JL, Luka SR, Deshpande AD, et al. Microscopic margins and patterns of treatment failure in resected pancreatic adenocarcinoma. Arch Surg 2012; 147(8):753–60.
84. Rupp CC, Linehan DC. Extended lymphadenectomy in the surgery of pancreatic adenocarcinoma and its relation to quality improvement issues. J Surg Oncol 2009;99(4):207–14.

85. Peparini N. Mesopancreas: a boundless structure, namely the rationale for dissection of the paraaortic area in pancreaticoduodenectomy for pancreatic head carcinoma. World J Gastroenterol 2015;21(10):2865–70.

86. Iqbal N, Lovegrove RE, Tilney HS, et al. A comparison of pancreaticoduodenectomy with extended pancreaticoduodenectomy: a meta-analysis of 1909 patients. Eur J Surg Oncol 2009;35(1):79–86.

87. Michalski CW, Kleeff J, Wente MN, et al. Systematic review and meta-analysis of standard and extended lymphadenectomy in pancreaticoduodenectomy for pancreatic cancer. Br J Surg 2007;94(3):265–73.

88. Watson K. Carcinoma of ampulla of Vater successful radical resection. Br J Surg 1944;31(124):368–73.

89. Traverso LW, Longmire WP Jr. Preservation of the pylorus in pancreaticoduodenectomy. Surg Gynecol Obstet 1978;146(6):959–62.

90. Diener MK, Fitzmaurice C, Schwarzer G, et al. Pylorus-preserving pancreaticoduodenectomy (pp Whipple) versus pancreaticoduodenectomy (classic Whipple) for surgical treatment of periampullary and pancreatic carcinoma. Cochrane Database Syst Rev 2011;(5):CD006053.

91. Diener MK, Fitzmaurice C, Schwarzer G, et al. Pylorus-preserving pancreaticoduodenectomy (pp Whipple) versus pancreaticoduodenectomy (classic Whipple) for surgical treatment of periampullary and pancreatic carcinoma. Cochrane Database Syst Rev 2014;(11):CD006053.

92. Kawai M, Tani M, Hirono S, et al. Pylorus ring resection reduces delayed gastric emptying in patients undergoing pancreatoduodenectomy: a prospective, randomized, controlled trial of pylorus-resecting versus pylorus-preserving pancreatoduodenectomy. Ann Surg 2011;253(3):495–501.

93. Gagner M, Pomp A. Laparoscopic pylorus-preserving pancreatoduodenectomy. Surg Endosc 1994;8(5):408–10.

94. Addeo P, Calabrese DP, Bachellier P. Robotic pancreaticoduodenectomy: fad or the future? Adv Robot Autom 2012;2168–9695.

95. Giulianotti PC, Addeo P, Buchs NC, et al. Early experience with robotic total pancreatectomy. Pancreas 2011;40(2):311–3.

96. Cirocchi R, Partelli S, Coratti A, et al. Current status of robotic distal pancreatectomy: a systematic review. Surg Oncol 2013;22(3):201–7.

97. Lai EC, Yang GP, Tang CN. Robot-assisted laparoscopic pancreaticoduodenectomy versus open pancreaticoduodenectomy–a comparative study. Int J Surg 2012;10(9):475–9.

98. Waters JA, Canal DF, Wiebke EA, et al. Robotic distal pancreatectomy: cost effective? Surgery 2010;148(4):814–23.

99. Palanivelu C, Jani K, Senthilnathan P, et al. Laparoscopic pancreaticoduodenectomy: technique and outcomes. J Am Coll Surg 2007;205(2):222–30.

100. Zeh HJ, Zureikat AH, Secrest A, et al. Outcomes after robot-assisted pancreaticoduodenectomy for periampullary lesions. Ann Surg Oncol 2012;19(3):864–70.

101. Wu W, He J, Cameron JL, et al. The impact of postoperative complications on the administration of adjuvant therapy following pancreaticoduodenectomy for adenocarcinoma. Ann Surg Oncol 2014;21(9):2873–81.

102. Valle JW, Palmer D, Jackson R, et al. Optimal duration and timing of adjuvant chemotherapy after definitive surgery for ductal adenocarcinoma of the pancreas: ongoing lessons from the ESPAC-3 study. J Clin Oncol 2014;32(6):504–12.

103. Gnerlich JL, Posner MC. More harm than good? Ann Surg Oncol 2014;21(9):2817–9.

104. Naritomi G, Tanaka M, Matsunaga H, et al. Pancreatic head resection with and without preservation of the duodenum: different postoperative gastric motility. Surgery 1996;120(5):831–7.

105. Tran TC, van Lanschot JJ, Bruno MJ, et al. Functional changes after pancreato-duodenectomy: diagnosis and treatment. Pancreatology 2009;9(6):729–37.

106. Courvoisier T, Donatini G, Faure JP, et al. Primary versus secondary delayed gastric emptying (DGE) grades B and C of the International Study Group of Pancreatic Surgery after pancreatoduodenectomy: a retrospective analysis on a group of 132 patients. Updates Surg 2015;67(3):305–9.

107. Wente MN, Bassi C, Dervenis C, et al. Delayed gastric emptying (DGE) after pancreatic surgery: a suggested definition by the International Study Group of Pancreatic Surgery (ISGPS). Surgery 2007;142(5):761–8.

108. El Nakeeb A, Askr W, Mahdy Y, et al. Delayed gastric emptying after pancrea-ticoduodenectomy. Risk factors, predictors of severity and outcome. A single center experience of 588 cases. J Gastrointest Surg 2015;19(6):1093–100.

109. Hartel M, Wente MN, Hinz U, et al. Effect of antecolic reconstruction on delayed gastric emptying after the pylorus-preserving Whipple procedure. Arch Surg 2005;140(11):1094–9.

110. Bell R, Pandanaboyana S, Shah N, et al. Meta-analysis of antecolic versus retro-colic gastric reconstruction after a pylorus-preserving pancreatoduodenectomy. HPB 2015;17(3):202–8.

111. Su AP, Cao SS, Zhang Y, et al. Does antecolic reconstruction for duodenojeju-nostomy improve delayed gastric emptying after pylorus-preserving pancreati-coduodenectomy? A systematic review and meta-analysis. World J Gastroenterol 2012;18(43):6315–23.

112. Robinson JR, Marincola P, Shelton J, et al. Peri-operative risk factors for delayed gastric emptying after a pancreaticoduodenectomy. HPB 2015;17(6):495–501.

113. Qu H, Sun GR, Zhou SQ, et al. Clinical risk factors of delayed gastric emptying in patients after pancreaticoduodenectomy: a systematic review and meta-analysis. Eur J Surg Oncol 2013;39(3):213–23.

114. Hu HL, Zhou XD, Zhang Q, et al. Factors influencing delayed gastric emptying after pancreaticoduodenectomy—a meta-analysis. Hepatogastroenterology 2014;61(134):1539–45.

115. Yeo CJ, Barry MK, Sauter PK, et al. Erythromycin accelerates gastric emptying after pancreaticoduodenectomy. A prospective, randomized, placebo-controlled trial. Ann Surg 1993;218(3):229–37 [discussion: 237–8].

116. Sturm A, Holtmann G, Goebell H, et al. Prokinetics in patients with gastropare-sis: a systematic analysis. Digestion 1999;60(5):422–7.

117. Machado NO. Pancreatic fistula after pancreatectomy: definitions, risk factors, preventive measures, and management-review. Int J Surg Oncol 2012;2012: 602478.

118. Bassi C, Falconi M, Molinari E, et al. Duct-to-mucosa versus end-to-side pan-creaticojejunostomy reconstruction after pancreaticoduodenectomy: results of a prospective randomized trial. Surgery 2003;134(5):766–71.

119. Tewari M, Hazrah P, Kumar V, et al. Options of restorative pancreaticoenteric anastomosis following pancreaticoduodenectomy: a review. Surg Oncol 2010; 19(1):17–26.

120. Orci LA, Oldani G, Berney T, et al. Systematic review and meta-analysis of fibrin sealants for patients undergoing pancreatic resection. HPB 2014;16(1):3–11.

121. Gurusamy KS, Koti R, Fusai G, et al. Somatostatin analogues for pancreatic sur-gery. Cochrane Database Syst Rev 2010;(2):CD008370.

122. Allen PJ, Gonen M, Brennan MF, et al. Pasireotide for postoperative pancreatic fistula. N Engl J Med 2014;370(21):2014–22.
123. Rajarathinam G, Kannan DG, Vimalraj V, et al. Post pancreaticoduodenectomy haemorrhage: outcome prediction based on new ISGPS Clinical severity grading. HPB 2008;10(5):363–70.
124. Yekebas EF, Wolfram L, Cataldegirmen G, et al. Postpancreatectomy hemorrhage: diagnosis and treatment: an analysis in 1669 consecutive pancreatic resections. Ann Surg 2007;246(2):269–80.
125. Limongelli P, Khorsandi SE, Pai M, et al. Management of delayed postoperative hemorrhage after pancreaticoduodenectomy: a meta-analysis. Arch Surg 2008; 143(10):1001–7 [discussion: 1007].
126. Rombouts SJ, Vogel JA, van Santvoort HC, et al. Systematic review of innovative ablative therapies for the treatment of locally advanced pancreatic cancer. Br J Surg 2015;102(3):182–93.
127. Gouma DJ, Busch OR, Van Gulik TM. Pancreatic carcinoma: palliative surgical and endoscopic treatment. HPB 2006;8(5):369–76.
128. Tarnasky PR, England RE, Lail LM, et al. Cystic duct patency in malignant obstructive jaundice. An ERCP-based study relevant to the role of laparoscopic cholecystojejunostomy. Ann Surg 1995;221(3):265–71.
129. Jeurnink SM, Steyerberg EW, van Hooft JE, et al. Surgical gastrojejunostomy or endoscopic stent placement for the palliation of malignant gastric outlet obstruction (SUSTENT study): a multicenter randomized trial. Gastrointest Endosc 2010;71(3):490–9.
130. Nagaraja V, Eslick GD, Cox MR. Endoscopic stenting versus operative gastrojejunostomy for malignant gastric outlet obstruction—a systematic review and meta-analysis of randomized and non-randomized trials. J Gastrointest Oncol 2014;5(2):92–8.
131. Gurusamy KS, Kumar S, Davidson BR. Prophylactic gastrojejunostomy for unresectable periampullary carcinoma. Cochrane Database Syst Rev 2013;(2):CD008533.
132. Kaufman M, Singh G, Das S, et al. Efficacy of endoscopic ultrasound-guided celiac plexus block and celiac plexus neurolysis for managing abdominal pain associated with chronic pancreatitis and pancreatic cancer. J Clin Gastroenterol 2010;44(2):127–34.
133. de Leon-Casasola OA. Critical evaluation of chemical neurolysis of the sympathetic axis for cancer pain. Cancer Control 2000;7(2):142–8.
134. Lussier D, Huskey AG, Portenoy RK. Adjuvant analgesics in cancer pain management. Oncologist 2004;9(5):571–91.
135. Ierardi AM, Lucchina N, Petrillo M, et al. Systematic review of minimally invasive ablation treatment for locally advanced pancreatic cancer. Radiol Med 2014; 119(7):483–98.

Adjuvant and Neoadjuvant Therapy for Pancreatic Cancer

 CrossMark

Daneng Li, MD[a], Eileen M. O'Reilly, MD[a,b],*

KEYWORDS

- Pancreas adenocarcinoma • Adjuvant therapy • Neoadjuvant therapy • Clinical trials

KEY POINTS

- Current international standards of care for adjuvant therapy for pancreas adenocarcinoma consist of 6 months of gemcitabine or 5-fluorouracil with leucovorin.
- Erlotinib does not provide additional benefit in the treatment of patients with resected or locally advanced pancreas adenocarcinoma.
- Neoadjuvant therapy provides theoretic advantages over standard adjuvant therapy including treatment of distant micrometastases, assessment of tumor response to treatment, and better selection of patients most appropriate for surgery.
- The use of combination cytotoxic therapy, targeted agents, incorporation of chemoradiation, and immunotherapy all represent approaches under active investigation for adjuvant and neoadjuvant treatment of pancreas adenocarcinoma.

INTRODUCTION

Patients diagnosed with pancreas adenocarcinoma have a poor prognosis with 5-year overall survival (OS) rates estimated to be 6%.[1] Although surgery for patients with localized resectable pancreas adenocarcinoma remains a potential curative modality, the risk of relapse remains substantial with local-regional recurrence rates from 50% to 80% and systemic recurrence rates of greater than 70%.[2] The value of adjuvant systemic therapy has been clearly established in terms of reducing the risk of recurrence and prolonging survival, albeit the risk of recurrence remains significant. The

Dr E.M. O'Reilly has received research funding and consulting fees from Sanofi Aventis and Celgene. The Andrea J. Will Foundation also provided funding support. Dr D. Li has no disclosures.
a Department of Medicine, Memorial Sloan Kettering Cancer Center, 1275 York Avenue, New York, NY 10065, USA; b Weill Cornell Medical College, 1300 York Avenue, New York, NY 10065, USA
* Corresponding author. Gastrointestinal Medical Oncology Service, Department of Medicine, Memorial Sloan-Kettering Cancer Center, 300 East 66th Street, New York, NY 10065.
E-mail address: oreillye@mskcc.org

determination of optimal adjuvant treatment modalities between the types of systemic therapy used, combined chemotherapy and radiation, and chemoradiation plus chemotherapy along with whether to pursue an adjuvant or neoadjuvant strategy remain areas of active investigation. Furthermore, neoadjuvant therapy provides an emerging paradigm with several theoretic advantages over adjuvant therapy. Although not based on randomized data but rather consensus opinion, neoadjuvant therapy before surgery is an emerging paradigm for patients with borderline resectable pancreas cancer.

HISTORIC ADJUVANT SYSTEMIC TRIALS

The major historic phase III trials of adjuvant therapy in pancreas adenocarcinoma are listed in **Table 1**. One of the earliest phase III trials was the Gastrointestinal Tumor Study Group (GITSG) trial.[3] Forty-three evaluable patients with surgically resected pancreas adenocarcinoma were randomized to receive adjuvant treatment with 5-fluorouracil (5-FU) concurrent with a split-course of radiation versus observation. Median survival was found to be significantly longer for the adjuvant treatment group at 20 months compared with 11 months for the observation group ($P = .035$). Although the GITSG study has been used by some as a basis for 5-FU-based chemoradiation in the adjuvant setting, other studies have challenged the value of chemoradiation inferring the benefit observed came from prolonged systemic therapy. The EORTC 40891 (European Organization for Research and Treatment of Cancer) trial was a large multicenter phase III study of patients with resected pancreatic head cancer and periampullary tumors.[4] Patients were randomized to either observation or postoperative chemoradiation with short-course infusional 5-FU with concurrent split-course radiation. A total of 120 patients (approximately >50% of the total study population) with resected pancreatic head cancer were evaluated as part of this study and the long-term follow-up analysis showed no significant difference in survival between the treatment and observation groups even when only the pancreatic head cancer group was evaluated, although a nonstatistically significant trend was in favor of adjuvant therapy.[5]

Along with EORTC 40891, the ESPAC-1 (European Study Group of Pancreatic Cancer) trial[6,7] further challenged the value of chemoradiation and rather suggested that chemotherapy alone provided a survival benefit in the adjuvant setting. This study used a complex 2 × 2 factorial study design to randomize patients undergoing curative resection for pancreas adenocarcinoma into four treatment arms: (1) chemoradiation consisting of an intravenous bolus of 5-FU with split-course radiation, (2) chemotherapy consisting of an intravenous bolus of leucovorin followed by intravenous bolus of 5-FU for a total of 6 months of therapy, (3) combination therapy consisting of chemoradiation followed by chemotherapy as described previously, or (4) observation. A total of 289 patients underwent randomization with results showing the 5-year survival rate was 21% among patients treated with chemotherapy versus 8% among patients not treated with chemotherapy ($P = .009$). In addition, the estimated 5-year survival rate was 10% for patients treated with chemoradiation compared with 20% for patients who did not receive chemoradiation ($P = .05$). These results ultimately lead to a path away from using chemoradiation in Europe and beyond in favor of systemic chemotherapy alone as the main adjuvant treatment choice for resected pancreas adenocarcinoma. However, in North America, debate over the radiation techniques used in the EORTC 40891 and ESPAC-1 studies underpin the ongoing controversies over the value of chemoradiation in the adjuvant setting, which continues to remain an area of ongoing investigation and is being evaluated as part of RTOG 0848 (NCT01013549; Radiation Therapy Oncology Group).

Table 1
Historic randomized phase III trials of adjuvant therapy in pancreas adenocarcinoma

Trial	Patients	Treatment Arms	Median Disease-Free Survival (Months)	Median Overall Survival (Months)
GITSG-9173[3]	43	1. 5-FU-based CRT with bolus 5-FU 500 mg/m² on Days 1–3 of Weeks 1 and 5 of radiation, given as a split course of 50 Gy with 2-wk break in the middle Maintenance 5-FU given weekly for 2 y or until recurrence 2. Observation	2 y survival: 48% vs 14%	21 vs 11 (P = .035)
EORTC-40891[4]	218	1. 5-FU-based CRT with infusional 5-FU at a dose of 25 mg/kg/d on Days 1–5 on Weeks 1 and 5 with concurrent split-course radiation totaling 40 Gy with 2-wk break between radiation blocks 2. Observation	17.4 vs 16 (P = .643)	24.5 vs 19 (P = .208)
ESPAC-1[7]	289	1. 5-FU chemotherapy consisting of intravenous bolus of leucovorin 20 mg/m² followed by intravenous bolus of 5-FU at 425 mg/m² Days 1–5 every 28 d for total of 6 mo 2. 5-FU-based CRT with intravenous bolus of 5-FU at 500 mg/m² on Days 1–3 of Weeks 1 and 5 of radiation, given as split course of 40 Gy with 2-wk break in the middle 3. 5-FU-based CRT followed by chemotherapy as described in treatment arms (1) and (2) 4. Observation	Chemo vs no chemo: 15.3 vs 9.4 (P = .02) CRT vs no CRT: 10.7 vs 15.2 (P = .04)	Chemo vs no chemo: 20.1 vs 15.5 (P = .009) CRT vs no CRT: 15.9 vs 17.9 (P = .05)
CONKO-001[8]	368	1. Gemcitabine given Days 1, 8, 15 q 4 wk of 1000 mg/m², for total of 6 cycles 2. Observation	13.4 vs 6.9 (P < .001)	22.8 vs 20.2 (P = .005)
RTOG 9704[10]	451	1. Gemcitabine (1000 mg/m²) for 3 wk -> CRT -> gemcitabine for 12 wk postradiation 2. 5-FU (continuous infusion of 250 mg/m² per day) -> CRT ->5-FU	No difference, NA	20.5 vs 16.9 (P = .09)
ESPAC-3 (v2)[12]	1088	1. Gemcitabine (1000 mg/m²) Days 1, 8, 15 q 4 wk for 6 mo 2. 5-FU (leucovorin 20 mg/m² intravenous bolus followed by 5-FU 425 mg/m² intravenous bolus given on Days 1–5 every 28 d) for 6 mo	14.3 vs 14.1 (P = .53)	23.6 vs 23.0 (P = .39)
JASPAC-01[14]	385	1. Gemcitabine (1000 mg/m² intravenous infusion once a week for 3 of every 4 wk) for 6 mo 2. S-1 (80–120 mg/day based on BSA for 4 wk followed by 2 wk of rest) for total of 6 mo	Relapse-free survival: 11.2 vs 23.2 (P < .0001)	25.5 vs 46.3 (P < .0001)

Abbreviations: 5-FU, 5-fluorouracil; BSA, body surface area; CRT, chemoradiation therapy.

Although ESPAC-1 demonstrated the benefit of adjuvant systemic chemotherapy alone in pancreas adenocarcinoma with intravenous 5-FU, the CONKO-001 (Charite Onkologie 001) trial was designed to compare adjuvant intravenous gemcitabine with observation alone in patients undergoing curative resection for pancreatic cancer.[8,9] A total of 368 patients were randomized to either observation or to receive 6 months of gemcitabine. The primary end point was disease-free survival (DFS) and the key result of the study was a significant DFS advantage of 13.4 months in the treatment group versus 6.7 months in the observation group ($P < .001$). In addition, patients in the treatment group were found to have significantly prolonged OS compared with those being observed ($P = .01$).[9] These findings from the CONKO-001 therefore provided strong level 1 evidence supporting the use of gemcitabine as a standard chemotherapy agent in the adjuvant setting.

In addition to CONKO-001, the RTOG 9704 study[10] was a US-based phase III trial to determine if the addition of gemcitabine to adjuvant fluorouracil-based chemoradiation improved survival in patients with resected pancreatic adenocarcinoma. A total of 451 patients were enrolled and randomized to chemotherapy with either 5-FU or gemcitabine for 3 weeks before chemoradiation therapy and for 12 weeks following chemoradiation therapy. With a key primary end point of OS for patients with pancreatic head tumors, the investigators reported a median survival of 20.5 months in the gemcitabine group versus a median survival of 16.9 months in the 5-FU group ($P = .09$). Although not statistically significant, the authors concluded that the addition of gemcitabine given before and after chemoradiation was associated with a survival trend in the adjuvant setting. Furthermore, stratification of postresctional carbohydrate antigen (CA) 19-9 demonstrated the use of CA 19-9 as a significant predictor of survival in patients treated with adjuvant chemoradiation.[11] As a result, CA 19-9 is now frequently being used as a key eligibility criteria or stratification factor in many pancreas cancer clinical trials.

The ESPAC investigators also began to build on results from their ESPAC-1 trial. The ESPAC-3 (v2) trial ultimately accrued a total of 1088 patients who received either 5-FU plus leucovorin or gemcitabine chemotherapy for 6 months in the adjuvant setting.[12] The final results revealed equivalency between the two different chemotherapy agents with a median survival of 23.0 months for patients treated with 5-FU plus leucovorin and 23.6 months for those patients treated with gemcitabine ($P = .39$). The study also reported that 14% of patients treated with 5-FU plus leucovorin developed serious (> grade 3) treatment-related adverse events compared with 7.5% of patients treated with gemcitabine ($P < .001$). Based on these results, the use of gemcitabine chemotherapy alone became favored as the predominant therapy in the adjuvant setting. However, these data also provide support for the use of 5-FU/leucovorin in settings where patients may be at risk or develop serious complications to gemcitabine.

Although gemcitabine chemotherapy alone is often recommended as a current standard adjuvant chemotherapy for resected pancreas adenocarcinoma, many trials under investigation are focused on adding either different chemotherapy or biologic agents to gemcitabine or the use of other agents. Recently, preliminary results of the 385-patient JASPAC-01 (Japan Adjuvant Study Group of Pancreatic Cancer) trial suggested that S-1 (an oral fluoropyrimidine)[13] seems to be not only noninferior to gemcitabine but was also superior to gemcitabine in the adjuvant setting for the Japanese patient subpopulation.[14] Although the initial results are impressive, it is unclear if the survival benefit with adjuvant S-1 will translate to a broader population because white persons receiving S-1 have been known to develop more severe gastrointestinal toxicities and therefore lower doses of S-1 may be required in a broader patient population, which may diminish the overall efficacy of the drug. Future results and publication of this trial are awaited.

CURRENT AND FUTURE AREAS OF INVESTIGATION IN ADJUVANT THERAPY

Currently, several approaches being explored in the adjuvant setting to improve outcomes include evaluating (1) the role of combination cytotoxic therapy, (2) the role of the addition of a targeted agent, (3) the role of chemoradiation therapy, and (4) the role of immunotherapeutic approaches. These selected areas of investigation are listed in **Table 2** and are described next.

In terms of combination cytotoxic therapies, ESPAC-4 (ISRCTN96397434) is a large randomized phase III trial comparing the addition of capecitabine plus gemcitabine to gemcitabine. The study is powered for OS with a target of 1080 patients. The study completed recruitment in late 2014 and results are awaited. In addition to capecitabine being added to gemcitabine, combination cytotoxic regimens with significant benefit in metastatic pancreas adenocarcinoma, such as FOLFIRINOX (5-FU, leucovorin, irinotecan, oxaliplatin)[15] and the combination of gemcitabine plus nab-paclitaxel,[16] are now currently under investigation in the adjuvant setting. For example, investigators from the PRODIGE group, which conducted the prior FOLFIRINOX study[15] in the metastatic setting, have now developed PRODIGE 24/ACCORD 24 (NCT01526135), which is a phase III trial comparing adjuvant chemotherapy with gemcitabine versus modified FOLFIRINOX (omission of bolus 5-FU) to treat resected pancreatic adenocarcinoma. The estimated enrollment will be 490 patients with the primary outcome being DFS at 3 years. Another key study, ABI-007-PANC-003

Table 2
Selected ongoing adjuvant phase III trials in pancreas adenocarcinoma

Trial	Patients	Trial Design	Primary End Point
ESPAC-4 (ISRCTN96397434)	1080	Gemcitabine + capecitabine vs gemcitabine	Overall survival
CONKO-005 (DRKS00000247)	436	Gemcitabine + erlotinib vs gemcitabine	Equivalent median 11.6 mo disease-free survival between groups reported ($P = .291$)
RTOG 0848 (NCT01013649)	952	First randomization: gemcitabine + erlotinib vs gemcitabine (now discontinued) Second randomization: chemoradiation vs no chemoradiation	Overall survival
PRODIGE/ACCORD 24 (NCT01526135)	490	Gemcitabine vs FOLFIRINOX	Disease-free survival at 3 y
APACT ABI-007-PANC-003 (NCT01964430)	800	Gemcitabine vs gemcitabine + nab-paclitaxel	Disease-free survival
NewLink Genetics Corporation (NCT01072981)	722	Gemcitabine (+/- chemoradiation) +/- hyperacute immunotherapy	Overall survival

Abbreviation: FOLFIRINOX, 5-fluorouracil, leucovorin, irinotecan, oxaliplatin.

(NCT01964430), the APACT trial, will compare the efficacy of nab-paclitaxel in combination with gemcitabine with gemcitabine alone as adjuvant treatment in patients with surgically resected pancreatic adenocarcinoma. This study will recruit 800 patients to evaluate the primary outcome of DFS.

Regarding targeted therapy, erlotinib is the agent that has been most extensively investigated in the adjuvant setting based on positive results reported in the locally advanced and metastatic treatment settings for pancreas adenocarcinoma.[17] The CONKO-005 (DRKS00000247) trial recently reported on the role of gemcitabine plus erlotinib compared with gemcitabine alone in patients with R0 resected pancreas cancer. The primary end point of the study was DFS. A total of 436 patients were accrued and results of this study were just recently presented at a median follow-up of 41 months; there was no significant difference between the two treatment groups in terms of median DFS (11.6 months for both groups; $P = .291$) and OS (24.6 months for gemcitabine plus erlotinib vs 26.5 months for gemcitabine; $P = .406$).[18] In addition to CONKO-005, RTOG 0848 (NCT01013549) is an active North American phase III trial also originally designed to evaluate the role of the addition of erlotinib in the adjuvant setting while also attempting to address the value of chemoradiation in the adjuvant setting. The study was originally designed for a target of 952 patients to be randomized to receive gemcitabine or gemcitabine plus erlotinib to complete a total of 6 months of adjuvant systemic therapy. Patients in this study will also undergo restaging after 5 months of chemotherapy and if found to have no recurrence, they will undergo a second randomization to the addition of chemoradiation versus no added therapy. In 2013, results from the LAP-07 phase III trial[19] were presented demonstrating that the addition of radiation did not improve outcomes following 4 months of systemic therapy in patients with locally advanced pancreas adenocarcinoma. In addition, there was no change in survival outcomes for patients in the LAP-07 study who were first randomized to receive gemcitabine alone versus gemcitabine plus erlotinib. Given these findings the RTOG 0848 study has since been amended, where patients will now only undergo one randomization to plus or minus the addition of fluoropyrimidine-based radiation to a single-agent gemcitabine cytotoxic backbone and the randomization to include erlotinib has been discontinued. Based on all of the previously mentioned studies, erlotinib seems to have no significant benefit in the treatment of patients with resected and locally advanced pancreas cancer.

Another area of increasing research interest in the adjuvant treatment of pancreas adenocarcinoma has been the development of the use of vaccinations and broad immunotherapeutic approaches. Although vaccinations targeting KRAS mutations,[20,21] the telomerase peptide vaccine GV1001,[22,23] and the allogenic whole cell vaccine GVAX (granulocyte-macrophage colony–stimulating factor gene-transfected tumor cell vaccine)[24,25] have yielded mixed results from prior studies, vaccine development using the concept of hyperacute rejection may have potential promise moving forward. A vaccine (algenpantucel-L) has been developed using genetically modified pancreas cancer cells with a mouse gene leading to foreign protein expression of α (1,3)-galactosyl (αGal). Pre-existing anti-αGal antibodies then trigger a significant immune response leading to proposed cell destruction of any tumor cells in patients undergoing treatment with this form of immunotherapy.[26,27] A phase II study evaluating the role of this form of algenpantucel-L immunotherapy in addition to therapy with gemcitabine with 5-FU-based chemoradiation in patients with resected pancreas adenocarcinoma showed a significant 1-year DFS of 63% and OS of 86%, which compares favorably with historical control subjects.[28] As a result, a phase III trial of chemotherapy and chemoradiotherapy with or without algenpatnucel-L immunotherapy in

722 subjects with surgically resected pancreatic cancer has recently completed recruitment and results are eagerly awaited (NCT01072981).

NEOADJUVANT THERAPY: AN EMERGING PARADIGM IN PANCREAS ADENOCARCINOMA

Neoadjuvant therapy has not yet been widely established or accepted as a standard of care for patients with borderline resectable pancreatic adenocarcinoma. However, it does offer an alternative to traditional upfront surgery and adjuvant therapy with several theoretic advantages including treating distant micrometastases not seen on initial staging radiographs, assessing tumor response to treatment, selecting patients most appropriate for surgery, and including radiation to improve margin negative resection (R0) rates.[29,30] In addition, up to an estimated 25% to 30% of patients are unable to receive adjuvant systemic therapy following surgical resection. Neoadjuvant therapy could potentially increase the overall exposure to systemic therapy for many patients by decreasing time off treatment during recovery after surgical resection.[31]

The National Comprehensive Cancer Network guidelines currently recommend neoadjuvant therapy for borderline resectable disease.[29,32] Although tumors have been typically classified as either resectable or unresectable, the concept of "borderline resectable disease" has recently emerged as a category clinically distinct from "resectable" or "locally advanced disease." However, consensus over the standardization of these individual categories remains a major challenge.[33] Furthermore, prior randomized studies exploring the role of neoadjuvant treatment in pancreas adenocarcinoma have been limited primarily to single institution patients often with various disease settings (resectable, borderline resectable, and locally advanced pancreas cancer).[34,35] Therefore, questions of when to administer neoadjuvant systemic therapy, what is the optimal therapy (systemic, systemic and chemoradiation, or chemoradiation), and duration of treatment remain unanswered and are areas of intense investigation.

NEOADJUVANT RADIATION THERAPY TRIALS

Ishikawa and colleagues[36] was one of the early investigators in a retrospective study to compare preoperative and postoperative radiation alone in resectable disease patients before a Whipple surgery. Although preoperative radiation significantly decreased local recurrence with a 1-year survival rate of 75% in the preoperative group, and 43% in the postoperative group ($P < .05$), the overall 5-year survival rates were not significant between the two groups (22% vs 26%). Similarly, studies using 5-FU-based chemoradiation performed by Staley and colleagues[37] and Spitz and colleagues[38] also showed a decrease in local recurrence for patients who received preoperative compared with postoperative chemoradiation. Interestingly, the Spitz study also found no difference in OS between the preoperative and postoperative treatment groups, whereas the Staley study found no incidences of pathologic complete response for those receiving preoperative chemoradiation.

Neoadjuvant gemcitabine-based radiation has also been studied (**Table 3**). Two phase II nonrandomized studies[39,40] found that patients with potentially resectable disease treated with neoadjuvant gemcitabine-based radiation had higher rates of R0 resection compared with previous studies using 5-FU-based therapy. However, the true beneficial value of chemoradiation in the neoadjuvant setting remains unclear, because Xu and colleagues[41] performed a meta-analysis with a total of 3088 patients

Table 3
Selected neoadjuvant trials in pancreas adenocarcinoma

Trial	Type	Patients	Initial Disease Stage	Therapy	Results
Talamonti et al,[40] 2006	Phase II	20	Resectable	Gemcitabine + RT	Resection rate 85% R0 rate 94% Median OS 26 mo (resected)
Evans et al,[39] 2008	Phase II	86	Resectable	Gemcitabine + RT	Resection rate 71% Median PFS 28.6 mo (resected) Median OS 34 mo (resected) vs OS 7 mo (unresectable)
Heinrich et al,[42] 2008	Phase II	28	Resectable	Gemcitabine + cisplatin	Resection rate 89% R0 rate 80% Median PFS 9.2 mo (resected) Median OS 26.5 mo (resected)
Sahora et al,[44] 2011	Phase II	33	Borderline resectable + locally advanced unresectable	Gemcitabine + oxaliplatin	Resection rate 39% R0 rate 69% Median PFS 10 mo (resected) Median OS 22 mo (resected) vs 12 mo (unresectable)
Sahora et al,[45] 2011	Phase II	25	Borderline resectable + locally advanced unresectable	Gemcitabine + docetaxel	Resection rate 32% R0 rate 87% Median PFS 12 mo (resected) Median OS 16.3 mo (resected) vs 12.2 mo (unresectable)
Motoi et al,[43] 2013	Phase II	35	Resectable + borderline resectable	Gemcitabine + S1	Resection rate 86% R0 rate 87% Median OS 34.7 mo (resected) vs OS 10 mo (unresectable)
Leone et al,[46] 2013	Phase II	39	Borderline resectable + locally advanced unresectable	Gemcitabine + oxaliplatin + gemcitabine-based RT	Resection rate 28% R0 rate 82% Median PFS 19.9 mo (resected) vs 7.6 mo (unresectable)
O'Reilly et al,[47] 2014	Phase II	38	Resectable	Gemcitabine + oxaliplatin	Resection rate 71% 18 mo OS 63% Median overall survival 27.2 mo

Abbreviations: PFS, progression free survival; R0, margin negative surgical resection; RT, radiation therapy.

with resectable pancreatic adenocarcinoma and found no significant difference in progression-free survival (PFS) and OS for patients who received either presurgical or postsurgical chemoradiation.

GEMCITABINE-BASED NEOADJUVANT SYSTEMIC THERAPY TRIALS

As gemcitabine-based regimens became widely accepted in the treatment of metastatic pancreas adenocarcinoma, numerous gemcitabine systemic combinations have been investigated preoperatively (see **Table 3**). Heinrich and colleagues[42] performed a phase II study using neoadjuvant gemcitabine and cisplatin systemic therapy in patients initially with resectable disease and found that 25 of 28 patients ultimately underwent surgery, of which 80% attained an R0 resection. Overall survival for the patients undergoing resection was 26.5 months, which was higher than the OS previously reported in 5-FU-based neoadjuvant studies.[37,38] The role of S1 in the neoadjuvant setting has also been explored. Motoi and colleagues[43] performed a phase II study with neoadjuvant gemcitabine plus S1 in 35 patients with resectable and borderline resectable disease. A total of 30 of 35 (85.7%) patients underwent resection with a median OS of 34.7 months for patients who had an R0 resection compared with 10 months for patients who could not undergo surgery or had resection with evidence of distant metastases.

Two prospective phase II trials by Sahora and colleagues[44,45] also examined the roles of neoadjuvant gemcitabine-based regimens with gemcitabine plus oxaliplatin and gemcitabine plus docetaxel in patients initially with borderline resectable and locally advanced disease. In the neoadjuvant trial with gemcitabine plus oxaliplatin, 13 of 33 (39%) patients underwent surgical resection after 6 weeks of neoadjuvant gemcitabine plus oxaliplatin. Median OS was 22 months for those who had surgical resection compared with 12 months for those without resection. Similarly, in the trial with neoadjuvant gemcitabine plus docetaxel, 8 of 25 (32%) patients underwent surgical resection after 8 weeks of neoadjuvant gemcitabine plus docetaxel. Median OS was 16.3 and 12.2 months for patients who did and did not undergo surgical resection, respectively. In addition to the Sahora studies, another prospective trial[46] explored the role of neoadjuvant gemcitabine plus oxaliplatin with gemcitabine-based chemoradiation for patients with borderline resectable and locally advanced unresectable disease, reporting similar results (28% patients ultimately underwent surgical resection with PFS advantage of 19.7 months compared with 7.6 months in favor of patients completing surgical resection). Furthermore, for patients with resectable disease, O'Reilly and colleagues[47] performed a single-arm prospective study with neoadjuvant gemcitabine plus oxaliplatin followed by adjuvant gemcitabine. A total of 27 of 38 (71%) patients underwent resection and an overall 18-month survival rate of 63% and a median OS of 27.2 months were observed. The American College of Surgeons Co-operative Oncology Group evaluated neoadjuvant gemcitabine and erlotinib in a single-arm nonrandomized design in resectable pancreas adenocarcinoma (NCT00773746). This trial, Z5041, used real-time central radiology review to adjudicate eligibility. This study was completed several years ago and results are awaited. Ultimately, although the number of patients in many neoadjuvant studies has been small to date, the potential benefit with respect to PFS and OS even for patients initially with borderline resectable or locally advanced disease has been encouraging. Investigation into the use of newer and more active systemic regimens in the neoadjuvant setting for the treatment of pancreas adenocarcinoma could potentially improve outcomes even further moving forward.

NEOADJUVANT THERAPY WITH FOLFIRINOX

FOLFIRINOX is an example of a multiagent cytotoxic systemic therapy currently established as a standard of care in the treatment of metastatic pancreas adenocarcinoma.[15] However, reports of its use in the neoadjuvant setting have currently been limited mainly to single institution experiences. One retrospective study of neoadjuvant FOLFIRINOX[48] in patients with both borderline resectable and locally advanced pancreas adenocarcinoma found that 11 of 21 (52%) patients underwent surgical resection. The authors also reported a 5% complete pathologic response and a 19% partial response rate following FOLFIRINOX treatment alone. Similarly, another retrospective study of neoadjuvant FOLFIRINOX[49] in patients with borderline resectable pancreas adenocarcinoma found that 12 of 18 (67%) patients undergoing treatment with FOLFIRINOX followed by gemcitabine- or capecitabine-based radiation therapy were able to undergo R0 resection. Even for locally advanced, unresectable disease, a retrospective single-institution study from the Massachusetts General Hospital noted that up to 20% of patients who received neoadjuvant FOLFIRINOX followed by 5-FU or capecitabine-based radiation therapy were converted from unresectable to resectable disease.[50] Given these findings, several ongoing prospective studies are examining the role of FOLFIRINOX in a neoadjuvant setting for resectable disease (**Table 4**). These include a single-arm nonrandomized trial evaluating preoperative and postoperative FOLFIRINOX in patients with resectable disease (NCT01660711) and the multicenter German randomized trial investigating adjuvant gemcitabine compared with neoadjuvant and adjuvant FOLFIRINOX (NCT02172976). For borderline resectable disease, the Alliance pilot trial A021101 (NCT01821612) represents an important study examining the role of neoadjuvant FOLFIRINOX and chemoradiation followed by surgery and adjuvant gemcitabine. The primary end points are R0/R1 resection rates, radiographic and pathologic response rates, time to local and distant recurrence, and OS. Initial results were recently presented showing 15 of 22 (68%) patients underwent successful R0/R1 resections after neoadjuvant treatment and 2 of 22 (9%) patients even achieved a pathologic complete response at time of resection.[51] Further follow-up is planned for this study and ongoing discussions are underway regarding designing a randomized phase II trial. This study also aims to further standardize the definition of borderline resectable disease, which will provide a better foundation and reference for future neoadjuvant trials involving patients with locally advanced disease.[52,53]

CURRENT AND EMERGING AREAS OF NEOADJUVANT INVESTIGATION

Given the dearth of randomized neoadjuvant trials, questions regarding neoadjuvant therapy strictly in resectable disease along with determination of the optimal therapeutic regimen remain areas of active investigation. Several emerging studies aimed to address these questions are summarized in **Table 4**.

The NEOPAC trial (NCT01521702) is a prospective randomized phase III trial comparing adjuvant gemcitabine with neoadjuvant gemcitabine and oxaliplatin in conjunction with surgery followed by adjuvant gemcitabine in patients with resectable head of pancreas adenocarcinoma. The study was initiated in 2011[54] with a target accrual of 310 patients and represents one of the largest randomized trials examining adjuvant and neoadjuvant gemcitabine-based therapy to date. The primary end point is PFS at 1 year and secondary end points are pathologic response to neoadjuvant therapy, OS, and postoperative complications. In addition to the NEOPAC trial, several other gemcitabine-based combination regimens are being explored with particular

Table 4
Select ongoing neoadjuvant trials for resectable pancreas adenocarcinoma

Trial	Type	Patients	Therapy	Primary Outcome
NEOPAC NCT01521702	Phase III	310	Neoadjuvant FOLFIRINOX -> surgery -> adjuvant gemcitabine vs adjuvant gemcitabine	5 y PFS
NCT01900327	Phase III	410	Neoadjuvant gemcitabine-based CRT -> surgery -> adjuvant gemcitabine vs adjuvant gemcitabine	3 y OS
NCT01771146	Phase II	100	Neoadjuvant FOLFIRINOX	PFS
NEONAX NCT02047513	Randomized phase II	166	Neoadjuvant gemcitabine + nab-paclitaxel -> surgery -> adjuvant gemcitabine + nab-paclitaxel vs adjuvant gemcitabine + nab-paclitaxel	18 mo DFS
NCT02172976	Randomized phase II/III	126	Adjuvant gemcitabine vs neoadjuvant FOLFIRINOX -> surgery -> adjuvant FOLFIRINOX	Median OS
NCT01150630	Randomized phase II/III	370	Adjuvant PEXG vs adjuvant gemcitabine vs neoadjuvant PEXG -> surgery -> adjuvant PEXG	1 y event-free survival
ACOSOG-Z5041 NCT00733746	Phase II	123	Neoadjuvant gemcitabine + erlotinib (completed; results pending)	2 y OS
NCT00727441	Phase II	87	GVAX +/- IV or oral cyclophosphamide -> surgery -> adjuvant gemcitabine + CRT	Safety, feasibility, and immune response
NCT02178709	Phase II	48	Neoadjuvant FOLFIRINOX	Pathologic complete response
GEMCAD1003 NCT01389440	Phase II	24	Neoadjuvant gemcitabine + erlotinib	R0 resection rate
NCT02243007	Randomized phase II	112	Neoadjuvant FOLFIRINOX vs gemcitabine + nab-paclitaxel	18 mo OS
NCT02030860	Pilot	15	Neoadjuvant gemcitabine + nab-paclitaxel +/- paricalcitol	Number of adverse events
NCT02305186	Randomized phase Ib/II	56	Neoadjuvant capecitabine based CRT +/- pembrolizumab (MK-3745)	Safety and immune response

Abbreviations: CRT, chemoradiation therapy; GVAX, granulocyte-macrophage colony-stimulating factor gene-transfected tumor cell vaccine; PEXG, cisplatin, epirubicin, capecitabine, gemcitabine; R0, margin-negative surgical resection.

interest with the combination of gemcitabine and nab-paclitaxel given its success in the metastatic setting. For example, several phase II trials investigating the neoadjuvant role of gemcitabine plus nab-paclitaxel in resectable (NCT02047513) and borderline/locally advanced disease (GAIN-1 study [NCT01470417] and trial [NCT02210559]) are currently under evaluation. Furthermore, neoadjuvant gemcitabine plus nab-paclitaxel are also being evaluated with oral hedgehog inhibitors, such as LDE-225 targeting the stroma (NCT01431794) or with paricalcitol targeting the vitamin D metabolic program (NCT02030860). These studies illustrate the opportunity for neoadjuvant trials to incorporate additional correlative and tissue evaluation that may ultimately provide a better understanding of the entire disease process.

IMMUNOTHERAPY TRIALS

The value of immunotherapeutic approaches is also an area of focused research in the neoadjuvant setting. Although the role of GVAX in metastatic pancreas adenocarcinoma has yet to be established, trial NCT00727441 is a randomized three-arm neoadjuvant study that has been completed and was designed to explore the role of neoadjuvant GVAX with and without cyclophosphamide for neoadjuvant and adjuvant treatment of 87 patients with resectable pancreatic adenocarcinoma. All patients in this study received standard adjuvant gemcitabine with chemoradiation. The primary end points are evaluating safety, immune infiltrate levels postvaccination, and changes in specific regulatory T-cell levels status-post GVAX and surgical resection. Secondary end points consist of disease-free and OS in those patients treated with GVAX. In addition to GVAX, algenpantucel-L is also being investigated in the adjuvant setting as previously discussed. In the neoadjuvant setting, the PILLAR trial (NCT01836432) is a phase III study developed to examine the effect of algenpantucel-L administered with either FOLFIRINOX or gemcitabine plus nab-paclitaxel in patients with borderline resectable or locally advanced pancreas adenocarcinoma. Neoadjuvant algenpantucel-L with stereotactic body radiation therapy following FOLFIRINOX will also be investigated in an upcoming phase II study in patients with borderline resectable pancreatic cancer (NCT02405585).

In addition to vaccines, modulating T-cell signaling through PD-1 (NCT02305186) or targeting the cell-surface CD40 cosignaling molecules using monoclonal ligands to affect an immune response against tumor antigens are additional areas of interesting investigation. For instance, Beatty and colleagues[55] reported a partial tumor response in 4 of 22 (18%) patients with advanced pancreas adenocarcinoma after the use of a CD40 agonist, CP-870893, combined with gemcitabine. Results from a follow-up phase I study (NCT01456585) examining the efficacy of neoadjuvant CP-870893 plus gemcitabine followed by postoperative 5-FU-based chemoradiation in 10 patients with resectable disease are pending. Further study evaluating the addition of CP-870893 to combinations, such as gemcitabine and nab-paclitaxel, in the neoadjuvant setting are being considered.

SUMMARY

The value of adjuvant systemic therapy in pancreas adenocarcinoma has been clearly established in terms of its ability to delay recurrence and enhance OS. Current international standards of care for adjuvant therapy consist of either 6 months of gemcitabine or 5-FU and leucovorin. The role of adjuvant chemoradiation has not yet been firmly established in the United States. Although not yet widely accepted as a standard of care for patients with resectable pancreatic adenocarcinoma, neoadjuvant chemotherapy provides theoretic advantages including most importantly selection of patients most appropriate for surgery. The roles of multiagent chemotherapy combinations, targeted agents, and immunotherapeutic approaches in the adjuvant and neoadjuvant settings remain areas of active investigation and represent opportunities for improved care in the treatment of pancreas adenocarcinoma.

REFERENCES

1. Siegel R, Ma J, Zou Z, et al. Cancer statistics, 2014. CA Cancer J Clin 2014;64: 9–29.
2. Garcea G, Dennison AR, Pattenden CJ, et al. Survival following curative resection for pancreatic ductal adenocarcinoma. A systemic review of the literature. JOP 2008;9:99–132.
3. Kalser MH, Ellenber SS. Pancreatic cancer. Adjuvant combined radiation and chemotherapy following curative resection. Arch Surg 1985;120:899–903.
4. Klinkenbijl JH, Jeekel J, Sahmoud T, et al. Adjuvant radiotherapy and 5-fluorouracil after curative resection of cancer of the pancreas and periampullary region: Phase III trial of the EORTC gastrointestinal tract cancer cooperative group. Ann Surg 1999;230:776–82.
5. Smeenk HG, van Eijck CH, Hop WC, et al. Long-term survival and metastatic pattern of pancreatic and periampullary cancer after adjuvant chemoradiation or observation. Long-term results of EORTC trial 40891. Ann Surg 2007;246:734–40.
6. Neoptolemos JP, Dunn JA, Stocken DD, et al. Adjuvant chemoradiotherapy and chemotherapy in resectable pancreatic cancer: a randomized controlled trial. Lancet 2001;358:1576–85.
7. Neoptolemos JP, Stocken DD, Friess H, et al. A randomized trial of chemoradiotherapy and chemotherapy after resection of pancreatic cancer. N Engl J Med 2004;350:1200–10.
8. Oettle H, Post S, Neuhaus P, et al. Adjuvant chemotherapy with gemcitabine vs observation in patients undergoing curative-intent resection of pancreatic cancer: a randomized controlled trial. JAMA 2007;297:267–77.
9. Oettle H, Neuhaus P, Hochhaus A, et al. Adjuvant chemotherapy with gemcitabine and long term outcomes among patients with resected pancreatic cancer. The CONKO-001 randomized trial. JAMA 2013;310:1473–81.
10. Regine WF, Winter KA, Abrams RA, et al. Fluorouracil vs gemcitabine chemotherapy before and after fluorouracil-based chemoradiation following resection of pancreatic adenocarcinoma: a randomized controlled trial. JAMA 2008;299: 1019–26.
11. Berger AC, Garcia M Jr, Hoffman JP, et al. Postresection Ca 19-9 predicts overall survival in patients with pancreatic cancer treated with adjuvant chemoradiation: a prospective validation by RTOG 9704. J Clin Oncol 2008;26:5918–22.
12. Neoptolemos JP, Stocken DD, Bassi C, et al. Adjuvant chemotherapy with fluorouracil plus folinic acid vs gemcitabine following pancreatic cancer resection: a randomized controlled trial. JAMA 2010;304:1073–81.
13. Saif MW, Syrigos KN, Katirzoglou NA. S-1: a promising new oral fluoropyrimidine derivative. Expert Opin Investig Drugs 2009;18:335–48.
14. Fukutomi A, Uesaka K, Boku N, et al. JASPAC 01: randomized phase III trial of adjuvant chemotherapy with gemcitabine versus S-1 for patients with resected pancreatic cancer. J Clin Oncol 2013;31 [meeting abstract: 4008].
15. Conroy T, Desseigne F, Ychou M, et al. FOLFIRINOX versus gemcitabine for metastatic pancreatic cancer. N Engl J Med 2011;364:1817–25.

16. Von Hoff DD, Ervin T, Arena FP, et al. Increased survival in pancreatic cancer with nab-paclitaxel plus gemcitabine. N Engl J Med 2013;369:1691–703.

17. Moore MJ, Goldstein D, Hamm J, et al. Erlotinib plus gemcitabine compared with gemcitabine alone in patients with advanced pancreatic cancer: a phase III trial of the National Cancer Institute of Canada clinical trials group. J Clin Oncol 2007; 25:1960–6.

18. Sinn M, Liersch T, Gellert K, et al. CONKO-005: adjuvant therapy in R0 resected pancreatic cancer patients with gemcitabine plus erlotinib versus gemcitabine for 24 weeks-A prospective randomized phase III study. J Clin Oncol 2015;33 [meeting abstract: 4007].

19. Hammel P, Huguet F, Van Laethem JL, et al. Comparison of chemoradiotherapy and chemotherapy in patients with a locally advanced pancreatic cancer controlled after 4 months of gemcitabine with or without erlotinib: final results of the international phase III LAP 07 study. J Clin Oncol 2013;31 [meeting abstract: 4003].

20. Weden S, Klemp M, Gladhaug IP, et al. Long term follow-up of patients with resected pancreatic cancer following vaccination against mutant K-ras. Int J Cancer 2011;128:1120–8.

21. Abou-Alfa GK, Champman PB, Feilchenfeldt J, et al. Targeting mutated K-ras in pancreatic adenocarcinoma using an adjuvant vaccine. Am J Clin Oncol 2011;3: 321–5.

22. Shaw VE, Naisbitt DJ, Costello E, et al. Current status of GV1001 and other telomerase vaccination strategies in the treatment of cancer. Expert Rev Vaccines 2010;9:1007–16.

23. Middleton GW, Valle JW, Wadsley J, et al. A phase III randomized trial of chemoimmunotherapy comprising gemcitabine and capecitabine with or without telomerase vaccine GV1001 in patients with locally advanced or metastatic pancreatic cancer. J Clin Oncol 2013;31 [meeting abstract: 4004].

24. Jaffee EM, Hruban RH, Biedrzycki B, et al. Novel allogeneic granulocyte-macrophage colony-stimulating factor-secreting tumor vaccine for pancreatic cancer: a phase I trial of safety and immune activation. J Clin Oncol 2001;19:145–56.

25. Lutz E, Yeo CJ, Lillemoe KD, et al. A lethally irradiated allogeneic granulocyte-macrophage colony stimulating factor-secreting tumor vaccine for pancreatic adenocarcinoma. A phase II trial of safety, efficacy, and immune activation. Ann Surg 2011;253:328–35.

26. Galili U, LaTemple DC. Natural anti-Gal antibody as a universal augmenter of autologous tumor vaccine immunogenicity. Immunol Today 1997;18:281–5.

27. LaTemple DC, Abrams JF, Zhang SY, et al. Increased immunogenicity of tumor vaccines complexed with anti-Gal: studies in knockout mice for alpha 1,3 glactosyltransferase. Cancer Res 1999;59:3417–23.

28. Hardacre JM, Mulcahy MF, Small W, et al. Addition of algenpantucel-L immunotherapy to standard of care adjuvant therapy for pancreatic cancer. J Clin Oncol 2012;30 [meeting abstract: 4049].

29. Belli C, Cereda S, Anand S, et al. Neoadjuvant therapy in resectable pancreatic cancer: a critical review. Cancer Treat Rev 2013;39:518–24.

30. Cooper AB, Tzeng CW, Katz MH. Treatment of borderline resectable pancreatic cancer. Curr Treat Options Oncol 2013;14:293–310.

31. Papavasiliou P, Chun YS, Hoffman JP. How to define and manage borderline resectable pancreatic cancer. Surg Clin North Am 2013;93:663–74.

32. Kelly KJ, Winslow E, Kooby D, et al. Vein involvement during pancreaticoduodenectomy: is there a need for redefinition of "borderline resectable disease"? J Gastrointest Surg 2013;17:1209–17.

33. Halperin DM, Varadhachary GR. Resectable, borderline resectable, and locally advanced pancreatic cancer: what does it matter? Curr Oncol Rep 2014;16:366.
34. He J, Page AJ, Weiss M, et al. Management of borderline and locally advanced pancreatic cancer: where do we stand? World J Gastroenterol 2014;20:2255–66.
35. Kang CM, Hwang HK, Choi SH, et al. Controversial issues of neoadjuvant treatment in borderline resectable pancreatic cancer. Surg Oncol 2013;22:123–31.
36. Ishikawa O, Ohigashi H, Imaoka S, et al. Is the long-term survival rate improved by preoperative irradiation prior to Whipple's procedure for adenocarcinoma of the pancreatic head? Arch Surg 1994;129:1075–80.
37. Staley CA, Lee JE, Cleary KR, et al. Preoperative chemoradiation, pancreatico-duodenectomy, and intraoperative radiation therapy for adenocarcinoma of the pancreatic head. Am J Surg 1996;171:118–24.
38. Spitz FR, Abbruzzese JL, Lee JE, et al. Preoperative and postoperative chemo-radiation strategies in patients treated with pancreaticoduodenectomy for adeno-carcinoma of the pancreas. J Clin Oncol 1997;15:928–37.
39. Evans DB, Varadhachary GR, Crane CH, et al. Preoperative gemcitabine-based chemoradiation for patients with resectable adenocarcinoma of the pancreatic head. J Clin Oncol 2008;26:3496–502.
40. Talamonti MS, Small W Jr, Mulcahy MF, et al. A multi-institutional phase II trial of preoperative full-dose gemcitabine and concurrent radiation for patients with potentially resectable pancreatic carcinoma. Ann Surg Oncol 2006;13:150–8.
41. Xu CP, Xue XJ, Liang N, et al. Effect of chemoradiotherapy and neoadjuvant chemoradiotherapy in resectable pancreatic cancer: a systematic review and meta-analysis. J Cancer Res Clin Oncol 2014;140:549–59.
42. Heinrich S, Pestalozzi BC, Schafer M, et al. Prospective phase II trial of neoadju-vant chemotherapy with gemcitabine and cisplatin for resectable adenocarci-noma of the pancreatic head. J Clin Oncol 2008;26:2526–31.
43. Motoi F, Ishida K, Fujishima F, et al. Neoadjuvant chemotherapy with gemcitabine and S-1 for resectable and borderline pancreatic ductal adenocarcinoma: results from a prospective multi-institutional phase 2 trial. Ann Surg Oncol 2013;20:3794–801.
44. Sahora K, Kuehrer I, Eisenhut A, et al. NeoGemOx: gemcitabine and oxaliplatin as neoadjuvant treatment for locally advanced, nonmetastasized pancreatic can-cer. Surgery 2011;149:311–20.
45. Sahora K, Kuehrer I, Schindl M, et al. NeoGemTax: gemcitabine and docetaxel as neoadjuvant treatment for locally advanced nonmetastasized pancreatic cancer. World J Surg 2011;35:1580–9.
46. Leone F, Gatti M, Massucco P, et al. Induction gemcitabine and oxaliplatin ther-apy followed by a twice-weekly infusion of gemcitabine and concurrent external-beam radiation for neoadjuvant treatment of locally advanced pancre-atic cancer: a single institutional experience. Cancer 2013;119:277–84.
47. O'Reilly EM, Perelshteyn A, Jarnagin WR, et al. A single-arm, nonrandomized phase II trial of neoadjuvant gemcitabine and oxaliplatin in patients with resect-able pancreas adenocarcinoma. Ann Surg 2014;260:142–8.
48. Boone BA, Steve J, Krasinskas AM, et al. Outcomes with FOLFIRINOX for border-line resectable and locally unresectable pancreatic cancer. J Surg Oncol 2013;108:236–41.
49. Christians KK, Tsai S, Mahmoud A, et al. Neoadjuvant FOLFIRINOX for borderline resectable pancreas cancer: a new treatment paradigm? Oncologist 2014;19:266–74.

50. Faris JE, Blaszkowsky LS, McDermott S, et al. FOLFIRINOX in locally advanced pancreatic cancer: the Massachusetts General Hospital Cancer Center experience. Oncologist 2013;18:543–8.
51. Katz MH, Shi Q, Ahmad SA, et al. Preoperative modified FOLFIRINOX (mFOLFIRINOX) followed by chemoradiation (CRT) for borderline resectable (BLR) pancreatic cancer (PDAC): initial results from Alliance Trial A021101. J Clin Oncol 2015;33 [meeting abstract: 4008].
52. Katz MH, Marsh R, Herman JM, et al. Borderline resectable pancreatic cancer: need for standardization and methods for optimal clinical trial design. Ann Surg Oncol 2013;20:2787–95.
53. Tempero MA, Malafa MP, Behrman SW, et al. Pancreatic adenocarcinoma, version 2.2014: featured updates to the NCCN guidelines. J Natl Compr Canc Netw 2014;12:1083–93.
54. Heinrich S, Pestalozzi B, Lesurtel M, et al. Adjuvant gemcitabine versus NEOadjuvant gemcitabine/oxaliplatin plus adjuvant gemcitabine in resectable pancreatic cancer: a randomized multicenter phase III study (NEOPAC study). BMC Cancer 2011;11:346.
55. Beatty GL, Torigian DA, Chiorean EG, et al. A phase I study of an agonist CD40 monoclonal antibody (CP-870,893) in combination with gemcitabine in patients with advanced pancreatic ductal adenocarcinoma. Clin Cancer Res 2013;19:6286–95.

Palliative Management of Unresectable Pancreas Cancer

Katherine E. Poruk, MD, Christopher L. Wolfgang, MD, PhD*

KEYWORDS

- Pancreatic adenocarcinoma • Unresectable • Metastatic • Biliary decompression
- Palliative bypass • Gastric outlet obstruction • Celiac plexus block

KEY POINTS

- Palliative surgical resection resulting in grossly positive margins offers no survival benefit and is not recommended for patients with unresectable or metastatic pancreatic cancer.
- Endoscopic biliary stenting and operative biliary bypass are both effective in relieving biliary obstruction without significant differences in mortality or overall survival.
- Prophylactic gastrojejunostomy should be performed at the time of hepaticojejunostomy, given a significant decrease in the incidence of postoperative gastric outlet obstruction without an associated increase in postoperative morbidity or mortality.
- Celiac plexus block improves pain control and decreases narcotic pain medication usage for patients with unresectable pancreatic cancer, resulting in few long-term adverse side effects.

BACKGROUND

Pancreatic adenocarcinoma (PDAC) is the fourth leading cause of cancer death in the United States with a 5-year all-stage overall survival of only 6%.[1] This dismal survival rate is in part attributed to a delay in diagnosis given limitations in disease screening and nonspecific symptoms. Most patients are often asymptomatic or present with vague, nonspecific symptoms, such as weight loss, abdominal pain, fatigue, or jaundice, so that when they are finally diagnosed, the disease is often progressed and has spread to distant organs, limiting treatment options.[2] Currently, surgical resection provides the best opportunity for survival, but is limited to patients with locally resectable

The authors have nothing to disclose.
Department of Surgery, The Sol Goldman Pancreatic Cancer Research Center, The Johns Hopkins University School of Medicine, 600 North Wolfe Street, Baltimore, MD 21287, USA
* Corresponding author. Department of Surgery, The Johns Hopkins University School of Medicine, 600 North Wolfe Street, Blalock 604, Baltimore, MD 21287.
E-mail address: cwolfga2@jhmi.edu

Surg Oncol Clin N Am 25 (2016) 327–337
http://dx.doi.org/10.1016/j.soc.2015.11.005
1055-3207/16/$ – see front matter © 2016 Elsevier Inc. All rights reserved.

tumors without distant metastases. As a result, only 15% to 20% of patients with pancreatic cancer present with tumors amenable to surgical resection, creating a large population of patients in whom treatment options are limited.[3] In addition, the local and distant spread of disease often creates symptomatic problems such as pain or obstruction, necessitating treatment for palliation of symptoms. This article reviews the current palliative treatment options in patients with unresectable pancreatic cancer, including palliative resection, surgical and endoscopic biliary and gastric decompression, and pain control with celiac plexus block.

CURRENT TREATMENT OF UNRESECTABLE PANCREATIC CANCER

Surgical resection offers the best opportunity for prolonged survival and the only chance for potential cure in patients with pancreatic adenocarcinoma. Five-year survival rates approach 25% in published series at specialized centers.[4,5] However, very few patients present with disease at a stage in which curative resection can be effectively offered. An analysis of 58,655 patients with pancreatic cancer diagnosed between 1977 and 2001 demonstrated only 8.9% had localized disease compared with 22.4% who presented with regional spread and 49.5% with distant metastases at the time of diagnosis, including an additional 19.4% who were unstaged.[6] Looking at the specific period between 1997 and 2001, only 7.4% presented with localized disease compared with a known 25.8% with regional disease and 49.8% with distant metastases.[6] Even without taking into account those with unstaged disease or delineating which patients with regional spread of disease were unresectable, at least half of all patients presenting with pancreatic cancer are unresectable at diagnosis because of the presence of distant metastases.

In addition to distant disease, current National Comprehensive Cancer Network guidelines define unresectable pancreatic tumors as those with greater than 180° encasement of the superior mesenteric artery or celiac artery, superior mesenteric vein or portal vein occlusion not amenable to reconstruction, invasion of the aorta, or the presence of nodal metastases beyond the field of resection.[7] Even in patients with small pancreatic cancers and no evidence of distant metastases, a proportion will be deemed unresectable based on the tumor's location to vital vasculature. Advances in surgical technique in recent years have allowed for pancreatic resection with portal vein resection and reconstruction at specialized centers in patients with borderline disease.[8] However, although this has increased the number of patients in whom pancreatic resection is possible, most patients are still not surgical candidates.

The main treatment currently for patients with locally unresectable and metastatic pancreatic adenocarcinoma is chemotherapy with or without radiation therapy.[9,10] Studies have shown a modest survival benefit with the addition of chemotherapy and radiation in these patients compared with no treatment. In patients with locally advanced, unresectable cancers, median survival ranges between 11 and 15 months in recent reports for patients undergoing treatment with chemotherapy and radiation.[11–15] In patients with metastatic pancreatic cancer, overall survival is much lower and 5-year survival is estimated at only 2%.[1] First-line treatment for metastatic pancreatic cancer often involves gemcitabine-based chemotherapy. Randomized trials of different chemotherapeutic regimens have not demonstrated much of a survival increase beyond a median survival of 5 to 8 months.[16] However, the addition of abraxane (nab-paclitaxel) before gemcitabine treatment in patients with metastatic pancreatic cancer has been shown in a randomized clinical trial to substantially increase median overall survival compared with gemcitabine alone (8.5 months vs 6.7 months, respectively).[17] In addition, patients treated with a gemcitabine-abraxane combination had significantly increased median progression-free survival compared with gemcitabine alone (5.5 months vs 3.7 months). Despite an increased incidence of side effects, the combination of gemcitabine and abraxane for metastatic pancreatic cancer has become a common therapy. Furthermore, a recent trial demonstrated significantly longer survival with FOLFIRINOX as compared with gemcitabine in patients with advanced-stage pancreatic cancer (11.1 months vs 6.8 months, $P<.001$).[18] Compared with the traditional median survival of only 3 to 6 months in this population, this outcome is remarkable and FOLFIRINOX has become a first-line treatment for metastatic pancreatic cancer.

PALLIATIVE RESECTION

Surgical options are limited for patients with locally advanced and metastatic pancreatic adenocarcinoma. Patients with stage IV disease are not considered candidates for surgical resection of the primary tumor. This is in comparison to other cancers, such as colorectal tumors in which a survival benefit has been shown after resection of the primary tumor and metastases.[19,20] However, there may be some survival benefit for resection in certain patients with recurrent distant disease after the initial pancreatic resection. An analysis of patients with pancreatic cancer with tumor recurrence to the lung demonstrated longer survival after pulmonary metastasectomy for isolated pulmonary metastases compared with a matched group that did not undergo lung resection (51 vs 23 months).[21] Although this study was a retrospective review of patients presenting with metastatic disease months after the initial pancreatic resection, it is an encouraging result for patients with stage IV disease limited to the lungs. In addition, case reports of concomitant pancreatic resection and hepatectomy for liver metastases for pancreatic adenocarcinoma have suggested a survival benefit, with one report including 3 patients alive 2 years after surgery.[22–25] However, these reports are limited to only a small number of carefully chosen patients. Whether there is a true benefit to resection for metastatic pancreatic cancer remains to be seen.

Even in patients without distant metastases, surgery is not attempted unless the tumor is felt to be completely resectable. Data have been mixed as to whether there is a survival benefit with resection with grossly positive margins, compared with palliative bypass for nonmetastatic, unresectable disease.[26,27] However, most studies show that there is no clear survival benefit to palliative resection. A retrospective review of 126 patients compared patients who underwent pancreaticoduodenectomy (PD) with negative margins, PD with a positive resection margin, or palliative bypass.[26] Most patients in the palliative bypass group had metastatic disease (75%). No significant difference in perioperative morbidity or mortality or readmission was noted among the 3 groups. Although no significant difference was noted between median survival for margin-negative PD or margin-positive PD, median and 1-year survival were lower after palliative bypass than margin-positive PD ($P<.05$). However, this survival difference was not seen when comparing margin-positive PD with palliative bypass in only those patients with locally advanced disease. Despite these findings, this study suggested that resection, even with positive margins, was preferable over palliative bypass in patients with unresectable disease.

A smaller retrospective review compared 64 patients undergoing PD with microscopic or grossly positive margins with 62 patients undergoing palliative bypass at a single institution.[28] There was no difference between groups with respect to perioperative morbidity or mortality. Length of hospital stay after operation was shorter in patients who underwent palliative bypass ($P<.05$). Overall survival was improved significantly in patients who underwent PD, even with positive margins, as compared with palliative bypass (P<.02). Given the benefit in survival, the investigators of this study suggested PD was superior to palliative bypass for patients with pancreatic adenocarcinoma. However, it is important to note that differentiation between microscopic (R1) and grossly (R2) positive surgical margins was not made, which could have biased the survival outcomes in this study.

A systemic review of 4 retrospective studies of 399 individuals with pancreatic cancer compared patients undergoing palliative resection with positive margins to palliative bypass.[27] Patients who underwent margin-positive PD had longer operative times and significantly increased rates of surgical morbidity and mortality compared with patients undergoing palliative bypass (P<.01 for all). Only one study included postoperative quality-of-life measurements, and patients who underwent palliative bypass were noted to have higher scores. Median survival times were 8.2 months for palliative resection with positive margins and 6.7 months for palliative bypass, comparable between both groups. This study noted the lack of any randomized control studies, but concluded that palliative resection was not advisable given increased hospital length of stay, operative times, morbidity, and mortality without any associated survival benefit. Based on this and other studies, palliative resection leading to grossly positive margins is not advised at this time as a surgical treatment for patients with unresectable or metastatic pancreatic cancer.

BILIARY DECOMPRESSION

Most patients with pancreatic adenocarcinoma have tumors located in the head of the pancreas.[29] This can lead to biliary and gastric obstruction over time due to tumor location or size, often causing symptoms such as jaundice, pruritus, nausea, and abdominal discomfort. As a result, many patients will require surgical or endoscopic intervention to relieve the obstruction, provide symptomatic relief, and improve quality of life. In patients who are surgical candidates or can tolerate operative intervention, this is accomplished through resection of the primary pancreatic tumor. In patients with known metastatic or unresectable disease or those unfit for anesthesia, however, this requires an alternative approach.

Biliary decompression can be accomplished by endoscopic placement of a stent in the biliary tree or surgical bypass. Endoscopic stenting involves the placement of a plastic or metallic stent into the biliary tree through the area of obstruction. Plastic stents were initially favored, as these could be easily replaced if necessary, but were prone to migration and occlusion. Newer, self-expandable metallic stents are being increasingly used given longer patency and decreased risk for occlusion; however, these cannot be removed after placement.[30] Alternatively, surgical bypass is performed by hepaticojejunostomy, cholecystojejunostomy, or choledochojejunostomy, effectively bypassing the obstruction and creating a direct link between the biliary tree and small bowel. Surgery also may involve concomitant gastrojejunostomy to bypass a gastric outlet obstruction. Although surgery provides definitive relief of the obstruction, it is reserved for patients fit for surgery, often those already undergoing attempted surgical resection, and those with severe symptoms in whom stenting cannot be performed.[31,32]

Comparisons of surgical bypass to endoscopic stenting demonstrate differences in outcomes but no clearly superior method (**Table 1**). Most studies are retrospective reviews with a limited number of patients, although a few early, randomized controlled trials were performed to directly compare outcomes between patients undergoing endoscopic stenting or palliative bypass. The first randomized trial of percutaneous biliary drainage and surgical bypass was in 1986, and demonstrated no difference

Table 1
Thirty-day mortality and overall median survival for major studies comparing endoscopic biliary stenting with palliative surgical bypass

Author, Year	Procedure	Patient Number	30-d Mortality, n (%)	Median Survival, wk
Bornman et al,[33] 1986	PTE stent	25	2 (8)	19
	Surgical bypass	25	5 (20)	15
Shepherd et al,[35] 1988	Endoscopic stenting	23	2 (9)	21.7
	Surgical bypass	25	5 (20)	17.7
Andersen et al,[36] 1989	Endoscopic stenting	25	5 (20)	12
	Surgical bypass	25	6 (24)	14.3
Smith et al,[34] 1994	Endoscopic stenting	100	8 (8)	21
	Surgical bypass	101	15 (15)	26
Nieveen et al,[37] 2003	Endoscopic stenting	14	0 (0)	Hospital free: 14.1
	Surgical bypass	13	0 (0)	Hospital free: 22
Scott et al,[38] 2009	Endoscopic stenting	33	6 (18.1)	19.2[a]
	Palliative bypass	23	1 (4.3)	54.5

Abbreviation: PTE, percutaneous transhepatic placement of biliary endoprosthesis.
[a] $P<.05$ between the 2 groups studied.

in perioperative morbidity or survival between groups.[33] Three further randomized trials were published before 2000, and continued to show no difference in perioperative mortality or overall survival.[34–36] However, recurrent symptoms, such as jaundice or cholangitis, were significantly higher at follow-up in patients who underwent stenting, whereas morbidity tended to be higher after palliative bypass and related to the operation. These studies were limited due to small numbers; all but one was limited to fewer than 50 patients total. The most recent randomized controlled trial from 2003 compared 13 patients undergoing surgical bypass for a periampullary cancer with 14 patients in whom endoscopic stenting was performed.[37] This study showed no significant difference among procedure-related morbidity, mortality, readmission, or complications. However, overall survival was longer in the surgical bypass group compared with patients undergoing stenting ($P = .05$).

A study of 56 patients with locally advanced pancreatic adenocarcinoma compared outcomes after either endoscopic stenting (n = 33) or surgical bypass with hepaticojejunostomy and gastrojejunostomy (n = 23).[38] Although there was no difference in complication or mortality rates between the 2 groups, hospital readmissions were higher in patients who underwent endoscopic stenting after excluding admissions for chemotherapy-related problems. Additionally, overall survival was greater in patients who underwent palliative bypass compared with endoscopic stenting (382 days vs 135 days, $P<.05$). This study concluded that surgical bypass represented an effective method of palliation for patients with locally advanced disease, impacting both readmission and survival. However, it was important to note that as a retrospective review, the exact rationale for the decision between stenting and surgical bypass in an individual patient was unknown, and patients who underwent endoscopic stenting may not have been fit for operative intervention.

In another study, surgical bypass with a Roux-en-Y biliary to enteric anastomosis with or without gastrojejunostomy (n = 41) and endoscopic placement of a metallic stent (n = 19) were retrospectively compared in 60 patients with jaundice due to unresectable pancreatic cancer.[39] Notably, patients who underwent surgical bypass had higher bilirubin levels before the procedure. No difference in 30-day mortality or overall survival was seen between groups. In addition, significantly shorter hospital stays after treatment ($P = .002$) and total hospital costs ($P = .0006$) were seen in the group undergoing metallic stenting. Patients who underwent surgical bypass were noted to have a higher, yet not significant, percentage of early complications ($P = .10$) related to surgical intervention, such as ileus, wound infection, and acute cholangitis. Conversely, a significantly higher number of late complications were noted in patients after endoscopic metallic stenting ($P = .04$), including duodenal obstruction, recurrence of jaundice, and acute cholangitis without biliary occlusion. This study concluded that the condition of the patient, including fitness for surgery and overall prognosis, should be considered before deciding to pursue either surgical bypass or endoscopic stenting.

A recent retrospective analysis of patients with unresectable pancreatic cancer compared readmission and reintervention rates between a matched cohort of patients undergoing endoscopic treatment (n = 219) and early surgical bypass (n = 241).[40] No difference was noted in readmission rates in this cohort, although patients in the endoscopic stenting group were more likely to require subsequent intervention ($P = .01$). However, median length of readmission and total readmission cost was significantly lower among patients who underwent endoscopic stenting as opposed to surgical bypass. This study suggested that some patients may benefit from early surgical bypass, but noted that, overall, patients are more likely to undergo endoscopic stenting as opposed to surgical intervention.

These studies demonstrate the risks and benefits associated with both procedures, although each has been shown to have a relatively low and equivalent perioperative morbidity and mortality. Endoscopic stenting is associated with a shorter hospital length of stay and total cost, but a higher incidence of long-term complications is seen. In addition, some studies suggest poorer survival after stent placement, although this may be biased due to selection of sicker patients for endoscopy who are poor candidates for surgical resection. Conversely, surgical resection is associated with fewer long-term complications but is associated with increased early complications associated with surgery, as well as longer hospital stay. These potential risks must be weighed individually for each patient to determine the best course of treatment for a patient who presents with unresectable pancreatic adenocarcinoma causing biliary obstruction.

GASTRIC DECOMPRESSION

Tumors, especially those in the head of the pancreas, can lead to symptoms of gastric outlet obstruction, often due to the tumor's size leading to compression of the duodenum or infiltration of the celiac nerve plexus leading to dysmotility.[41] Gastric outlet obstruction can lead to symptoms of persistent nausea and vomiting, leading to pain, an inability to eat, and decreased quality of life.[42] Although surgical resection can remove the tumor and alleviate symptoms in resectable patients, management of obstruction in unresectable and metastatic patients often requires other techniques.

In patients who undergo exploratory laparotomy and are found to be unresectable, gastric bypass by gastrojejunostomy is often performed in conjunction with biliary decompression for palliation. Two randomized controlled trials have been performed to assess the benefits and risks of concomitant gastrojejunostomy with biliary decompression. The first compared 87 patients with an unresectable periampullary malignancy without concern for gastric outlet obstruction to either gastrojejunostomy with biliary bypass (n = 44) or biliary bypass (n = 43) alone at the time of exploratory laparotomy.[43] This study demonstrated no differences in rates of perioperative morbidity or mortality, hospital length of stay, or overall survival. No patient who underwent palliative gastrojejunostomy had symptoms of gastric outlet obstruction. However, 19% (8 of 43 patients) of those who did not have a prophylactic gastrojejunostomy developed late gastric outlet obstruction requiring intervention with either gastrojejunostomy (n = 7) or endoscopic duodenal stent placement (n = 1). This study recommended routine gastrojejunostomy at the time of biliary bypass to reduce the incidence of late gastric outlet obstruction.

In the second randomized study, 65 patients with unresectable periampullary cancer at the time of laparotomy were randomized to double bypass (hepaticojejunostomy and gastrojejunostomy; n = 36) or hepaticojejunostomy alone (n = 29).[44] Gastric outlet obstruction developed in only 2 patients (5.5%) who underwent double bypass as compared with 12 patients (41.4%) treated with hepaticojejunostomy alone (P = .001). Six patients in the single bypass group eventually required gastrojejunostomy, whereas only 1 patient undergoing double bypass required operative revision of the gastric bypass (P = .04). There was no significant difference in median postoperative hospital stay, postoperative morbidity, or overall survival between the 2 groups. This trial, similar to the first, concluded that prophylactic gastrojejunostomy should be performed at the time of hepaticojejunostomy in all patients undergoing surgical palliation given a significant decrease in the incidence of postoperative gastric outlet obstruction without any increase in postoperative morbidity or mortality.

Recent studies have demonstrated that duodenal stenting is a potential method for treatment of obstruction, particularly those patients who may not be surgical candidates. Self-expandable metal stents are placed in the duodenum endoscopically, with a success rate between 90% and 100% and a low complication rate reported in several case series.[45–47] However, questions remained as to the superiority of endoscopic stenting when compared with surgical bypass. A recent meta-analysis reviewed studies comparing patients with gastric outlet obstruction who underwent gastrojejunostomy or endoscopic stent placement.[48] Twenty studies were included, including only 3 randomized controlled trials. These randomized controlled trials demonstrated a lower rate of major and minor complications after stent placement when compared with surgical bypass. Additionally, significantly shorter hospital stays were noted after endoscopic stent placement, and these patients also trended toward a shorter time to tolerating oral intake. These findings were similar to those found in the nonrandomized controlled trials included in this meta-analysis. There was no significant difference noted in hospital costs, mortality, or median survival between both patient groups in the nonrandomized controlled trial studies. Although this study demonstrated that endoscopic duodenal stent placement has outcomes comparable to gastrojejunostomy with a shorter hospital length of stay, it noted that confounding variables could not be studied, which may result in bias. In addition, one of the included studies noted a higher incidence of reintervention in patients who underwent endoscopic stenting as compared with gastrojejunostomy.[49] Thus, as with endoscopic biliary stenting, it is likely that stenting for gastric outlet obstruction is most beneficial in carefully chosen patients, including those unable to tolerate operative intervention or who do not want to undergo surgery.

PAIN CONTROL

Adequate pain control remains a challenge in many patients with inoperable or metastatic pancreatic cancer. Abdominal and back pain related to tumor size and location can significantly reduce a patient's quality of life. Goals remain providing adequate pain relief with the use of narcotic and non-narcotic pain medications in conjunction with alternative mechanisms. Celiac plexus block has become a popular procedure in recent years for the alleviation of pain in this population, especially given the potential adverse effects of both narcotic and non-narcotic pain medications. Celiac plexus block involves the destruction of the celiac ganglia and/or splanchnic nerves with alcohol or other neurolytic solutions by fluoroscopic guidance, endoscopic ultrasound (EUS), or computed tomography (CT).[50,51] In some cases, this procedure also may be performed intraoperatively during a palliative bypass. A recent meta-analysis of 6 studies including 358 patients comparing celiac plexus block with standard narcotic pain medication found significantly lower pain scores in those undergoing the block after 4 and 8 weeks.[50] In addition, patients who underwent a celiac plexus block required significantly less narcotic medication than the control group and also had a significant reduction in narcotic-related adverse events, such as constipation. An older meta-analysis of 24 studies, including 2 randomized controlled trials, involving 1145 patients, demonstrated partial to complete pain relief in upwards of 90% of patients at 3 months and 70% to 90% of patients until death after celiac plexus block.[52] Adverse effects related to the plexus block, such as local pain, diarrhea, or hypotension, were transient, and most patients did not experience long-term adverse events. Both reviews noted that celiac plexus block was a safe method for pain reduction in patients with pancreatic cancer, and as a result this procedure has become central to providing pain control to patients with unresectable tumors.

SUMMARY

Pancreatic adenocarcinoma remains a dismal diagnosis with a 5-year survival of only 6%. Currently, more than half of all patients will present with metastatic or unresectable disease, removing the possibility of curative resection. Palliative resection, which once seemed promising, has not demonstrated an increased survival in this patient population. Although research aims to identify mechanisms for early detection and improve treatment to prolong survival, current management focuses on the palliation of symptoms in the patients who present with unresectable or metastatic disease. Biliary obstruction can be alleviated either with surgical palliation through hepaticojejunostomy or choledochojejunostomy at the time of surgical exploration or through endoscopic stent placement. Gastric outlet obstruction can be managed with either concurrent gastrojejunostomy at the time of biliary bypass or endoscopic duodenal stent placement. Although outcomes, including survival, appear similar for the surgical and endoscopic groups, specific patient management will likely depend on an individual's overall prognosis and health status at the time of intervention. Adequate pain control is a challenge in unresectable pancreatic cancer, but the use of CT-guided or EUS-guided celiac plexus block has been shown to provide long-term pain relief while reducing the need for narcotic medications. Advances in medical care have allowed for improved management of symptoms in this patient cohort, and the future holds great promise with regard to new methods of treatment to prolong survival in patients with unresectable pancreatic cancer.

REFERENCES

1. Siegel R, Ma J, Zou Z, et al. Cancer statistics, 2014. CA Cancer J Clin 2014;64(1): 9–29.
2. Porta M, Fabregat X, Malats N, et al. Exocrine pancreatic cancer: symptoms at presentation and their relation to tumour site and stage. Clin Transl Oncol 2005;7(5):189–97.

3. Wagner M, Redaelli C, Lietz M, et al. Curative resection is the single most important factor determining outcome in patients with pancreatic adenocarcinoma. Br J Surg 2004;91(5):586–94.

4. Sener SF, Fremgen A, Menck HR, et al. Pancreatic cancer: a report of treatment and survival trends for 100,313 patients diagnosed from 1985-1995, using the National Cancer Database. J Am Coll Surg 1999;189(1):1–7.

5. Winter JM, Cameron JL, Campbell KA, et al. 1423 pancreaticoduodenectomies for pancreatic cancer: a single-institution experience. J Gastrointest Surg 2006; 10(9):1199–210 [discussion: 1210–1].

6. Shaib YH, Davila JA, El-Serag HB. The epidemiology of pancreatic cancer in the United States: changes below the surface. Aliment Pharmacol Ther 2006;24(1): 87–94.

7. Tempero MA, Malafa MP, Behrman SW, et al. Pancreatic adenocarcinoma, version 2.2014: featured updates to the NCCN guidelines. J Natl Compr Canc Netw 2014;12(8):1083–93.

8. Yekebas EF, Bogoevski D, Cataldegirmen G, et al. En bloc vascular resection for locally advanced pancreatic malignancies infiltrating major blood vessels: perioperative outcome and long-term survival in 136 patients. Ann Surg 2008; 247(2):300–9.

9. Burris HA 3rd, Moore MJ, Andersen J, et al. Improvements in survival and clinical benefit with gemcitabine as first-line therapy for patients with advanced pancreas cancer: a randomized trial. J Clin Oncol 1997;15(6):2403–13.

10. Park JK, Yoon YB, Kim YT, et al. Survival and prognostic factors of unresectable pancreatic cancer. J Clin Gastroenterol 2008;42(1):86–91.

11. Lee JL, Kim SC, Kim JH, et al. Prospective efficacy and safety study of neoadjuvant gemcitabine with capecitabine combination chemotherapy for borderline-resectable or unresectable locally advanced pancreatic adenocarcinoma. Surgery 2012;152(5):851–62.

12. Loehrer PJ Sr, Feng Y, Cardenes H, et al. Gemcitabine alone versus gemcitabine plus radiotherapy in patients with locally advanced pancreatic cancer: an Eastern Cooperative Oncology Group trial. J Clin Oncol 2011;29(31):4105–12.

13. Chauffert B, Mornex F, Bonnetain F, et al. Phase III trial comparing intensive induction chemoradiotherapy (60 Gy, infusional 5-FU and intermittent cisplatin) followed by maintenance gemcitabine with gemcitabine alone for locally advanced unresectable pancreatic cancer. Definitive results of the 2000-01 FFCD/SFRO study. Ann Oncol 2008;19(9):1592–9.

14. Mamon HJ, Niedzwiecki D, Hollis D, et al. A phase 2 trial of gemcitabine, 5-fluorouracil, and radiation therapy in locally advanced nonmetastatic pancreatic adenocarcinoma: Cancer and Leukemia Group B (CALGB) 80003. Cancer 2011;117(12):2620–8.

15. Mukherjee S, Hurt CN, Bridgewater J, et al. Gemcitabine-based or capecitabine-based chemoradiotherapy for locally advanced pancreatic cancer (SCALOP): a multicentre, randomised, phase 2 trial. Lancet Oncol 2013;14(4):317–26.

16. Poruk KE, Firpo MA, Adler DG, et al. Screening for pancreatic cancer: why, how, and who? Ann Surg 2013;257(1):17–26.

17. Von Hoff DD, Ervin T, Arena FP, et al. Increased survival in pancreatic cancer with nab-paclitaxel plus gemcitabine. N Engl J Med 2013;369(18):1691–703.

18. Conroy T, Desseigne F, Ychou M, et al. FOLFIRINOX versus gemcitabine for metastatic pancreatic cancer. N Engl J Med 2011;364(19):1817–25.

19. Choti MA, Sitzmann JV, Tiburi MF, et al. Trends in long-term survival following liver resection for hepatic colorectal metastases. Ann Surg 2002;235(6):759–66.

20. Kopetz S, Chang GJ, Overman MJ, et al. Improved survival in metastatic colorectal cancer is associated with adoption of hepatic resection and improved chemotherapy. J Clin Oncol 2009;27(22):3677–83.
21. Arnaoutakis GJ, Rangachari D, Laheru DA, et al. Pulmonary resection for isolated pancreatic adenocarcinoma metastasis: an analysis of outcomes and survival. J Gastrointest Surg 2011;15(9):1611–7.
22. Howard JM. Pancreatoduodenectomy (Whipple resection) with resection of hepatic metastases for carcinoma of the exocrine pancreas. Arch Surg 1997; 132(9):1044.
23. Yamada H, Hirano S, Tanaka E, et al. Surgical treatment of liver metastases from pancreatic cancer. HPB (Oxford) 2006;8(2):85–8.
24. Yamada H, Katoh H, Kondo S, et al. Hepatectomy for metastases from non-colorectal and non-neuroendocrine tumor. Anticancer Res 2001;21(6A): 4159–62.
25. Takada Y, Otsuka M, Seino K, et al. Hepatic resection for metastatic tumors from noncolorectal carcinoma. Hepatogastroenterology 2001;48(37):83–6.
26. Lavu H, Mascaro AA, Grenda DR, et al. Margin positive pancreaticoduodenectomy is superior to palliative bypass in locally advanced pancreatic ductal adenocarcinoma. J Gastrointest Surg 2009;13(11):1937–46 [discussion: 1946–7].
27. Gillen S, Schuster T, Friess H, et al. Palliative resections versus palliative bypass procedures in pancreatic cancer–a systematic review. Am J Surg 2012;203(4): 496–502.
28. Lillemoe KD, Cameron JL, Yeo CJ, et al. Pancreaticoduodenectomy. Does it have a role in the palliation of pancreatic cancer? Ann Surg 1996;223(6):718–25 [discussion: 725–8].
29. Artinyan A, Soriano PA, Prendergast C, et al. The anatomic location of pancreatic cancer is a prognostic factor for survival. HPB (Oxford) 2008;10(5):371–6.
30. Kaassis M, Boyer J, Dumas R, et al. Plastic or metal stents for malignant stricture of the common bile duct? Results of a randomized prospective study. Gastrointest Endosc 2003;57(2):178–82.
31. Sohn TA, Lillemoe KD, Cameron JL, et al. Surgical palliation of unresectable periampullary adenocarcinoma in the 1990s. J Am Coll Surg 1999;188(6):658–66 [discussion: 666–9].
32. Di Fronzo LA, Cymerman J, Egrari S, et al. Unresectable pancreatic carcinoma: correlating length of survival with choice of palliative bypass. Am Surg 1999; 65(10):955–8.
33. Bornman PC, Harries-Jones EP, Tobias R, et al. Prospective controlled trial of transhepatic biliary endoprosthesis versus bypass surgery for incurable carcinoma of head of pancreas. Lancet 1986;1(8472):69–71.
34. Smith AC, Dowsett JF, Russell RC, et al. Randomised trial of endoscopic stenting versus surgical bypass in malignant low bile duct obstruction. Lancet 1994; 344(8938):1655–60.
35. Shepherd HA, Royle G, Ross AP, et al. Endoscopic biliary endoprosthesis in the palliation of malignant obstruction of the distal common bile duct: a randomized trial. Br J Surg 1988;75(12):1166–8.
36. Andersen JR, Sorensen SM, Kruse A, et al. Randomised trial of endoscopic endoprosthesis versus operative bypass in malignant obstructive jaundice. Gut 1989;30(8):1132–5.
37. Nieveen van Dijkum EJ, Romijn MG, Terwee CB, et al. Laparoscopic staging and subsequent palliation in patients with peripancreatic carcinoma. Ann Surg 2003; 237(1):66–73.

38. Scott EN, Garcea G, Doucas H, et al. Surgical bypass vs. endoscopic stenting for pancreatic ductal adenocarcinoma. HPB (Oxford) 2009;11(2):118–24.
39. Maosheng D, Ohtsuka T, Ohuchida J, et al. Surgical bypass versus metallic stent for unresectable pancreatic cancer. J Hepatobiliary Pancreat Surg 2001;8(4): 367–73.
40. Bliss L, Kent T, Watkins A, et al. Early surgical bypass versus endoscopic stent placement in pancreatic cancer [abstract]. J Clin Oncol 2015;22(Suppl 3) [abstract: 391].
41. Thor PJ, Popiela T, Sobocki J, et al. Pancreatic carcinoma-induced changes in gastric myoelectric activity and emptying. Hepatogastroenterology 2002; 49(43):268–70.
42. DiMagno EP, Reber HA, Tempero MA. AGA technical review on the epidemiology, diagnosis, and treatment of pancreatic ductal adenocarcinoma. American Gastroenterological Association. Gastroenterology 1999;117(6):1464–84.
43. Lillemoe KD, Cameron JL, Hardacre JM, et al. Is prophylactic gastrojejunostomy indicated for unresectable periampullary cancer? A prospective randomized trial. Ann Surg 1999;230(3):322–8 [discussion: 328–30].
44. Van Heek NT, De Castro SM, van Eijck CH, et al. The need for a prophylactic gastrojejunostomy for unresectable periampullary cancer: a prospective randomized multicenter trial with special focus on assessment of quality of life. Ann Surg 2003;238(6):894–902 [discussion: 902–5].
45. Maire F, Hammel P, Ponsot P, et al. Long-term outcome of biliary and duodenal stents in palliative treatment of patients with unresectable adenocarcinoma of the head of pancreas. Am J Gastroenterol 2006;101(4):735–42.
46. Nassif T, Prat F, Meduri B, et al. Endoscopic palliation of malignant gastric outlet obstruction using self-expandable metallic stents: results of a multicenter study. Endoscopy 2003;35(6):483–9.
47. Adler DG, Baron TH. Endoscopic palliation of malignant gastric outlet obstruction using self-expanding metal stents: experience in 36 patients. Am J Gastroenterol 2002;97(1):72–8.
48. Nagaraja V, Eslick GD, Cox MR. Endoscopic stenting versus operative gastrojejunostomy for malignant gastric outlet obstruction—a systematic review and meta-analysis of randomized and non-randomized trials. J Gastrointest Oncol 2014;5(2):92–8.
49. Khashab M, Alawad AS, Shin EJ, et al. Enteral stenting versus gastrojejunostomy for palliation of malignant gastric outlet obstruction. Surg Endosc 2013;27(6): 2068–75.
50. Arcidiacono PG, Calori G, Carrara S, et al. Celiac plexus block for pancreatic cancer pain in adults. Cochrane Database Syst Rev 2011;(3):CD007519.
51. Si-Jie H, Wei-Jia X, Yang D, et al. How to improve the efficacy of endoscopic ultrasound-guided celiac plexus neurolysis in pain management in patients with pancreatic cancer: analysis in a single center. Surg Laparosc Endosc Percutan Tech 2014;24(1):31–5.
52. Eisenberg E, Carr DB, Chalmers TC. Neurolytic celiac plexus block for treatment of cancer pain: a meta-analysis. Anesth Analg 1995;80(2):290–5.

Spectrum and Classification of Cystic Neoplasms of the Pancreas

Jonathan B. Greer, MD[a], Cristina R. Ferrone, MD[b],*

KEYWORDS

- Cystic neoplasms of the pancreas • Mucinous cystic neoplasm
- Serous cystic neoplasm • Cystic pancreatic endocrine neoplasm
- Solid pseudopapillary neoplasm • Intraductal papillary mucinous neoplasm

KEY POINTS

- Cystic neoplasms of the pancreas are an increasingly recognized clinical entity, now in up to 10% of patients older than 70 years.
- Management of these lesions, particularly intraductal papillary mucinous neoplasm, remains controversial.
- Many of these neoplasms can be managed safely with surgical resection at high-volume pancreatic centers, whereas an increasing number of subgroups may be watched safely. Accurate diagnosis is paramount.
- The revised Sendai guidelines seem to provide a safe framework for management of mucinous cystic neoplasm and intraductal papillary mucinous neoplasm.
- Ongoing research will likely better stratify the underlying risk of invasive cancers in these patients.

INTRODUCTION

The incidental finding of pancreatic cysts creates significant concern for the clinician given the grave prognosis for patients with pancreatic ductal adenocarcinoma (PDAC). The increasing use of axial imaging has contributed to the surge in the diagnosis of pancreatic cystic lesions. In asymptomatic patients, up to 2.5% are found to have pancreatic cysts, a number that increases to 10% in patients older than 70 years.[1,2] Fortunately, more sophisticated understanding of these clinical entities

---

Disclosure Statement: The authors have nothing to disclose.
[a] General Surgery, Department of Surgery, Massachusetts General Hospital, Harvard Medical School, 55 Fruit Street, GRB-425, Boston, MA 02114, USA; [b] Department of Surgery, Massachusetts General Hospital, Harvard Medical School, 15 Parkman Street, Boston, MA 02114, USA
* Corresponding author.
E-mail address: cferrone@mgh.harvard.edu

Surg Oncol Clin N Am 25 (2016) 339–350
http://dx.doi.org/10.1016/j.soc.2015.11.002
surgonc.theclinics.com

has allowed for more nuanced management in recent years, which has obviated many unnecessary and morbid operations. However, despite our improved understanding of pancreatic cysts, there is still ongoing debate regarding management of these lesions. We aim to provide a guide to the diagnosis and management of cystic neoplasms of the pancreas (CNPs).

For cystic lesions of the pancreas, there is a spectrum from benign to malignant. Benign entities include pancreatic pseudocysts, infectious cystic lesions of the pancreas, congenital cysts, pancreatic duplication cysts, retention cysts, and lymphoepithelial cysts.[3,4] There are several rare nonepithelial neoplasms, including lymphangiomas, epidermoid cysts in an intrapancreatic spleen, cystic pancreatic hamartomas, and mesothelial cysts.[4] Of the epithelial neoplasms, the most common are mucinous cystic neoplasms (MCNs), serous cystic neoplasms (SCNs), cystic pancreatic endocrine neoplasms (CPENs), solid pseudopapillary neoplasms (SPNs), and intraductal papillary mucinous neoplasms (IPMNs). These 5 clinical entities are discussed in this review. Another notable cystic neoplasm is a PDAC with cystic degeneration, but this comprises less than 1% of resected specimens and is not discussed here.[5] Overall, the number of invasive cancers in this epithelial group of cystic neoplasms has significantly declined over the last 40 years, from 41% in the 1970s and 1980s to 12% in the 2000s, consistent with earlier diagnosis and treatment of incidentally discovered and presumably premalignant lesions.[5] It is predicted that this number will continue to decline as our diagnostic capabilities improve.[4]

MUCINOUS CYSTIC NEOPLASMS
Introduction

MCNs make up approximately 23% of the resected cystic tumors of the pancreas.[5] To make the diagnosis of an MCN, the cyst must contain ovarian-type stroma.[6,7] MCNs occur almost exclusively in women, as solitary lesions in the body or tail of the pancreas.[6,8–13] The median age of diagnosis is mid-to-late 40s.[6,8–13] Given the risk of invasive disease, current guidelines recommend resection for all patients with MCN who are fit enough to undergo an operation.[6]

Clinical Presentation

Many of the patients with an MCN are symptomatic at the time of presentation, with nonspecific abdominal pain as the most common symptom.[8–13] Other less-common symptoms include fatigue, weight loss, abdominal mass, and pancreatitis, and jaundice is exceedingly rare.[8–13] The remaining MCNs are found incidentally on imaging or on final pathology.[8–13] The mean size at resection in our series of 199 patients was 4.4 cm.[5]

Pathophysiology

The mechanism of MCN development remains under investigation. Recent reports implicate the KRAS pathway[14,15] and the canonical Wnt pathway.[16] Activation of the canonical Wnt pathway promotes development of the pathognomonic ovarianlike stroma in a mouse model of MCN.[16]

Pathology/Classification

The histologic hallmark of MCN is an inner epithelial layer, consisting of mucin-secreting cuboidal epithelium, and an outer layer of ovarianlike stroma.[6,7] The cysts often lack a connection to the duct.[10,11] There is a spectrum of disease from benign (mucinous cystadenoma) to malignant (mucinous cystadenocarcinoma), with invasive carcinoma present in 5% to 16% of MCNs.[8–13] Factors associated with a higher likelihood of invasive carcinoma include the presence of greater than 1 cm intracystic papillary nodules, increased size (>3 cm), and increased serum CA19-9 level.[9–13] Additional studies have posited that age itself is a risk factor for malignant versus benign MCN.[9]

Diagnosis

The diagnosis of MCN is made by confirmation of the aforementioned histologic characteristics. Suggestive radiologic features include a solitary cyst with thick walls, septations, calcifications, and mural nodules.[4] The presence of these findings in a middle-age woman is highly suggestive of MCN.[6] MCNs are most often found in the body or tail of the pancreas.[8–13] endoscopic ultrasound scan (EUS) can be performed and a high carcinoembryonic antigen (CEA) level in the cyst fluid aspirate is expected for mucinous lesions.[4]

Management

Given the risk of malignant disease, definitive surgical management is the current standard of care for all suspected MCNs.[6] Some investigators advocate for a watchful waiting approach,[13] whereas others suggest that smaller lesions (<4-cm tumors without nodules) do not require a radical resection.[12] This approach is similar to the approach advocated by the Sendai Consensus guidelines for brand duct intraductal papillary mucinous neoplasms (BD-IPMN).[13] Patients whose benign, noninvasive MCN has been resected have an excellent survival rate, whereas once invasive or malignant tumors have developed, the 5-year survival rate decreases dramatically, ranging from 0% to 75% in various studies.[9–13]

SEROUS CYSTIC NEOPLASM
Introduction

Serous cystadenomas or SCNs are benign cystic tumors of the pancreas and represent approximately 16% of resected pancreatic cystic neoplasms.[5] These tumors occur more frequently in women (75%) at a mean age of 50 to 60 years.[17–23] Rare case reports document serous cystadenocarcinomas. SCNs grow slowly, and most are found incidentally on imaging. Operative intervention is reserved for symptomatic patients.[4]

Clinical Presentation

In most large series, patients present with symptoms.[17–23] Abdominal pain is the most common presenting symptom, with fullness/palpable mass. Jaundice and diabetes are seen less frequently.[17–23] Mean size at presentation is variable, ranging from 2.9 to 5.1 cm.[17–23]

Pathophysiology

The pathophysiology of SCNs is unknown, although some sporadic SCNs are found to have modifications of the VHL-related genes.[24] Von Hippel-Lindau syndrome is a known risk factor for SCN.[20,21]

Pathology/Classification

SCNs are benign, slow-growing cystic lesions without predilection for a particular part of the pancreas. They are classically described as having many tiny glycogen-rich cysts, a cuboidal epithelial lining resembling a honeycomb, and a central scar.[4] A recent classification of 4 variants has been proposed: microcystic, macrocystic, mixed, and solid.[23] The cutoff between microcystic and macrocystic is 2 cm for the dominant cyst.[18] A mixed type contains elements of both. Microcystic is the most common variant (45%), followed by macrocystic (32%), mixed (18%), and solid (5%).[19] There are rare cases of malignant SCNs, serous cystadenocarcinoma, with 28 published cases since 1989.[19,22,25] Of the 3 patients in a series of 2622, 2 had hepatic metastases and 1 had a positive portal lymph node.[19] These tumors tended to be large (7.1–17 cm) and all were symptomatic.[19] In the same study, of the 1590 patients undergoing resection, 18 tumors were locally aggressive, based on the definition from the Hopkins group.[19,22] Most common sites of invasion were the peripancreatic vessels (8 of 18) and regional organs (6 of 18).[19]

Diagnosis

The diagnosis of SCN is often made by radiologic appearance.[4] The classic appearance of a microcystic SCN is of a honeycomb that is multilobular with central calcifications or scar in 16% to 26%.[20,21] The diagnosis is more difficult in oligocystic or solid variants, as these appear similar to MCN or branch duct IPMN.[4] EUS with fluid analysis can be performed but may be difficult in microcystic disease. These nonmucinous cysts typically have low CEA levels in the cyst fluid.[4]

Management

The largest multicenter series found only 3 serous adenocarcinomas of 2622 patients, confirming the benign natural history of this entity.[19] As such, symptoms remain the cardinal indication for operation.[4] The growth rate is 4 to 6 mm/y,[17,19] with increased rates of growth after 7 years of observation[18] or in tumors 4 cm.[17] Given the variability of the data regarding size and symptoms, it seems that symptoms are paramount in determining the necessity of an intervention. It would logically follow that a younger patient will likely undergo resection at some point, and it may be wise to intervene before the procedure becomes more difficult.[4] Lastly, diagnostic certainty must be in place before a trial of watchful waiting is undertaken,[4] which is more difficult to obtain in cases of the oligocystic variant. In the aforementioned large retrospective series, over the course of 26 years, 61% of all patients eventually underwent resection with less than 1% perioperative or disease-specific mortality.[19]

CYSTIC PANCREATIC ENDOCRINE NEOPLASMS
Introduction

CPENs are an uncommon variant of solid pancreatic neuroendocrine tumors (PNET) and account for 7% of all resected cystic pancreatic neoplasms[5] and 12% to 17% of all resected PNETs.[26,27] For many years, CPENs were considered similar in behavior to their solid counterparts, but more recent series suggest a difference in presentation and biology.[26] CPENs are divided equally by sex and have a slight predilection for the body or tail of the pancreas.[26–29] Mean age at presentation is in the 50s.[26,27,29] Current recommendations are for surgical resection given the risk of invasive cancer.[4]

Clinical Presentation

Symptoms are present in 32% to 73% of patients.[26–29] The most common symptoms are abdominal and back pain, whereas less common symptoms are weight loss, anemia, weakness, palpable mass, and pancreatitis.[26–29] CPENs are more likely to be nonfunctional compared with solid PNETs (80% vs 50%), with 67% of functional CPENs being insulinomas.[26] These tumors tended to be larger than PNETs, with a mean size of 4.9 cm versus 2.4 cm,[26] however, in another series, CPENs were smaller than other cystic pancreatic neoplasms (2.1 cm vs 3.0 cm).[27] Perhaps this difference in size at presentation explains the lower incidence of symptoms at presentation in the latter study (32% vs 73%).[26,27]

Pathophysiology

The pathophysiology of CPENs remains unknown, although several series show a significant association with multiple endocrine neoplasia type 1,[26–28] an autosomal dominant genetic disorder associated with parathyroid hyperplasia, endocrine tumors of the pancreas, pituitary adenomas, and carcinoid tumors.[28]

Pathology/Classification

CPENs can be described as either purely cystic (34%) or partially cystic (66%).[26] CPENs classically have prominent septations.[26–29] The cystic nature of these tumors was thought to be from degeneration of solid PNET, but on pathologic examination, necrosis is uncommon.[26] The diagnosis is made with immunohistochemical staining for synaptophysin (100%), chromogranin A (82%), pancreatic polypeptide (74%), and glucagon (>50%).[26] In terms of biologic activity, nearly all CPENs had low mitotic rates,[28,29] although the rate of metastasis was similar to that of solid PNETs (7.8% vs 10%).[26] CK19, a marker of aggressive behavior in PNET, was present in only 24% of cases of CPEN.[26,30]

Diagnosis

The appearance on imaging is variable, with many showing prominent septations and arterial enhancement.[26–29] The Massachusetts General Hospital (MGH) series found that an accurate preoperative diagnosis was only made in 23% of patients but increased to 71% if preoperative cytology was used.[26,31] Memorial Sloan Kettering Cancer Center reported a 61% accuracy based on preoperative studies, including cytologic evaluation.[27] Cyst aspiration classically finds a low cyst CEA level.[4]

Management

The risk of aggressive biology or metastatic disease is variable, anywhere from 0% to 14%.[26–29] As such, the current recommendation is for surgical resection. The 5-year outcomes are excellent, with survival rates in excess of 87%, which is not statistically significantly different from those of PNETs of the same size.[26,27]

SOLID PSEUDOPAPILLARY NEOPLASM
Introduction

SPNs are the most rare of the 5 major types of cystic neoplasms of the pancreas, making up just 3% of resected specimens.[5] SPN is a tumor of young women, with the mean age at presentation in the fourth decade of life.[32,33] SPNs are most commonly found in the tail of the pancreas.[32,33] Given the potential for advanced or metastatic disease, surgical resection remains the recommended treatment modality.[4]

Clinical Presentation

Most patients are symptomatic (84%–87%), with abdominal pain being the most common symptom (84%).[32,33] Other symptoms include nausea/vomiting (19%), pancreatitis (10%), and weight loss (10%).[32,33] Jaundice is variably reported.[32,33] The median size at the time of resection is 4.5 to 4.9 cm.[32,33]

Pathophysiology

The adenomatous polyposis coli/β-catenin pathway has been implicated in the pathophysiology of SPN, whereas K-ras mutations and DPC4 inactivation were uniformly absent.[34] The exact mechanism is unknown.

Pathology/Classification

SPNs are on a spectrum from mostly solid to mostly cystic. SPNs are easily distinguishable from surrounding tissue and can have hemorrhage present.[33] Histologically, there are uniform discohesive polygonal cells that envelop small blood vessels.[4,32–34] Approximately 10% to 20% of these patients have locoregional spread, often to the lymph nodes, with some patients having direct invasion of the superior mesenteric artery, portal vein, or duodenum.[33] There are rare cases of liver metastases or otherwise widely metastatic disease.[32,33] Tumor size is found to correlate with aggressive behavior.[33]

Diagnosis

Computed tomography findings are consistent with the pathologic spectrum from mostly solid to mostly cystic, with peripheral arterial enhancement and central calcification in 16% of lesions.[32] EUS/fine-needle aspiration may be helpful, but the diagnosis was only made in 62% of patients undergoing cytologic analysis.[33] In a series of both transperitoneal and endoscopic biopsy techniques, preoperative diagnosis was only made 56% of the time.[32] Cytology results often show necrotic cells, and CEA level is low on fluid analysis.[4]

Management

Given the high frequency of symptoms and the 10% to 20% risk of aggressive biology, the treatment is principally surgical.[4,32,33] There are rare recurrences after operative intervention, which are treated with either an operation or systemic chemotherapy, or both.[32,33] Despite the risk of malignancy and locoregional spread, most patients do well, and the long-term survival rate is excellent, well in excess of 80% to 90%.[32,33]

INTRADUCTAL PAPILLARY MUCINOUS NEOPLASM
Introduction

IPMNs are divided into 2 main entities, main duct (M-IPMN) and branch duct (BD-IPMN), with a third group, mixed IPMN, behaving more closely to M-IPMN (and often included in that group). These lesions are differentiated by the extent of involvement of the main pancreatic duct, if any, present on radiographic or EUS studies preoperatively and pathologic examination postoperatively. As a whole, these lesions make up approximately 38% of resected CNPs,[5] although given the percentage of BD-IPMNs that are managed nonoperatively, this number likely significantly underrepresents the true incidence of IPMNs as a whole.

M-IPMNs present at a median age of 66 years.[35] In most studies, there is a slight male predominance, but interestingly, this increases to a 3:1 male-to-female ratio in Asia.[36,37] M-IPMNs (including mixed IPMNs) account for 60% of all resected IPMNs from a large multicenter database,[35] and around 40% in the Sendai guidelines (as this included tumors that were not resected).[4,6,23] Approximately two-thirds were in the proximal pancreas.[35] Eight percent were diffuse along the main pancreatic duct, but none were multifocal.[35] Given the risk of invasive cancer in excess of 40% and underlying malignant features in greater than 58%, the current guidelines recommend surgical resection for all M-IPMNs and mixed IPMNs.[6]

BD-IPMNs are the most common type of IPMN.[4,6] The median age at diagnosis is also 66 years.[35] As opposed to M-IPMN, there is a slight female predominance, although once again in Asia, there is a male predominance.[35,36] Although BD-IPMS made up roughly 40.9% of resected tumors in one large series, this number increased to 56.8% in the Sendai guidelines, and the true incidence is likely much higher.[4,6,35] These lesions are found to have a predilection for the proximal pancreas (52%) but can be diffuse (25%) and multifocal (23%).[35] The Sendai guidelines recommend a selective strategy for operative interventions based on "worrisome features" and "high-risk stigmata" (see later discussion).[6]

Clinical Presentation

Most patients with M-IPMN are symptomatic at the time of diagnosis, with abdominal pain present in more than half of patients.[35] Other symptoms include weight loss, most commonly, followed by jaundice, acute pancreatitis, and diabetes mellitus.[35] This symptomatic nature is in contrast to BD-IPMN, which more commonly presents as an incidental finding.[35] Most patients do not have abdominal pain at presentation, and weight loss tends to be less prevalent.[35]

Pathophysiology

IPMNs are thought to represent a step along the adenoma to carcinoma transition, similar to pancreatic intraepithelial neoplasia in PDAC.[4] It has been proposed that IPMN represents a "field defect" that places the pancreatic ductal cells at risk for both IPMN and PDAC, as both PDAC derived from IPMN and pancreatic intraepithelial neoplasia synchronous with and separate from IPMN have been described.[38]

Pathology/Classification

IPMNs are defined by some degree of ductal dilatation and papillary overgrowth of ductal epithelia.[4] M-IPMNs have an intestinal phenotype and express lineage markers such as CDX2 and MUC2.[39] Carcinomas arising from within M-IPMNs have a colloid phenotype that is more indolent than that of PDAC.[40,41] On the contrary, BD-IPMNs have mostly a gastric phenotype, MUC5AC$^+$ and MUC1$^-$, whereas MUC2 staining is not prominent.[42] BD-IPMN can also have other phenotypes such as oncocytic, intestinal, and pancreaticobiliary.[41,42] Gastric phenotype IPMN is associated with the tubular adenocarcinoma histologic variant, which is less common but has a poor prognosis similar to PDAC.[40]

The underlying risk of carcinoma is the driving force behind the differentiation between M-IPMN and BD-IPMN and has been extensively studied. In the MGH/Verona study, the risks of adenoma, borderline carcinoma, carcinoma in situ, and invasive carcinoma for M-IPMN were 11%, 21%, 20%, and 48%, respectively.[35] The risks for mixed type were 8%, 30%, 20%, and 42%, respectively, and for B-IPMN risks were 44%, 34%, 11%, and 11%, respectively.[35] The risks for lymph node metastases in those patients with invasive cancer were 33%, 48.5%, and 23.5% for M-IPMN, mixed type IPMN, and B-IPMN, respectively.[35] The Sendai guidelines aggregated 20 studies and found a risk of malignant tumors or invasive tumors to be 40.4% and 30.8% for all IPMNs, greater than 62.2% and 43.6% for M-IPMN, greater than 57.6% and 45.3% for mixed IPMN, and greater than 24.4% and 16.6% for BD-IPMN, respectively.[6]

Diagnosis

The diagnosis of IPMN is made radio graphically or histologically. The Sendai guidelines call for imaging for all cysts $\geq$1 cm to look for high-risk features (see Management section).[6] Radiographically, M-IPMNs are defined by either segmental or diffuse dilation of the main pancreatic duct, greater than 5 mm, with no other etiology for the ductal obstruction (ie, stones, proximal tumor, stricture).[6] The guidelines suggest that a main pancreatic ductal dilation of 5 to 9 mm is a "worrisome feature" and ≥10 mm is a "high-risk stigmata."[6] BD-IPMN is defined as a pancreatic cyst greater than 5 mm that communicates with branches of the main pancreatic duct but does not appear to be arising directly from it.[6] A cystic lesion that combines features of both M-IPMN and BD-IPMN are considered mixed type, and, as stated earlier, these tumors are considered to behave more like M-IPMN biologically.

The diagnostic modalities used most often for diagnosis are multidetector computed tomography scans and magnetic resonance cholangiopancreatography, which has largely replaced endoscopic retrograde cholangiopancreatography.[6] The classic endoscopic retrograde cholangiopancreatography finding was that of multiple filling defects in the main pancreatic duct.[4] The solid aspect of the tumor may be present in the duct wall or in the lumen itself.[39] Calcifications may be present, and the rest of the pancreas can have a heterogeneous appearance.[39] The pathognomonic finding on upper endoscopy of a so-called bulging papilla-extruding mucus is only seen in a third of cases.[4]

EUS is used to locate nodular components of the tumor and perform cyst fluid aspiration or biopsy.[4] Elevated cyst fluid CEA is present in 80% of cases.[4] Cytology can confer the degree of atypia.[4] Newer adjunctive studies, such as the monoclonal antibody mDas-1, are helping to differentiate high-risk or malignant IPMNs with high specificity in both tissue and cyst fluid.[43]

Management

The management of IPMN, particularly BD-IPMN, remains an active area of controversy among pancreatic surgeons. The Sendai guidelines set the indications for resection in all patients with M-IPMN or positive margins after resection of M-IPMN (ideally done with frozen section in the operating room until the margin returns at most moderate-grade dysplasia).[6] For BD-IPMN, indications for resection include worrisome features or high-risk stigmata.[6] Symptoms, although not explicitly defined by the guidelines, are also an indication for resection.[4] Worrisome features include a cyst ≥3 cm, thickened and radiographically enhanced cyst walls, nonenhanced mural nodules, main pancreatic duct size of 5 to 9 mm, an abrupt change in the main pancreatic duct caliber with distal pancreatic atrophy, and lymphadenopathy.[6] High-risk stigmata include an enhanced solid component and a main pancreatic duct size of ≥10 mm.[6] All cysts with high-risk stigmata should be resected.[6] All cysts ≥3 cm without worrisome features and cysts ≤3 cm with worrisome features should undergo diagnostic workup as above, including EUS.[6] Cysts that are ≤3 cm without worrisome features can be observed with close follow-up (recommendations are suggested in the Sendai guidelines).[6]

Localization of tumors, particularly multifocal tumors, can be difficult and may require intraoperative pancreatoscopy or repeated frozen section for confirmation of an adequate resection.[4,39] In patients that have had long-standing pancreatitis, resection may be difficult, so the risks and benefits of any operation must be weighed with that of underlying malignancy.[4]

The importance of the revised Sendai guidelines is that some pancreatic cystic neoplasms can be safely watched. However, these guidelines rely heavily on a correct preoperative diagnosis. Certainly, management at a high-volume pancreatic center is paramount. But, even in such a center, only 68% of cases were correctly diagnosed before surgical resection.[44] In that particular study, 20% of the presumed BD-IPMNs were actually M-IPMNs.[44] A recent German study found similar diagnostic accuracy with 29% of suspected BD-IPMNs having involvement of the main pancreatic duct.[45] However, a large series both retrospective and prospective from the MGH, in an attempt to validate the revised guidelines, found that only 1 patient of 378 followed up for BD-IPMN subsequently had invasive cancer without worrisome features (0.26%).[46] The investigators did note, however, that high-grade dysplasia did occur in 9% of resected cysts without worrisome features, with only half of these cysts larger than 3 cm, highlighting again the importance of close long-term follow-up.[46] Further complicating this picture is another recent report from the MGH that challenges the categorization of mixed IPMN with M-IPMN, as the investigators found some mixed IPMN with only minimal main duct involvement to behave similar to BD-IPMN and perhaps make up yet another group that perhaps could be safely watched.[47]

The revised Sendai guidelines recommend that patients without high-risk stigmata undergo early radiographic follow-up (3-6 months) to establish trajectory of the tumor followed by yearly examinations.[6] In patients that are progressing toward high-risk features, close follow-up is recommended.[6] A note is made that patients with a family history of PDAC and an IPMN may need closer follow-up,[6] as again the field defect concept does place them at higher risk for development of a second PDAC.

SUMMARY

CNPs are a heterogeneous group of tumors with very different biology. The increasing use of axial imaging will demand wider knowledge of CNPs by physicians to allow for proper triage. Nonoperative management relies greatly on excellent radiologic and cytologic analysis, and management of these tumors should be undertaken at experienced pancreatic centers. IPMN in particular continues to be a source of ongoing debate, but recent evidence suggests that following the revised Sendai guidelines is safe. As with the last 5 years, surely the next 5 years will bring even further delineation of which groups are particularly high and low risk and which patients ultimately need an operation.

REFERENCES

1. de Jong K, Nio CY, Mearadji B, et al. Disappointing interobserver agreement among radiologists for a classifying diagnosis of pancreatic cysts using magnetic resonance imaging. Pancreas 2012;41(2):278–82.
2. Laffan TA, Horton KM, Klein AP, et al. Prevalence of unsuspected pancreatic cysts on MDCT. AJR Am J Roentgenol 2008;191(3):802–7.
3. Konstantinidis IT, Kambadakone A, Catalano OA, et al. Lymphoepithelial cysts and cystic lymphangiomas: under-recognized benign cystic lesions of the pancreas. World J Gastrointest Surg 2014;6(7):136–41.
4. Farrell JJ, Fernandez-del Castillo C. Pancreatic cystic neoplasms: management and unanswered questions. Gastroenterology 2013;144(6):1303–15.
5. Valsangkar NP, Morales-Oyarvide V, Thayer SP, et al. 851 resected cystic tumors of the pancreas: a 33-year experience at the Massachusetts General Hospital. Surgery 2012;152(3 Suppl 1):S4–12.
6. Tanaka M, Fernández-del Castillo C, Adsay V, et al. International consensus guidelines 2012 for the management of IPMN and MCN of the pancreas. Pancreatology 2012;12(3):183–97.
7. Bosman FT, Carneiro F, Hruban RH, et al. WHO classification of tumours of the digestive system. Lyon (UK): IARC; 2010.

8. Sarr MG, Carpenter HA, Prabhakar LP, et al. Clinical and pathologic correlation of 84 mucinous cystic neoplasms of the pancreas: can one reliably differentiate benign from malignant (or premalignant) neoplasms? Ann Surg 2000;231(2): 205–12.

9. Le Baleur Y, Couvelard A, Vullierme MP, et al. Mucinous cystic neoplasms of the pancreas: definition of preoperative imaging criteria for high-risk lesions. Pancreatology 2011;11(5):495–9.

10. Park JW, Jang JY, Kang MJ, et al. Mucinous cystic neoplasm of the pancreas: is surgical resection recommended for all surgically fit patients? Pancreatology 2014;14(2):131–6.

11. Yamao K, Yanagisawa A, Takahashi K, et al. Clinicopathological features and prognosis of mucinous cystic neoplasm with ovarian-type stroma: a multi-institutional study of the Japan pancreas society. Pancreas 2011;40(1): 67–71.

12. Crippa S, Salvia R, Warshaw AL, et al. Mucinous cystic neoplasm of the pancreas is not an aggressive entity: lessons from 163 resected patients. Ann Surg 2008; 247(4):571–9.

13. Jang KT, Park SM, Basturk O, et al. Clinicopathologic characteristics of 29 invasive carcinomas arising in 178 pancreatic mucinous cystic neoplasms with ovarian-type stroma: implications for management and prognosis. Am J Surg Pathol 2015;39(2):179–87.

14. Wu J, Jiao Y, Dal Molin M, et al. Whole-exome sequencing of neoplastic cysts of the pancreas reveals recurrent mutations in components of ubiquitin-dependent pathways. Proc Natl Acad Sci U S A 2011;108(52):21188–93.

15. Wu J, Matthaei H, Maitra A, et al. Recurrent GNAS mutations define an unexpected pathway for pancreatic cyst development. Sci Transl Med 2011;3(92): 92ra66.

16. Sano M, Driscoll DR, De Jesus-Monge WE, et al. Activated wnt signaling in stroma contributes to development of pancreatic mucinous cystic neoplasms. Gastroenterology 2014;146(1):257–67.

17. Tseng JF, Warshaw AL, Sahani DV, et al. Serous cystadenoma of the pancreas: tumor growth rates and recommendations for treatment. Ann Surg 2005;242(3): 413–9 [discussion: 419–21].

18. Malleo G, Bassi C, Rossini R, et al. Growth pattern of serous cystic neoplasms of the pancreas: observational study with long-term magnetic resonance surveillance and recommendations for treatment. Gut 2012;61(5):746–51.

19. Jais B, Rebours V, Malleo G, et al. Serous cystic neoplasm of the pancreas: a multinational study of 2622 patients under the auspices of the International Association of Pancreatology and European Pancreatic Club (European Study Group on Cystic Tumors of the Pancreas). Gut 2016;65(2):305–12.

20. Bassi C, Salvia R, Molinari E, et al. Management of 100 consecutive cases of pancreatic serous cystadenoma: wait for symptoms and see at imaging or vice versa? World J Surg 2003;27(3):319–23.

21. Le Borgne J, de Calan L, Partensky C. Cystadenomas and cystadenocarcinomas of the pancreas: a multiinstitutional retrospective study of 398 cases. French Surgical Association. Ann Surg 1999;230(2):152–61.

22. Galanis C, Zamani A, Cameron JL, et al. Resected serous cystic neoplasms of the pancreas: a review of 158 patients with recommendations for treatment. J Gastrointest Surg 2007;11(7):820–6.

23. Kimura W, Moriya T, Hirai I, et al. Multicenter study of serous cystic neoplasm of the Japan pancreas society. Pancreas 2012;41(3):380–7.

24. Panarelli NC, Park KJ, Hruban RH, et al. Microcystic serous cystadenoma of the pancreas with subtotal cystic degeneration: another neoplastic mimic of pancreatic pseudocyst. Am J Surg Pathol 2012;36(5):726–31.

25. Wasel BA, Keough V, Huang WY, et al. Histological percutaneous diagnosis of stage IV microcystic serous cystadenocarcinoma of the pancreas. BMJ Case Rep 2013;2013:1–7.

26. Bordeianou L, Vagefi PA, Sahani D, et al. Cystic pancreatic endocrine neoplasms: a distinct tumor type? J Am Coll Surg 2008;206(3):1154–8.

27. Gaujoux S, Tang L, Klimstra D, et al. The outcome of resected cystic pancreatic endocrine neoplasms: a case-matched analysis. Surgery 2012;151(4):518–25.

28. Ligneau B, Lombard-Bohas C, Partensky C, et al. Cystic endocrine tumors of the pancreas: clinical, radiologic, and histopathologic features in 13 cases. Am J Surg Pathol 2001;25(6):752–60.

29. Boninsegna L, Partelli S, D'Innocenzio MM, et al. Pancreatic cystic endocrine tumors: a different morphological entity associated with a less aggressive behavior. Neuroendocrinology 2010;92(4):246–51.

30. Deshpande V, Fernandez-del Castillo C, Muzikansky A, et al. Cytokeratin 19 is a powerful predictor of survival in pancreatic endocrine tumors. Am J Surg Pathol 2004;28(9):1145–53.

31. Morales-Oyarvide V, Yoon WJ, Ingkakul T, et al. Cystic pancreatic neuroendocrine tumors: the value of cytology in preoperative diagnosis. Cancer Cytopathol 2014; 122(6):435–44.

32. Butte JM, Brennan MF, Gönen M, et al. Solid pseudopapillary tumors of the pancreas. Clinical features, surgical outcomes, and long-term survival in 45 consecutive patients from a single center. J Gastrointest Surg 2011;15(2):350–7.

33. Reddy S, Cameron JL, Scudiere J, et al. Surgical management of solid-pseudopapillary neoplasms of the pancreas (Franz or Hamoudi tumors): a large single-institutional series. J Am Coll Surg 2009;208(5):950–7 [discussion: 957–9].

34. Abraham SC, Klimstra DS, Wilentz RE, et al. Solid-pseudopapillary tumors of the pancreas are genetically distinct from pancreatic ductal adenocarcinomas and almost always harbor beta-catenin mutations. Am J Pathol 2002;160(4):1361–9.

35. Crippa S, Fernández-Del Castillo C, Salvia R, et al. Mucin-producing neoplasms of the pancreas: an analysis of distinguishing clinical and epidemiologic characteristics. Clin Gastroenterol Hepatol 2010;8(2):213–9.

36. Ingkakul T, Warshaw AL, Fernandez-Del Castillo C. Epidemiology of intraductal papillary mucinous neoplasms of the pancreas: sex differences between 3 geographic regions. Pancreas 2011;40(5):779–80.

37. Marchegiani G, Mino-Kenudson M, Sahora K, et al. IPMN involving the main pancreatic duct: biology, epidemiology, and long-term outcomes following resection. Ann Surg 2015;261(5):976–83.

38. Yamaguchi K, Kanemitsu S, Hatori T, et al. Pancreatic ductal adenocarcinoma derived from IPMN and pancreatic ductal adenocarcinoma concomitant with IPMN. Pancreas 2011;40(4):571–80.

39. Fernandez-del Castillo C, Adsay NV. Intraductal papillary mucinous neoplasms of the pancreas. Gastroenterology 2010;139(3):708–13, 713.e1–2.

40. Mino-Kenudson M, Fernández-del Castillo C, Baba Y, et al. Prognosis of invasive intraductal papillary mucinous neoplasm depends on histological and precursor epithelial subtypes. Gut 2011;60(12):1712–20.

41. Sadakari Y, Ohuchida K, Nakata K, et al. Invasive carcinoma derived from the nonintestinal type intraductal papillary mucinous neoplasm of the pancreas has

a poorer prognosis than that derived from the intestinal type. Surgery 2010; 147(6):812–7.

42. Furukawa T, Klöppel G, Volkan Adsay N, et al. Classification of types of intraductal papillary-mucinous neoplasm of the pancreas: a consensus study. Virchows Arch 2005;447(5):794–9.

43. Das KK, Xiao H, Geng X, et al. mAb Das-1 is specific for high-risk and malignant intraductal papillary mucinous neoplasm (IPMN). Gut 2014;63(10):1626–34.

44. Correa-Gallego C, Ferrone CR, Thayer SP, et al. Incidental pancreatic cysts: do we really know what we are watching? Pancreatology 2010;10(2–3):144–50.

45. Fritz S, Klauss M, Bergmann F, et al. Pancreatic main-duct involvement in branch-duct IPMNs: an underestimated risk. Ann Surg 2014;260(5):848–55 [discussion: 855–6].

46. Sahora K, Mino-Kenudson M, Brugge W, et al. Branch duct intraductal papillary mucinous neoplasms: does cyst size change the tip of the scale? A critical analysis of the revised international consensus guidelines in a large single-institutional series. Ann Surg 2013;258(3):466–75.

47. Sahora K, Fernández-del Castillo C, Dong F, et al. Not all mixed-type intraductal papillary mucinous neoplasms behave like main-duct lesions: implications of minimal involvement of the main pancreatic duct. Surgery 2014;156(3):611–21.

Therapeutic Approach to Cystic Neoplasms of the Pancreas

Mohammad Al Efishat, MD[a,b], Peter J. Allen, MD[a],*

KEYWORDS

- Pancreatic cysts • IPMN • Serous cystadenoma • Mucinous cystic neoplasms
- Pancreatectomy

KEY POINTS

- Resection should be considered whenever the risk of malignancy is higher than the risk of the operation.
- Serous cystadenomas are considered benign and should be followed radiographically, unless symptomatic.
- Mucinous cystic neoplasms are typically resected as they are most frequently seen in young women and typically occur in the pancreatic body or tail.
- Management of branch duct IPMN is selective with resection indicated for symptomatic lesions and those with high risk or worrisome features.
- Main duct IPMN should generally be resected as there is presumed risk of high-grade dysplasia or invasive disease.

INTRODUCTION

Cystic neoplasms of the pancreas are being diagnosed more frequently given the widespread use of high-quality imaging studies (computed tomography [CT] and MRI). The reported prevalence of incidental pancreatic cysts is about 2.6% on CT imaging and has been reported as high as 13.5% on MRI.[1,2]

The 3 most common subtypes of cystic neoplasms are serous cystadenoma (SCA), mucinous cystic neoplasm (MCN), and intraductal papillary mucinous neoplasm (IPMN). The latter represent most neoplastic cystic lesions and are of particular

The authors have nothing to disclose.
[a] Department of Surgery, Memorial Sloan-Kettering Cancer Center, 1275 York Avenue, New York, NY 10021, USA; [b] Department of Surgery, Johns Hopkins Hospital, 600 N Wolfe Street, Baltimore, MD 21287, USA
* Corresponding author.
E-mail address: allenp@mskcc.org

importance to surgeons because these lesions are considered precancerous. IPMN and MCN represent the only radiographically identifiable precursor lesions of pancreatic cancer.[3] For detailed discussion of the different classifications, subtypes, and diagnostic evaluation of cystic neoplasms, (See Ferrone CR: Spectrum and classification of cystic lesions of the pancreas, in this issue).

Management of cystic neoplasms of the pancreas is challenging because it involves decision making in the setting of imperfect diagnostic information. The decision between operative resection and radiographic surveillance must balance the risk of a significant operative procedure that has measurable associated mortality with the risk of malignant progression if radiographic surveillance is chosen.

Resection of all pancreatic cysts is no longer appropriate. The vast majority of lesions now identified are asymptomatic, small (<2 cm), and benign. The risk of malignant progression in this group of patients is lower than the risk of operative resection.[3]

This article focuses on the therapeutic approach to the 3 major subtypes of cystic neoplasms of the pancreas (IPMN, MCN, and SCA), with the understanding that determining the histopathology of a given cystic lesion, based on imaging and cyst fluid analysis, is considered the cornerstone for managing these cysts. Treatment recommendations are usually based on the natural history, biological behavior, and risk of malignancy for each histologic subtype (**Fig. 1**). Histopathology of small cysts can be hard to determine without resection and represent a clinical dilemma.

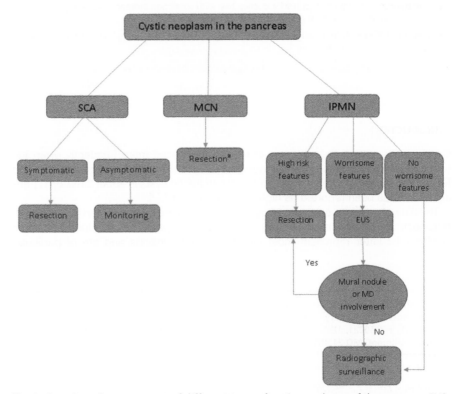

Fig. 1. Overview of management of different types of cystic neoplasms of the pancreas. EUS, endoscopic ultrasound; MD, main duct. [a] Monitoring in elderly with no worrisome features.

SEROUS CYSTADENOMA

Serous cystic neoplasms of the pancreas are considered benign slow-growing tumors (typically<5 mm/y) with very rare malignant transformation. There have been approximately 30 reported cases of malignant transformation of SCA in the world literature and these malignant SCA reports typically describe locally invasive lesions rather than metastatic disease.[4]

Asymptomatic SCAs should be managed conservatively with radiographic monitoring.[5] Monitoring with MRI or high-resolution triphasic CT should typically be repeated within 3 to 6 months of initial diagnosis, both to confirm the confidence of the diagnosis and to confirm radiographic stability. Once this has been performed, either annual or biennial imaging is appropriate. A recent observational study of 145 subjects with SCA concluded that surveillance for SCA should not be more frequent than every 2 years based on the slow observed growth rate.[6] This study also showed that the rate of growth depends on the age of the cyst rather than the original size at presentation because growth dramatically increased after the first 7 years of surveillance regardless of the original size. Other factors that increased the rate of growth were oligocystic or macrocystic pattern, and a personal history of other tumors.

The exact growth rate of these lesions is unclear because a previous study by Tseng and colleagues[7] reported that there was a difference in the growth rate of lesions less than 4 cm (0.48 cm/y) compared with those equal to or greater than 4 cm (1.98 cm/y). These investigators also reported that cysts greater than 4 cm were more likely to be symptomatic; hence, they recommended resection for asymptomatic patients with SCAs greater than 4 cm. These latter findings have not been observed in patients followed for SCA at the authors' institution; therefore, we do not use the size of the lesion at presentation as a factor in treatment decision making.[8]

We generally recommend resection in lesions that are clearly symptomatic and for large lesions that are marginally resectable at presentation. Rapid growth, which is rarely observed, is another situation that may warrant resection.

Outcome and Long-Term Recommendations

Following resection, survival is only affected by operative mortality and postoperative complications, rather than the disease itself. In our series of 469 subjects who underwent resection of pancreatic cysts (of all subtypes), the 30-day mortality rate was between 0.5% and 1%.[3] Postoperative surveillance following resection of SCA is generally not indicated. There is no evidence of an increased risk of pancreatic cancer in this group of patients.[9]

MUCINOUS CYSTIC NEOPLASMS (CYSTADENOMA AND CYSTADENOCARCINOMA)

Similar to other cystic neoplasms, the clinical features and natural history of mucinous cysts dictates management as well as the surgical procedure of choice. These lesions are usually identified in women in their 40s or 50s as a solitary cyst in the body or tail of the pancreas. Characteristic radiographic features include a single cyst in the body or tail of the pancreas without significant papillary solid component. Eggshell calcifications may also be present. Cyst fluid analysis typically shows an elevated carcinoembryonic antigen level (mucin production) and low amylase (no communication with the pancreatic duct).[10,11]

It is known that MCNs have the potential to transform into malignancy and because these typically occur in the tail of the pancreas in young women, surgical resection is often recommended. Given that these lesions are typically unifocal, resection is considered curative because the pancreatic remnant has not been found to be at increased risk for the development of carcinoma. The risk of carcinoma in situ or invasive disease in published series of resected lesions has been reported around 17%.[12] Other features that reportedly increase the likelihood of invasive disease and thus warrant surgical resection are: symptomatic cysts, large size (>4 cm), elevated tumor marker, and presence of solid component or mural nodule.[13,14]

In elderly patients with multiple medical comorbidities that preclude surgical resection, monitoring of the lesion with serial imaging is an option, especially if there are no worrisome features (MCNs of<4 cm without mural nodules). This is generally done by MRI with MR cholangiopancreatography (MRCP), or triphasic multidetector CT with 2 mm cuts through the pancreas. Once stability has been determined, annual imaging is appropriate. Notably, multiple studies have demonstrated that invasive MCN usually occurs in older patients, without distinctive imaging characteristics. This is further evidence that we currently are unable to identify invasive MCN before it progresses from noninvasive precursor. Thus, resection should be considered in most patients.[15]

Distal pancreatectomy with lymph node dissection with or without splenectomy is the most common procedure for MCN because most of these cysts are located in the body or tail of the pancreas. Parenchyma-sparing resections (central pancreatectomy) may be performed in small MCNs without features of invasive disease. A recent meta-analysis showed that, compared with distal pancreatectomy, central pancreatectomy is associated with higher morbidity, including higher pancreatic fistula, but lower rate of postoperative endocrine insufficiency.[16] This latter finding is a factor that should be considered because many patients with MCN are in their 30s or 40s at the time of resection. Pancreatic enucleation is also an option and is generally associated with less morbidity, shorter operative time, and lower incidence of endocrine and exocrine pancreatic insufficiency.[17] Enucleation for these lesions, however, is typically quite challenging because they are often greater than 4 cm in diameter and often thoroughly embedded within the parenchyma with an associated inflammatory infiltrate.

Laparoscopic resection with spleen preservation is feasible and safe for MCNs.[14] Laparoscopic distal pancreatectomy has been thought to be associated with shorter hospital stay, less blood loss, and decreased overall complications compared with the open approach.[18] Endoscopic ultrasound (EUS)-guided ablation is still considered investigational and is not recommended for patients with MCN.[14]

Outcome and Long-Term Recommendations

Noninvasive MCN has no risk for distant recurrence after resection and there is no increased risk of pancreatic cancer in the remaining pancreas, with a 5-year survival close to 100%. Thus, these patients do not usually require long-term radiographic surveillance following resection.[15,19] However, those who are found to have invasive MCN after resection are at risk for distant recurrence. Reported recurrence rates range from 37% to 83% at 5 years,[4] whereas 5-year survival was reported as 57% in a large series of 163 resected MCNs.[15] Per the 2012 international consensus guidelines, recommended follow-up for invasive MCN is similar to resected pancreatic cancer and usually consists of high-quality CT scan (pancreas-protocol scan) every 6 months for the first 2 years and then annually afterward.[14]

INTRADUCTAL PAPILLARY MUCINOUS NEOPLASMS OF THE PANCREAS

IPMNs are a heterogeneous group of neoplasms that arise in the ductal system of the pancreas and may involve the pancreatic main duct (MD) -IPMN, branch duct (BD)-IPMN, or both (mixed-IPMN). Since the recognition of this entity 2 decades ago,

IPMNs have been gaining increased attention because they are the most common radiographically identifiable precursor lesion of pancreatic cancer and are presumed to progress from low-grade dysplasia to high-grade dysplasia to carcinoma. This pathway of progression to pancreatic cancer is believed to represent between 20% and 30% of pancreatic cancers. Approximately 40% to 70% of resected IPMN lesions will have either high-grade dysplasia or invasive carcinoma identified at the time of resection.[20,21]

The 2 main histopathological subtypes of invasive IPMN that have been described are colloid carcinoma, which typically arises in the setting of intestinal-type IPMN, and tubular carcinoma, which generally arises in the setting of pancreatobiliary-type IPMN. There are currently no means of differentiating between these 2 subtypes preoperatively; however, recent studies have suggested that GNAS mutations are strongly associated with colloid carcinoma and KRAS mutations associated with tubular carcinoma.[22] Preoperative distinction between these subtypes may be important because the outcomes following resection differ significantly with reported 5-year survival following resection of colloid carcinoma approximating 75%, whereas resected tubular invasive IPMN has a reported 5-year survival similar to that of conventional pancreatic cancer (15%–25%).[23,24]

Generally, management of IPMN depends on the result of the initial CT or MRI-MRCP, which will determine whether the patient needs further evaluation with EUS, surveillance, or should undergo surgical resection. Per the 2012 Fukuoka consensus guidelines, high-risk features include an enhancing solid component or MD size equal to or greater than 10 mm. Cysts with either of these features should be resected. Worrisome features include pancreatitis (clinically), cyst equal to or greater than 3 cm, thickened enhanced cyst walls, nonenhanced mural nodules, MD size of 5 to 9 mm, abrupt change in the MD caliber with distal pancreatic atrophy, and lymphadenopathy. Presence of any of these features warrants further work-up with EUS to evaluate for mural nodules or MD involvement. If none of these features are present, no further work-up is indicated but radiographic surveillance is still warranted.[14]

Branch Duct Intraductal Papillary Mucinous Neoplasms

BD-IPMN is defined as a pancreatic cyst of greater than 5 mm in diameter with communication with the MD without associated MD dilation. BD-IPMN is more common in the elderly and less likely to harbor high-grade dysplasia or invasive disease compared with MD-IPMN. The annual risk of malignancy has been estimated to be between 2% to 3%.[25,26]

For small, less than 3 cm, BD-IPMN with no high-risk or worrisome features, radiographic monitoring is generally recommended, with resection reserved for symptomatic patients or those who develop worrisome features. The typical follow-up schedule at the authors' institution for those undergoing nonoperative management includes a short interval scan (3–6 months) to determine stability, followed by either annual imaging or imaging every 6 months. Every 6 month imaging is generally reserved for patients for whom there is some degree of concern, such as a larger BD-IPMN or in the setting of minimal MD dilation (<1 cm).

Indications for resection include the presence of symptoms or any of the high-risk stigmata or worrisome features previously described. The procedure of choice is segmental pancreatectomy or enucleation, depending on the location of the lesion (**Fig. 2**). A standard resection with lymphadenectomy should be performed for segmental resections. Limited or focal nonanatomic resection is an option as long as there are no preoperative or intraoperative concerns for malignancy.

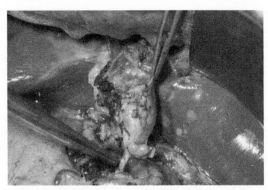

Fig. 2. Enucleation of a cystic tumor in the head of the pancreas. Note the preservation of the gastroduodenal artery (*arrow*).

EUS-guided ablation of pancreatic cysts by ethanol or ethanol followed by paclitaxel are investigational methods that have been used in unilocular or oligolocular cysts less than 2 cm, cysts with no radiographic communication with the MD, and in patients who refuse to undergo resection or are poor candidates for surgery.[27–31] A recent meta-analysis of 7 studies that performed EUS-guided ethanol ablation of pancreatic cysts showed a pooled complete cyst resolution of 56% and partial cyst resolution of 24%. Related complications included abdominal pain in 6.5% of patients and pancreatitis in 3.9%.[32] Concerns related to this approach are numerous, including the inability to perform surveillance on collapsed cysts, the high risk of cyst recurrence, and the unknown effects of alcohol on incompletely ablated IPMN epithelium.[33]

For multifocal BD-IPMN, the number of lesions has not been demonstrated to correlate with the risk of invasive disease. Interestingly, a report showed that symptomatic unifocal BD-IPMN had a higher risk of malignancy compared with multifocal BD-IPMN (18% vs 7%).[34] Treatment includes segmental pancreatectomy for high-risk lesions, with an attempt at avoiding total pancreatectomy whenever the lesions are confined to one pancreatic region.[14] The decision to proceed with total pancreatectomy is an extremely important one; careful patient selection is essential. The long-term morbidity of total pancreatectomy is measurable and this procedure should only be considered for BD-IPMN when there is diffuse whole-gland involvement of high-risk lesions.[14,35]

Main Duct Intraductal Papillary Mucinous Neoplasms

The 2012 Fukuoka consensus guidelines lowered the threshold for pancreatic dilation to 5 mm from 10 mm as this would increase the sensitivity for radiologic diagnosis of MD-IPMN without compromising specificity. The recommendation for operative resection in MD-IPMN is less controversial than other cystic lesions because resection is typically indicated in all radiologically or endoscopically confirmed MD-IPMN given the high incidence of invasive and malignant disease. Because our ability to define the site of high-grade dysplasia or invasive disease in MD-IPMN is limited, the greater challenge in MD-IPMN is not whether an operation should be done but, instead, which operation should be done.[36]

The authors' typical approach to MD-IPMN is to assess for the presence of an invasive lesion and to evaluate the pancreas for the predominant radiographic or endosonographic site of disease. When an invasive lesion is identified, partial pancreatectomy is performed to resect the site of invasive disease. In the absence of an invasive lesion, and in the setting of a clear radiographic predominance of disease in an isolated portion of the gland, a partial pancreatectomy is typically performed to remove the area of radiographic predominance. Intraoperative frozen section is typically performed to rule out high-grade dysplasia at the resection margin. If high-grade dysplasia is present, further resection should be performed. Frozen section requires intact epithelium at the margin to be able to evaluate for the degree of dysplasia. The accuracy of frozen section, however, is limited with positive predictive value for frozen section of about 50% and a negative predictive value of up to 74%.[37]

In a study by the authors' group at Memorial Sloan Kettering Cancer Center (MSKCC), local recurrence in the remnant gland occurred in 8% of subjects after a median of 36 months of follow-up. Thus, all patients who have been resected for IPMN should be considered for long-term radiographic surveillance. High-grade dysplasia and a margin positive for IPMN have been identified as risk factors for this recurrence and should be considered when the interval of follow-up is being determined.[37]

In cases of diffuse ductal dilation without focal lesions on imaging, further work-up with endoscopic retrograde cholangiopancreatography (ERCP) or EUS should be performed to confirm the diagnosis and to exclude an occult invasive lesion.[14,38] In the absence of invasive disease, and in the absence of a site of predominant disease, total pancreatectomy should be considered. This operation should be reserved for selected patients with obvious diffuse disease or to those in whom the intraoperative finding of high-grade dysplasia on frozen section dictates completion pancreatectomy. This selective approach is important given the significant morbidity of total pancreatectomy with the inevitable endocrine and exocrine insufficiency. This morbidity was demonstrated in a series of 47 subjects from the Mayo Clinic who underwent total pancreatectomy for noninvasive IPMN. Within this group, the reported 30-day major morbidity and mortality rates were 19% and 2%, respectively. There were significant reported metabolic derangements, exocrine insufficiency, weight loss, diabetes, and a high readmission rate.[39]

Outcome and Long-Term Follow-up

Noninvasive IPMN should be at no risk for distant recurrence. Recurrence and survival following resection of invasive lesions depends on histologic subtype. In a recent multi-institutional study of 70 small IPMN-associated invasive carcinomas (≤2 cm), the overall recurrence rate was 24% and the median time to recurrence was 16 months (range 4–132 months). Median and 5-year survival rates were 99 months and 59%, respectively. Recurrence of invasive disease was local in 35%, distant in 47%, and both in 18% of subjects. Lymphatic spread and T3 stage were predictive of recurrence, whereas tubular carcinoma subtype was the strongest predictor of poor overall survival.[40]

For resected noninvasive MD-IPMN, variable recurrence rates have been reported in the literature (5%–20%)[37,40–42] but close radiographic follow-up is recommended because these patients are presumed to have a higher risk of developing a new IPMN. This was demonstrated in a recent study from Johns Hopkins that found that these patients have a 25% chance of developing a new IPMN in the 5 years following surgery for noninvasive IPMN. The risk of developing pancreatic cancer was 7% and 38% at 5 and 10 years, respectively.[41]

Another study of 78 subjects who had undergone resection of noninvasive IPMN at MSKCC, found that 8% had recurrence in the pancreatic remnant at 36 months of median follow-up and the 5-year recurrence rate was 13%. Local recurrence increased with positive margins; however, most subjects with positive margins have not developed local recurrence. Furthermore, recurrence in the pancreatic remnant was the same for both MD-IPMN and BD-IPMN, at 8%.[37]

LESS COMMON CYSTIC NEOPLASMS OF THE PANCREAS
Solid Pseudopapillary Neoplasms

Solid pseudopapillary neoplasms (SPNs) are uncommon cystic lesions of the pancreas and represent less than 4% of resected pancreatic cystic lesions. SPNs are more commonly reported in the literature. They can occur throughout the pancreas but more commonly occur in the body or tail. On imaging, SPNs appear as large, well-demarcated, solitary, mixed solid, and cystic heterogeneous masses.[43]

Given the malignant potential of these lesions, surgical resection is typically recommended. The goal of resection is to obtain negative margins. The procedure of choice depends on the location of the lesion (pancreaticoduodenectomy, distal pancreatectomy, or enucleation).

Despite locally aggressive features, and even in the presence of metastatic disease, SPNs have a favorable prognosis following resection with 5-year survival rates of greater than 95%. The recurrence rate is reported to be less than 5% and the mean time to tumor recurrence has been reported to be 4 years. There are currently no recommendations regarding surveillance but patients should be typically followed for at least 5 years. Male patients, those with atypical histopathology, large tumors greater than 5 cm, and patients with incomplete resection may have increased risk of recurrence and warrant closer follow-up.[43,44]

Cystic Endocrine Neoplasms

These lesions are considered malignant and behave similar to noncystic endocrine tumors for which treatment and outcome is beyond the scope of this article. Endocrine tumors are typically indolent tumors but have metastatic potential. Resection is recommended for all surgically fit patients, especially for patients with lesions greater than 2 cm in size. Despite the potential for metastasis, overall prognosis is excellent with reported postresection 1-year and 5-year survival of 97% and 87%, respectively.[45]

SUMMARY

Management of cystic neoplasms will continue to evolve as our ability to diagnose and accurately identify histopathologic subtype and the degree of dysplasia improves. SCAs are usually benign and only resected if symptomatic, whereas MCN and IPMN are considered premalignant and selective resection is indicated. Management of BD-IPMN depends on the presence of high-risk or worrisome features. Currently, segmental pancreatectomy is the procedure of choice for mucinous lesions that have a malignancy risk that is greater than the risk of resection. MD-IPMN is typically treated with resection because of the higher risk of high-grade dysplasia or invasive disease.

In the absence of invasive disease, prognosis is excellent for resected lesions, whereas the presence of invasive disease with tubular histology in IPMN signifies a poor prognosis. Lifelong follow-up, for resected IPMN, is indicated regardless of the presence of invasion. Future research efforts should be focused on improving our ability to accurately diagnose the different histopathologic subtypes of pancreatic cysts and to identify high-risk disease in patients with mucinous lesions because this will result in better risk stratification and appropriate management.

REFERENCES

1. Laffan TA, Horton KM, Klein AP, et al. Prevalence of unsuspected pancreatic cysts on MDCT. AJR Am J Roentgenol 2008;191:802–7.
2. Lee KS, Sekhar A, Rofsky NM, et al. Prevalence of incidental pancreatic cysts in the adult population on MR imaging. Am J Gastroenterol 2010;105: 2079–84.
3. Gaujoux S, Brennan MF, Gonen M, et al. Cystic lesions of the pancreas: changes in the presentation and management of 1,424 patients at a single institution over a 15-year time period. J Am Coll Surg 2011;212:590–600 [discussion: 600-3].
4. Robinson SM, Scott J, Oppong KW, et al. What to do for the incidental pancreatic cystic lesion? Surg Oncol 2014;23:117–25.
5. Galanis C, Zamani A, Cameron JL, et al. Resected serous cystic neoplasms of the pancreas: a review of 158 patients with recommendations for treatment. J Gastrointest Surg 2007;11:820–6.
6. Malleo G, Bassi C, Rossini R, et al. Growth pattern of serous cystic neoplasms of the pancreas: observational study with long-term magnetic resonance surveillance and recommendations for treatment. Gut 2012;61:746–51.
7. Tseng JF, Warshaw AL, Sahani DV, et al. Serous cystadenoma of the pancreas. Trans Meet Am Surg Assoc Am Surg Assoc 2005;123:111–8.
8. Allen PJ, D'Angelica M, Gonen M, et al. A selective approach to the resection of cystic lesions of the pancreas: results from 539 consecutive patients. Ann Surg 2006;244:572–82.
9. Katz MH, Mortenson MM, Wang H, et al. Diagnosis and management of cystic neoplasms of the pancreas: an evidence-based approach. J Am Coll Surg 2008;207:106–20.
10. Yoon WJ, Brugge WR. Pancreatic cystic neoplasms: diagnosis and management. Gastroenterol Clin North Am 2012;41:103–18 [Systamtic review].
11. Cizginer S, Turner BG, Bilge AR, et al. Cyst fluid carcinoembryonic antigen is an accurate diagnostic marker of pancreatic mucinous cysts. Pancreas 2011;40: 1024–8.
12. Crippa S, Fernandez-Del Castillo C, Salvia R, et al. Mucin-producing neoplasms of the pancreas: an analysis of distinguishing clinical and epidemiologic characteristics. Clin Gastroenterol Hepatol 2010;8:213–9.
13. Reddy RP, Smyrk TC, Zapiach M, et al. Pancreatic mucinous cystic neoplasm defined by ovarian stroma: demographics, clinical features, and prevalence of cancer. Clin Gastroenterol Hepatol 2004;2:1026–31.
14. Tanaka M, Fernandez-Del Castillo C, Adsay V, et al. International consensus guidelines 2012 for the management of IPMN and MCN of the pancreas. Pancreatology 2012;12:183–97 [Systamtic review].
15. Crippa S, Salvia R, Warshaw AL, et al. Mucinous cystic neoplasm of the pancreas is not an aggressive entity: lessons from 163 resected patients. Ann Surg 2008; 247:571–9.
16. Iacono C, Verlato G, Ruzzenente A, et al. Systematic review of central pancreatectomy and meta-analysis of central versus distal pancreatectomy. Br J Surg 2013;100:873–85 [Meta-analysis].
17. Cauley CE, Pitt HA, Ziegler KM, et al. Pancreatic enucleation: improved outcomes compared with resection. J Gastrointest Surg 2012;16:1347–53.
18. Kooby DA, Gillespie T, Bentrem D, et al. Left-sided pancreatectomy: a multicenter comparison of laparoscopic and open approaches. Ann Surg 2008; 248:438–46.

19. Yamao K, Yanagisawa A, Takahashi K, et al. Clinicopathological features and prognosis of mucinous cystic neoplasm with ovarian-type stroma: a multi-institutional study of the Japan pancreas society. Pancreas 2011;40:67–71.

20. Marchegiani G, Mino-Kenudson M, Sahora K, et al. IPMN involving the main pancreatic duct: biology, epidemiology, and long-term outcomes following resection. Ann Surg 2015;261:976–83.

21. Sohn TA, Yeo CJ, Cameron JL, et al. Intraductal papillary mucinous neoplasms of the pancreas: an increasingly recognized clinicopathologic entity. Ann Surg 2001;234:313–21 [discussion: 321–2].

22. Tan MC, Basturk O, Brannon AR, et al. GNAS and KRAS mutations define separate progression pathways in intraductal papillary mucinous neoplasm-associated carcinoma. J Am Coll Surg 2015;220:845–54.e1.

23. Furukawa T, Kloppel G, Volkan Adsay N, et al. Classification of types of intraductal papillary-mucinous neoplasm of the pancreas: a consensus study. Virchows Arch 2005;447:794–9.

24. Adsay NV, Merati K, Basturk O, et al. Pathologically and biologically distinct types of epithelium in intraductal papillary mucinous neoplasms: delineation of an "intestinal" pathway of carcinogenesis in the pancreas. Am J Surg Pathol 2004;28:839–48.

25. Kang MJ, Jang JY, Kim SJ, et al. Cyst growth rate predicts malignancy in patients with branch duct intraductal papillary mucinous neoplasms. Clin Gastroenterol Hepatol 2011;9:87–93.

26. Levy P, Jouannaud V, O'Toole D, et al. Natural history of intraductal papillary mucinous tumors of the pancreas: actuarial risk of malignancy. Clin Gastroenterol Hepatol 2006;4:460–8.

27. Oh HC, Seo DW, Kim SC, et al. Septated cystic tumors of the pancreas: is it possible to treat them by endoscopic ultrasonography-guided intervention? Scand J Gastroenterol 2009;44:242–7.

28. Oh HC, Seo DW, Lee TY, et al. New treatment for cystic tumors of the pancreas: EUS-guided ethanol lavage with paclitaxel injection. Gastrointest Endosc 2008; 67:636–42.

29. Oh HC, Seo DW, Song TJ, et al. Endoscopic ultrasonography-guided ethanol lavage with paclitaxel injection treats patients with pancreatic cysts. Gastroenterology 2011;140:172–9.

30. Gan SI, Thompson CC, Lauwers GY, et al. Ethanol lavage of pancreatic cystic lesions: initial pilot study. Gastrointest Endosc 2005;61:746–52.

31. DeWitt J, McGreevy K, Schmidt CM, et al. EUS-guided ethanol versus saline solution lavage for pancreatic cysts: a randomized, double-blind study. Gastrointest Endosc 2009;70:710–23.

32. Kandula M, Moole H, Cashman M, et al. Success of endoscopic ultrasound-guided ethanol ablation of pancreatic cysts: a meta-analysis and systematic review. Indian J Gastroenterol 2015;34:193–9 [Meta-analysis].

33. Tanaka M. Controversies in the management of pancreatic IPMN. Nat Rev Gastroenterol Hepatol 2011;8:56–60.

34. Schmidt CM, White PB, Waters JA, et al. Intraductal papillary mucinous neoplasms: predictors of malignant and invasive pathology. Ann Surg 2007;246: 644–51 [discussion: 651–4].

35. Shi C, Klein AP, Goggins M, et al. Increased Prevalence of Precursor Lesions in Familial Pancreatic Cancer Patients. Clin Cancer Res 2009;15:7737–43.

36. Maker AV, Katabi N, Qin LX, et al. Cyst fluid interleukin-1beta (IL1beta) levels predict the risk of carcinoma in intraductal papillary mucinous neoplasms of the pancreas. Clin Cancer Res 2011;17:1502–8.

37. White R, D'Angelica M, Katabi N, et al. Fate of the remnant pancreas after resection of noninvasive intraductal papillary mucinous neoplasm. J Am Coll Surg 2007;204:987–93 [discussion: 993–5].
38. Jana T, Shroff J, Bhutani MS. Pancreatic cystic neoplasms: review of current knowledge, diagnostic challenges, and management options. J Carcinog 2015; 14:3 [Systamtic review].
39. Stauffer JA, Nguyen JH, Heckman MG, et al. Patient outcomes after total pancreatectomy: a single centre contemporary experience. HPB (Oxford) 2009;11: 483–92.
40. Winter JM, Jiang W, Basturk O, et al. Recurrence and survival after resection of small intraductal papillary mucinous neoplasm-associated carcinomas (</=20-mm Invasive Component): a multi-institutional analysis. Ann Surg 2015; 00:1–9.
41. He J, Cameron JL, Ahuja N, et al. Is it necessary to follow patients after resection of a benign pancreatic intraductal papillary mucinous neoplasm? J Am Coll Surg 2013;216:657–65 [discussion: 665–7].
42. Marchegiani G, Mino-Kenudson M, Ferrone CR, et al. Patterns of recurrence after resection of IPMN: Who, When, and How? Ann Surg 2015;262(6):1108–14.
43. Law JK, Ahmed A, Singh VK, et al. A systematic review of solid-pseudopapillary neoplasms: are these rare lesions? Pancreas 2014;43:331–7 [Systamtic review].
44. Reddy S, Cameron JL, Scudiere J, et al. Surgical management of solid-pseudopapillary neoplasms of the pancreas (Franz or Hamoudi tumors): a large single-institutional series. J Am Coll Surg 2009;208:950–7 [discussion: 957–9].
45. Gaujoux S, Tang L, Klimstra D, et al. The outcome of resected cystic pancreatic endocrine neoplasms: a case-matched analysis. Surgery 2012;151:518–25.

Clinical Presentation and Diagnosis of Pancreatic Neuroendocrine Tumors

Carinne W. Anderson, MD*, Joseph J. Bennett, MD

KEYWORDS

- Pancreatic neuroendocrine tumor • Nonfunctional pancreatic neuroendocrine tumor
- Insulinoma • Gastrinoma • Glucagonoma • VIPoma • Somatostatinoma

KEY POINTS

- Pancreatic neuroendocrine tumors are a rare group of neoplasms, most of which are nonfunctioning.
- Functional pancreatic neoplasms secrete hormones that produce unique clinical syndromes.
- The key management of these rare tumors is to first suspect the diagnosis; to do this, clinicians must be familiar with their clinical syndromes.

Pancreatic neuroendocrine tumors (PNETs) are a rare group of neoplasms that arise from multipotent stem cells in the pancreatic ductal epithelium. Most PNETs are nonfunctioning, but they can secrete various hormones resulting in unique clinical syndromes. Clinicians must be aware of the diverse manifestations of this disease, as the key step to management of these rare tumors is to first suspect the diagnosis. In light of that, this article focuses on the clinical features of different PNETs. Surgical and medical management will not be discussed here, as they are addressed in other articles in this issue.

EPIDEMIOLOGY
Classification

PNETs are classified clinically as nonfunctional or functional, based on the properties of the hormones they secrete and their ability to produce a clinical syndrome. Nonfunctional PNETs (NF-PNETs) do not produce a clinical syndrome simply because they do not secrete hormones or because the hormones that are secreted do not

The authors have nothing to disclose.
Department of Surgery, Helen F. Graham Cancer Center, 4701 Ogletown-Stanton Road, S-4000, Newark, DE 19713, USA
* Corresponding author.
E-mail address: Carinne.Wright@gmail.com

cause specific symptoms. NF-PNETs are discovered incidentally on imaging or are detected as a result of symptoms related to tumor mass, invasion of adjacent structures, or metastatic disease. Functional PNETs (F-PNETs) are much less common and present with specific clinical syndromes related to their hormonal secretions. Diagnosis of F-PNETs is based on the presence of this clinical syndrome and diagnostic hormonal and functional studies; diagnosis is not based on immunocytochemistry. Both F-PNETs and NF-PNETs may secrete multiple peptides. **Table 1** reviews the characteristics of the 9 commonly recognized PNETs. In addition to these 9, other rare PNETs have been described and new syndromes proposed but in not enough patients to result in a well-defined syndrome. The biologically active peptides secreted from rare F-PNETs in the literature include luteinizing hormone,[1,2] erythropoietin,[3] insulinlike growth factor II,[4] enteroglucagon,[5] renin,[3,6] glucagon-like peptide–1,[7,8] glucagon-like peptide–2,[8] and pancreatic polypeptide.[8] In addition, there are peptides

Table 1
Characteristics of recognized PNETs

Tumor (Syndrome)	Hormone	Clinical Presentation	Location	Malignancy
NF-PNETs	Eg, Pancreatic polypeptide, chorionic gonadotropin alpha, neuron-specific enolase	Related to tumor mass, invasion of adjacent structures, or metastatic disease	Pancreas 100%	60%–90%
Insulinoma	Insulin	Whipple's triad; neuroglycopenic, sympathetic	Pancreas 100%	<10%
Gastrinoma (Zollinger-Ellison)	Gastrin	Peptic ulcer disease, gastroesophageal reflux disease, diarrhea	Duodenum 70%, pancreas 25%, other 5%	60%–90%
Glucagonoma	Glucagon	NME, DM, gastrointestinal symptoms, deep vein thrombosis, neurologic symptoms	Pancreas 100%	>60%
VIPoma (Verner-Morrison)	VIP	WHDA	Pancreas 90%, other 10%	70%–90%
Somatostatinoma (SSoma)	Somatostatin	Tumor mass related, DM, gallbladder disease, weight loss, diarrhea, anemia	Pancreas 50%, duodenum and jejunum 50%	60%–70%
GRFoma	Growth hormone–releasing factor	Acromegaly	Pancreas, lung, small intestine	30%–50%
ACTHoma	ACTH	Cushing syndrome	Pancreas 100%	95%
PTHrp-oma	PTHrp	Hypercalcemia	Pancreas 100%	>85%
PNET causing carcinoid syndrome	Serotonin, tachykinins	Carcinoid syndrome	Pancreas 100%	60%–90%

Abbreviations: DM, diabetes melitus; WHDA, watery diarrhea, hypokalemia, and achlorhydria.

known to be secreted from NF-PNETs with the theoretic potential to produce a clinical syndrome, although they have never been described as doing so. These peptides include calcitonin, neurotensin, pancreatic polypeptide, ghrelin, and subunits of human gonadotropin.[9–11]

Pathology, Staging, and Grading

PNETs make up a heterogeneous group of tumors not only in their clinical features but also in their pathology. PNETs were previously referred to as *islet cell tumors* because of their resemblance to the islets of Langerhans. Although it was once thought that these tumors arose from neuroendocrine cells that migrated from the neural crest, it is now apparent that enteropancreatic neuroendocrine cells originate from multipotent stem cells that give rise to all epithelial cell types in the pancreas and gastrointestinal tract.[12]

Lack of a uniform pathologic classification system has contributed to our lack of understanding of PNETs. Per recent consensus guidelines shared by the European and North American Neuroendocrine Tumor Societies and the World Health Organization, PNETs are now graded and staged separately.

In the 2010 World Health Organization classification system, PNETs are divided into 3 grades based on 2 factors: mitotic count and ki-67 labeling index. The system further divides PNETs into well-differentiated neuroendocrine tumors, made up of grade 1 and 2, and poorly differentiated neuroendocrine tumors, comprising grade 3.[13] This finding reflects an increasing belief that poorly differentiated PNETs should be regarded as a completely separate entity from ordinary, well-differentiated PNETs.

There are several current staging systems for PNETs. The combined American Joint Commission on Cancer/Union of International Cancer Control/College of American Pathologists TNM staging system is similar to that used for exocrine tumors. It defines T3 tumors as those with peripancreatic spread.[14,15] Unfortunately, most PNETs protrude from the pancreas even when small. The European Neuroendocrine Tumor Society TNM staging system relies more on tumor size for T stage.[16]

Incidence

Pancreatic neuroendocrine tumors have an incidence of 1 to 5 per million per year. Autopsy studies suggest a greater frequency, occurring in 0.5% to 1.5% of the population.[9] PNETs make up only 1% to 2% of pancreatic neoplasms; however, their incidence is increasing. NF-PNETs in particular may be increasing in incidence and are increasingly diagnosed in earlier stages of disease. This early diagnosis is likely because of increased incidental detection on imaging studies performed for another reason.[9,17,18] The order of frequency of PNETs from most to least frequent is NF-PNETs, insulinoma, gastrinoma, glucagonoma, VIPoma, and others.[9,19] Pancreatic neuroendocrine tumors are most frequently seen in adults but can rarely occur in children, and in these instances they are likely to have a hereditary predisposition.[20] PNETs most often manifest in the fourth to sixth decades, occurring equally between the sexes, although poorly differentiated PNETs may have a higher incidence in men.

Etiology and Inherited Pancreatic Neuroendocrine Tumors Syndromes

Most PNETs are sporadic, but they are also seen in association with a few specific hereditary syndromes, including multiple endocrine neoplasia type 1 (MEN1), von Hippel–Lindau syndrome (VHL), neurofibromatosis type 1 (NF1), and tuberous sclerosis.

Almost all patients with MEN1 will have PNETs, most commonly microscopic and clinically insignificant NF-PNETs; however, F-PNETs also occur in MEN1. Of those with F-PNETS, 54% will have gastrinomas, 18% will have insulinomas, and less than 5% will have other types. These F-PNETs occur at an earlier age in patients with MEN1 than in sporadic cases and are more likely to be multiple.[21]

PNETs develop in 10% to 17% of patients with VHL, almost always NF-PNETs. The mean age of PNET diagnosis in this population is 29 to 38 years, and 67% to 70% have a single PNET.[21]

NF1, also known as Von Recklinghausen disease, has an uncommon incidence of PNETs, reported in up to 10%. These are almost exclusively duodenal somatostatinomas, usually occurring in the periampullary region. The behavior of duodenal somatostatinomas in patients with NF1 is similar to that of sporadic duodenal somatostatinomas in most respects.[21]

Less than 1% of patients with tuberous sclerosis, also known as Bourneville disease, subsequently have PNETs. Both F-PNETs and NF-PNETs have been reported.[9,21]

CLINICAL BEHAVIORS AND DIAGNOSIS OF SPECIFIC PANCREATIC NEUROENDOCRINE TUMORS
Nonfunctional Pancreatic Neuroendocrine Tumors

NF-PNETs frequently synthesize more than one peptide, but they do not produce a specific syndrome. For this reason, they are either incidentally discovered, or their presenting symptoms are related to tumor mass, invasion of adjacent structures, or metastatic disease. These symptoms may include abdominal pain, weight loss, anorexia, nausea, and jaundice. Patients may also present with a palpable mass. Historically, NF-PNETs presented late in the disease course, with 70% being greater than 5 cm and more than 60% presenting with synchronous liver metastases.[9] Currently, however, the incidental discovery of these tumors seems to be increasing because of the increased use of computed tomography imaging for other indications.

Hormones secreted by NF-PNETs include pancreatic polypeptide, chromogranin A, neuron-specific enolase, ghrelin, neurotensin, and subunits of human chorionicgonadotropin. If an NF-PNET is suspected, initial workup should include serum levels of chromogranin A, which is elevated in 88% to 100% of PNETs, with a diagnostic sensitivity of 60% to 100% in patients with metastatic disease but less than 50% in patients with localized disease. Other possible PNET markers include serum neuron-specific enolase, which is elevated in 83% to 100% of PNETs, and pancreatic polypeptide, elevated in 50% to 100%. Somatostatin receptor scintigraphy may also be of use in the workup of suspected NF-PNET. A confirmed diagnosis requires histologic analysis.[22–26] **Table 2** reviews recommended diagnostic tests for various PNETs.

Insulinoma

Insulinomas are the most common F-PNET, with an incidence of 0.1 to 0.3 per million per year.[27] They are also the most benign F-PNET, with less than 10% reported to be malignant on diagnosis and greater than 95% amenable to surgical cure.[28] All insulinomas are found within the pancreas, and they are equally distributed throughout the organ. Insulinomas are usually small tumors (82%–90% <2 cm) and 90% are solitary.[27,29] Ninety percent are sporadic, although 5% to 10% are associated with MEN1, and in this population they are also predominantly multiple.[21] Insulinomas most commonly present between ages of 40 and 45 years, and there is a slight female predominance.[30]

Insulinomas secrete insulin, and their clinical syndrome is from the resulting hypoglycemia caused by elevated insulin levels. Hypoglycemia causes neuroglycopenic symptoms in 90%, and autonomic symptoms, which occur in 60% to 70% of patients.[31] Neuroglycopenia includes psychiatric and neurologic manifestations of

Table 2 Diagnostic workup of PNETs	
Tumor	**Diagnostic Tests**
NF-PNETs	Chromogranin A
Insulinoma	Blood glucose, insulin, C-peptide, proinsulin, β-hydroxybutyrate, plasma and urine sulfonylurea metabolites 72H fast; genetic testing for MEN1 is recommended if there is a personal or family history of endocrinopathy, or if there are multiple tumors
Gastrinoma	FSG level, gastric pH, BAO, and secretin test; genetic testing for MEN1 is recommended for all gastrinomas
Glucagonoma	Serum glucagon level
VIPoma	Plasma VIP level
Somatostatinoma	Serum SS level; genetic testing for NF1 is recommended for all duodenal and periampullary SSomas
GRFoma	Serum GH-releasing factor level
ACTHoma	24-hour urinary cortisol, midnight plasma or salivary cortisol, dexamethasone suppression tests as needed
PTHrp-oma	Serum ionized calcium, serum PTH, serum PTHrp
PNET causing carcinoid syndrome	Serum serotonin, urine 5-HIAA

Abbreviations: BAO, basal acid output; FSG, fasting serum gastrin; SS, somatostatin.

hypoglycemia, including confusion, visual disturbances, amnesia, coma, altered consciousness, behavioral changes, headache, and seizures. Hypoglycemia also results in catecholamine excess and autonomic symptoms including sweating, weakness, palpitations, tremor, paresthesias, and hunger. These symptoms are more likely to be present when the body is substrate deficient, such as during exercise or while fasting. This point is important to keep in mind when differentiating patients with potential insulinomas from the growing population of patients with hypoglycemia occurring after bariatric surgery, whose hypoglycemic symptoms are more often postprandial. There is usually a delay in diagnosis of insulinoma, and as a result weight gain is also frequently present as patients learn from their symptoms that these episodes of hypoglycemia can be prevented with frequent oral intake.

Insulinoma should be suspected in any patient with the classically described Whipple's triad: (1) symptoms of hypoglycemia while fasting, (2) documented hypoglycemia, and (3) relief of symptoms with administration of exogenous glycose.[32] The classical gold standard for establishing the diagnosis of is a 72-hour fast.[33] The diagnosis of insulinoma is absolutely established using the following 6 criteria: (1) documented blood glucose levels $\leq$2.2 mmol/L ($\leq$40 mg/dL), (2) concomitant insulin levels $\geq$6 μU/mL ($\geq$36 pmol/L; $\geq$3 U/L by immunochemiluminescent assay), (3) C-peptide levels $\geq$200 pmol/L, (4) proinsulin levels $\geq$5 pmol/L, (5) β-hydroxybutyrate levels $\leq$2.7 mmol/L, and (6) absence of sulfonylurea(metabolites) in the plasma or urine.[28]

Gastrinoma

Gastrinomas are the second most common F-PNET, with an incidence of 0.5 to 2 per 100,000 per year.[9,28,34,35] They are classically located in the gastrinoma triangle, which is bound by the junction of the cystic and common bile ducts, the junction of the second and third parts of the duodenum, and the junction of the neck and body of the pancreas. Seventy percent of gastrinomas are located in the duodenum, 25% are found in the pancreas, and 5% are found in adjacent tissues.[36] Duodenal gastrinomas are smaller and more likely to be multiple compared with pancreatic gastrinomas, which are larger and more likely to be metastatic on diagnosis.[35] Sixty percent to 90% of gastrinomas are malignant, and one-third present with metastatic disease at the time of diagnosis, most commonly to the liver.[19] Twenty percent to 30% of gastrinomas are associated with MEN1; therefore, it is recommended that all patients with gastrinoma undergo screening for MEN1.[28,37]

Gastrinomas produce a clinical syndrome known as Zollinger-Ellison syndrome (ZES), which results from tumor production of excessive gastrin. High gastrin levels produce high gastric acid output. As a result patients develop peptic ulcer disease (PUD) or gastroesophageal reflux disease, leading to abdominal pain in 75% to 98% of cases. Other symptoms include diarrhea (30%–73%), bleeding (44%–75%), and weight loss (7%–53%).[28,35,37,38] Chronic hypergastrinemia also has trophic effects on the gastric mucosa. As a result, prominent gastric folds have been described in up to 92% of patients with gastrinomas, and this diagnosis should be suspected whenever seen on endoscopy.[28,31,37,38] Gastrinoma should also be suspected in any patient with recurrent, severe, or familial PUD; PUD without *Helicobacter pylori* or other risk factors; PUD with diarrhea, especially if diarrhea resolves with treatment with proton pump inhibitors (PPIs); and finally PUD associated with personal or family history of endocrinopathies or hypercalcemia. Patients with multiple ulcers, ulcers in unusual locations, and complications of PUD (obstruction, perforation, bleeding) are also classically highly suspicious for gastrinoma, although these presentations may be declining with the efficacy of current PPI therapy.[28,31,37,38]

The recent increase in the use of PPIs has implications for both the presentation and diagnosis of gastrinomas. Unlike H2 blockers, PPIs are effective at controlling the symptoms of acid hypersecretion seen in gastrinomas, potentially masking or delaying the diagnosis. Additionally, PPIs result in hypergastrinemia in patients without gastrinoma and thus must be stopped 1 week before diagnostic testing to avoid false-positive results.[9,39–42]

Once gastrinoma is suspected, a combination of laboratory studies can establish the diagnosis: fasting serum gastrin (FSG) level, gastric pH, basal acid output (BAO), and secretin test. FSG is usually the first study performed when gastrinoma is suspected. It is a great screening test, as FSG is elevated in greater than 98% of all gastrinomas.[31,38,42] However, there are other causes of elevated gastrin, so FSG alone cannot confirm the diagnosis. The next test to order after elevated FSG is confirmed is a gastric pH level. A gastric pH of greater than 2 excludes gastrinoma.[37–39] In 40% of patients, FSG levels are greater than 10-fold elevated. If in these patients gastric pH is also found to be less than 2, the diagnosis of gastrinoma is confirmed. For the 60% of patients whose FSG is less than 10 fold elevated and gastric pH is less than 2, the next step we recommend is a BAO and a secretin test. The diagnosis of gastrinoma is supported by a BAO of greater than 15 mEq/h in patients without prior vagotomy or gastrectomy.[43] The addition of a positive secretin test confirms the diagnosis. Secretin should normally decrease gastrin levels by an inhibitory feedback loop, but when a gastrinoma is present then secretin stimulation causes paradoxic elevation in the gastrin levels.[44]

Glucagonoma

Glucagonomas are rare even among F-PNETs, with an incidence of 0.04 to 0.12 per million per year.[45] Glucagonomas are typically diagnosed in the fifth decade and are equally distributed between the sexes.[46] All glucagonomas occur in the pancreas and are found most frequently in the tail.[47] Glucagonomas are usually large tumors (>5 cm), more than 60% are malignant, and 50% to 80% present with metastatic liver disease.[48,49]

Glucagonoma syndrome is characterize by weight loss (60%–90%); diabetes mellitus (40%–95%); gastrointestinal symptoms such as diarrhea (10%–25%), constipation, abdominal pain, and anorexia; and neurologic symptoms such as ataxia, dementia, depression, optic atrophy, and proximal muscle weakness.[9,31,48,49] Glucagonoma syndrome also causes a specific dermatitis in up to 90% of patients, called *necrolytic migratory erythema* (NME). NME is characterized by erythematous macules, papules, or plaques that progressively enlarge, necrose, and then form pigmented scars. The mucous membranes may be similarly affected, producing glossitis, cheilitis, stomatitis, and blepharitis.[9,19,31,48,49] Thromboembolism has been reported in up to 50% of patients with glucagonoma.[19,50,51] The glucagonoma syndrome has been referred to as the *4Ds syndrome*, referencing the symptoms of dermatitis, diabetes, depression, and deep vein thrombosis.[50,51]

Laboratory studies frequently find anemia (30%–90%), and hypoaminoacidemia (30%–100%).[48,49] Diagnosis requires serum glucagon levels of greater than 500 pg/mL, although this is not specific to glucagonoma, as other disease entities can cause hyperglucagonemia.[9,31] NME is also not specific to glucagonoma. A combination of high glucagon levels, abnormal imaging, and symptoms make the diagnosis.

VIPoma

VIPoma is another rare F-PNET, with an incidence of 1 per ten million per year.[19] VIPomas are most often sporadic, solitary lesions greater than 3 cm in diameter. Eighty-five percent to 95% form in the pancreas, with 75% found in the tail. Vasoactive intestinal peptide (VIP)-secreting tumors have also been found in the bronchus, colon, adrenals, and liver.[19] In children, VIPomas are commonly seen in extrapancreatic ganglioneuromas.[9,49] Seventy percent to 90% are malignant, and 60% to 80% are metastatic on diagnosis.[19]

VIPomas produce a clinical syndrome known as *Verner-Morrison syndrome*, WDHA syndrome (watery diarrhea, hypokalemia, and achlorhydria), or pancreatic cholera syndrome. Excessive VIP produces a large volume of watery diarrhea. Stool volume is greater than 3 L/d in 70% to 80% and continues even during fasting, as it is secretory in nature.[9,49] This watery diarrhea leads to dehydration (45%–95%), hypokalemia (70%–100%), and achlorhydria (35%–76%) (hence, WDHA syndrome).[9] Other electrolyte abnormalities include metabolic acidosis, hypercalcemia (25%–50%), and hyperglycemia (20%–50%).[9] Other symptoms result from vasodilation, including flushing (15%–30%) and hypotension and from dehydration and hypokalemia, including lethargy, nausea, vomiting, and muscle cramps and weakness.[49,52]

Diagnosis is established with a large volume of watery diarrhea (>700 mL/d) that is secretory in nature (no osmolar gap in stool fluid) in addition to plasma VIP level greater than 500 pg/mL. Most patients also have clear evidence on imaging of tumor mass.[9,49]

Somatostatinoma

Somatostatinomas (SSomas) are rare PNETs, occurring in less than one in 40 million people.[53] As a result of their rarity, their presentation is poorly defined. About half occur in the pancreas and the other half in the duodenum and jejunum. Sixty percent to 70% are malignant, and pancreatic SSomas are more often malignant than duodenal SSomas.[54] These tumors can rarely occur in association with VHL or MEN1 and in up to 10% of NF1 patients.[21,54] In NF1 patients SSomas are found almost exclusively in the duodenum, characteristically in the periampullary region.[21] Most

SSomas, however, are found incidentally. The most common symptoms of SSomas are caused by tumor mass effect. A true SSoma syndrome is seen in less than 10% of patients with these tumors. This rare syndrome is characterized by diabetes, gallbladder disease, weight loss, diarrhea, steatorrhea, and anemia. Pancreatic SSomas are more likely to produce this SSoma syndrome, whereas 90% to 98% of small bowel SSomas do not.[9,49,54]

The diagnosis of SSoma is rarely made before surgery or biopsy. Diagnosis is most strongly supported by a pancreatic or duodenal mass and an elevated serum SS level. Currently, there is no confirmatory test for patients with typical symptoms but no visible mass. If a duodenal or periampullary SSoma is found, genetic screening for NF1 is recommended, as this genetic syndrome accounts for 48% of all duodenal SSomas reported in the literature.[21]

GRFoma

GRFomas are so rare that their incidence is unknown. They are malignant in 30% to 50% of cases.[55] GRFomas arise in several organs including the pancreas (30%–57%), lung (50%–54%), small intestine (8%–75%), and other rare locations including the adrenal glands.[9,19,31,55]

GRFomas present with acromegaly that is clinically indistinguishable from that seen with pituitary adenomas. GRFomas account for less than 1% of all acromegaly.[55] GRFomas should be suspected in patients with acromegaly without pituitary adenoma, with an abdominal mass, or with a paradoxic response to thyroid-stimulating hormone or glucose-load. The diagnosis is confirmed by elevated serum growth hormone–releasing factor level.

ACTHoma

ACTHomas secrete adrenocorticotropic hormone (ACTH) and produce Cushing's syndrome. ACTHomas are rare and malignant in 95% of cases.[19,56,57] ACTHomas are located in the pancreas and appear to be distributed evenly throughout the organ[57] and are more frequent in women than in men, with a mean age of diagnosis of 42 years.[57,58] ACTHomas make up 4% to 25% of all ectopic Cushing's syndrome. ACTHomas may occur concurrently in patients with ZES. One series reported an incidence of ACTHoma in 8% of patients with ZES.[56] The incidence of gastrin production in ACTHomas has been reported from 26% to 80%.[57] Because these tumors tend to be large, one study has suggested that once the diagnosis of ectopic ACTH production has been made, if pancreatic-specific imaging fails to depict a pancreatic mass or liver metastases, an ACTH-secreting PNET can be ruled out as a potential source of ACTH production.[57]

PTHrp-oma

Parathyroid hormone–related peptide–secreting PNETs (PTHrp-omas) are rare but are being recognized as an F-PNET. PTHrp-omas are found in the pancreas, appear to be low grade in most cases, and are malignant in greater than 85%.[19,59,60] They cause hypercalcemia and resultant symptoms. PTHrp-omas should be considered in the differential diagnosis of patients with pancreatic lesions with hypercalcemia and a disproportionately low PTH.

Pancreatic Neuroendocrine Tumors Causing Carcinoid Syndrome

There are less than 50 reported cases of pancreatic carcinoids. These pancreatic carcinoids are found in the pancreatic body or tail in 70% of cases[61] and are usually large tumors and mostly malignant on diagnosis (60%–90%).[19,62] As a result, they are associated with a high incidence of carcinoid syndrome. They account for less than 1% of gastrointestinal carcinoids and have less favorable outcomes than other gastro-intestinal carcinoids.[61,62]

Pancreatic carcinoids may oversecrete serotonin or tachykinins. The most common symptoms are abdominal pain and diarrhea. The diarrhea results from pancreatic exocrine insufficiency and the action of serotonin on the intestine. Diagnosis requires serum serotonin or measurement of its derivative, 5-HIAA, in urine.

TUMOR BEHAVIOR AND PROGNOSIS

PNETs are a heterogeneous group of tumors in their clinical behavior, pathology, loca-tion, malignant potential, and survival rates. It is a challenge to understand the natural history of PNETs for this and many other reasons. Identification of prognostic factors in PNETs is currently evolving. Metastases usually first develop in regional lymph nodes followed by the liver. Liver metastases seem to be a better predictor of prog-nosis than lymph node disease and in general are a poor prognostic factor for PNETs.[9,28] Low-grade (G1 and G2) PNETs have an overall 10-year survival rate of 60% to 70%. G1 T1N0M0 tumors have a good prognosis, with a 10-year survival rate of greater than 95%. Poorly differentiated PNETs, G3, have a worse prognosis.[63]

SUMMARY

PNETs account for a growing proportion of pancreatic tumors. Nonfunctional PNETs are being detected more frequently because of the widespread use of high-quality im-aging to evaluate other diseases. Functional PNETs are rare, but the surgeon needs to be aware of the various signs and symptoms that may occur in a patient being eval-uated with a pancreatic mass. The surgeon should be capable of ordering targeted hormone studies to make the diagnosis of an F-PNET. Many patients have had symp-toms for years before diagnosis, and being cognizant that other medical issues even as common as PUD or diabetes can occur from F-PNETs is excellent clinical practice.

REFERENCES

1. Piaditis G, Angellou A, Kontogeorgos G, et al. Ectopic bioactive luteinizing hor-mone secretion by a pancreatic endocrine tumor, manifested as luteinized gran-ulosathecal cell tumor of the ovaries. J Clin Endocrinol Metab 2005;90:2097–103.
2. Brignardello E, Manti R, Papotti M, et al. Ectopic secretion of LH by an endocrine pancreatic tumor. J Endocrinol Invest 2004;27:361–5.
3. Samyn I, Fontaine C, Van Tussenbroek F, et al. Paraneoplastic syndromes in can-cer: case 1. Polycythemia as a result of ectopic erythropoietin production in met-astatic pancreatic carcinoid tumor. J Clin Oncol 2004;22:2240–2.
4. Chung JO, Hong SI, Cho DH, et al. Hypoglycemia associated with the production of insulin-like growth factor II in a pancreatic islet cell tumor: a case report. En-docr J 2008;55:607–12.
5. Stevens FM, Flanagan RW, O'Gorman D, et al. Glucagonoma syndrome demon-strating giant duodenal villi. Gut 1984;25:351–4.
6. Ruddy MC, Atlas SA, Salerno FG. Hypertension associated with a renin-secreting adenocarcinoma of the pancreas. N Engl J Med 1982;307:993–7.
7. Roberts RE, Zhao M, Whitelaw BC, et al. GLP-1 and glucagon secretion from a pancreatic neuroendocrine tumor causing diabetes and hyperinsulinemic hypo-glycemia. J Clin Endocrinol Metab 2012;97:3039–45.

8. Byrne MM, McGregor GP, Barth P, et al. Intestinal proliferation and delayed intestinal transit in a patient with a GLP-1-, GLP-2 and PYY-producing neuroendocrine carcinoma. Digestion 2001;63:61–8.

9. Metz DC, Jensen RT. Gastrointestinal neuroendocrine tumors: pancreatic endocrine tumors. Gastroenterology 2008;135:1469–92.

10. Vinik AI, Strodel WE, Eckhauser FE, et al. Somatostatinomas, PPomas, neurotensinomas. Semin Oncol 1987;14:263–81.

11. Wang HS, Oh DS, Ohning GV, et al. Elevated serum ghrelin exerts an orexigenic effect that may maintain body mass index in patients with metastatic neuroendocrine tumors. J Mol Neurosci 2007;33:225–31.

12. Barker N, van Es JH, Kuipers J, et al. Identification of stem cells in small intestine and colon by marker gene Lgr5. Nature 2007;449:1003–7.

13. Klimstra D, Arnold R, Capella C, et al. Neuroendocrine neoplasms of the pancreas. In: Bosman F, Carneiro F, Hruban R, et al, editors. WHO classification of tumours of the digestive system. 3rd edition. Lyon (France): IARC; 2010. p. 322–6.

14. AJCC. Cancer staging manual. 7th edition. New York: Springer; 2010.

15. Sobin L, Gospodarowicz M, Wittekind C. UICC: TNM classification of malignant tumors. 7th edition. Oxford (United Kingdom): Wiley-Blackwell; 2009.

16. Rindi G, Kloppel G, Alhman H, et al. TNM staging of foregut (neuro)endocrine tumors: a consensus proposal including a grading system. Virchows Arch 2006; 449(4):395–401.

17. Ito T, Sasano H, Tanaka M, et al. Epidemiological study of gastroenteropancreatic neuroendocrine tumors in Japan. J Gastroenterol 2010;45:234–43.

18. Gullo L, Migliori M, Falconi M, et al. Nonfunctioning pancreatic endocrine tumors: a multicenter clinical study. Am J Gastroenterol 2003;98:2435–9.

19. Grozinsky-Glasberg S, Mazeh H, Gross DJ. Clinical features of pancreatic neuroendocrine tumors. J Hepatobiliary Pancreat Sci 2015;22(8):578–85.

20. Marchegiani G, Crippa S, Malleo G, et al. Surgical treatment of pancreatic tumors in childhood and adolescence: uncommon neoplasms with favorable outcome. Pancreatology 2011;11:383–9.

21. Jensen RT, Berna MJ, Bingham DB, et al. Inherited pancreatic endocrine tumor syndromes: advances in molecular pathogenesis, diagnosis, management, and controversies. Cancer 2008;113:1807–43.

22. de Herder WW. Biochemistry of neuroendocrine tumours. Best Pract Res Clin Endocrinol Metab 2007;21:33–41.

23. Nobels FR, Kwekkeboom DJ, Coopmans W, et al. Chromogranin A as serum marker for neuroendocrine neoplasia: comparison with neuron-specific enolase and the alpha-subunit of glycoprotein hormones. J Clin Endocrinol Metab 1997;82:2622–8.

24. Campana D, Nori F, Piscitelli L, et al. Chromogranin A: is it a useful marker of neuroendocrine tumors? J Clin Oncol 2007;25:1967–73.

25. Zatelli MC, Torta M, Leon A, et al. Chromogranin A as a marker of neuroendocrine neoplasia: an Italian Multicenter Study. Endocr Relat Cancer 2007;14: 473–82.

26. Baudin E. Gastroenteropancreatic endocrine tumors: clinical characterization before therapy. Nat Clin Pract Endocrinol Metab 2007;3:228–39.

27. de Herder WW, Niederle B, Scoazec JY, et al. Well-differentiated pancreatic tumor/carcinoma:insulinoma. Neuroendocrinology 2006;84:183–8.

28. Jensen RT, Cadiot G, Brandi ML, et al, Barcelona Consensus Conference Participants. ENETS consensus guidelines for the management of patients with

digestive neuroendocrine neoplasms: functional pancreatic endocrine tumor syndromes. Neuroendocrinology 2012;95:98–119.

29. Finlayson E, Clark OH. Surgical treatment of insulinomas. Surg Clin North Am 2004;84:775–85.

30. Vezzosi D, Bennet A, Fauvel J, et al. Insulin, C-peptide and proinsulin for the biochemical diagnosis of hypoglycaemia related to endogenous hyperinsulinism. Eur J Endocrinol 2007;157:75–83.

31. Ito T, Igarashi H, Jensen RT. Pancreatic neuroendocrine tumors: clinical features, diagnosis and medical treatment: advances. Best Pract Res Clin Gastroenterol 2012;26:737–53.

32. Whipple AO, Frantz VK. Adenoma of islet cells with hyperinsulinism: a review. Ann Surg 1935;101:1299–335.

33. Grant CS. Insulinoma. Best Pract Res Clin Gastroenterol 2005;19:783–98.

34. Oberg K. Pancreatic endocrine tumors. Semin Oncol 2010;37:594–618.

35. Ellison EC, Johnson JA. The Zollinger-Ellison syndrome: a comprehensive review of historical, scientific, and clinical considerations. Curr Probl Surg 2009;46: 13–106.

36. Zogakis TG, Gibril F, Libutti SK, et al. Management and outcome of patients with sporadic gastrinoma arising in the duodenum. Ann Surg 2003;238:42–8.

37. Grimaldi F, Fazio N, Attanasio R, et al. Italian association of clinical endocrinologists (AME) position statement: a stepwise clinical approach to the diagnosis of gastroenteropancreatic neuroendocrine neoplasms. J Endocrinol Invest 2014;37: 875–909.

38. Roy PK, Venzon DJ, Shojamanesh H, et al. Zollinger-Ellison syndrome. Clinical presentation in 261 patients. Medicine (Baltimore) 2000;79:379–411.

39. Banasch M, Schmitz F. Diagnosis and treatment of gastrinoma in the era of proton pump inhibitors. Wien Klin Wochenschr 2007;119:573–8.

40. Osefo N, Ito T, Jensen RT. Gastric acid hyper-secretory states: recent insights and advances. Curr Gastroenterol Rep 2009;11:433–41.

41. O'Toole D, Grossman A, Gross D, et al. ENETS consensus guidelines for the standards of care in neuroendocrine tumors: biochemical markers. Neuroendocrinology 2009;90:194–202.

42. Ito T, Cadiot G, Jensen RT. Diagnosis of Zollinger-Ellison syndrome: increasingly difficult. World J Gastroenterol 2012;18:5495–503.

43. Roy PK, Venzon DJ, Feigenbaum KM, et al. Gastric secretion in Zollinger-Ellison syndrome: correlation with clinical expression, tumor extent and role in diagnosis - A prospective NIH study of 235 patients and review of the literature in 984 cases. Medicine (Baltimore) 2001;80:189–222.

44. Berna MJ, Hoffmann KM, Long SH, et al. Serum gastrin in Zollinger- Ellison syndrome: II. Prospective study of gastrin provocative testing in 293 patients from the National Institutes of Health and comparison with 537 cases from the literature. Evaluation of diagnostic criteria, proposal of new criteria, and correlations with clinical and tumoral features. Medicine (Baltimore) 2006;85:331–64.

45. Halfdanarson TR, Rubin J, Farnell MB, et al. Pancreatic endocrine neoplasms: epidemiology and prognosis of pancreatic endocrine tumors. Endocr Relat Cancer 2008;15:409–27.

46. Kindmark H, Sundin A, Granberg D, et al. Endocrine pancreatic tumors with glucagon hyper- secretion: a retrospective study of 23 cases during 20 years. Med Oncol 2007;24:330–7.

47. Wermers RA, Fatourechi V, Wynne AG, et al. The glucagonoma syndrome. Clinical and pathologic features in 21 patients. Medicine (Baltimore) 1996;75:53–63.

48. Wermers RA, Fatourechi V, Kvols LK. Clinical spectrum of hyperglucagonemia associated with malignant neuroendocrine tumors. Mayo Clin Proc 1996;71: 1030–8.

49. Jensen RT, Norton JA. Endocrine tumors of the pancreas and gastrointestinal tract. In: Feldman M, Friedman LS, Brandt LJ, editors. Sleisenger and Fordtran's gastrointestinal and liver disease. Philadelphia: Saunders; 2010. p. 491–522.

50. Vinik A, Feliberti E, Perry RR. Glucagonoma syndrome. In: De Groot LJ, Beck-Peccoz P, Chrousos G, et al, editors. Endotext [Internet]. South Dartmouth (MA): MDText.com, Inc; 2014. 2000.

51. de Wilde RF, Edil BH, Hruban RH, et al. Well-differentiated pancreatic neuroendocrine tumors: from genetics to therapy. Nat Rev Gastroenterol Hepatol 2012;9: 199–208.

52. Mekhjian HS, O'Dorisio TM. VIPoma syndrome. Semin Oncol 1987;14:282–91.

53. House MG, Yeo CJ, Schulick RD. Periampullary pancreatic somatostatinoma. Ann Surg Oncol 2002;9:869–74.

54. Nesi G, Marcucci T, Rubio CA, et al. Somatostatinoma: clinico-pathological features of three cases and literature reviewed. J Gastroenterol Hepatol 2008;23: 521–6.

55. Garby L, Caron P, Claustrat F, et al. Clinical characteristics and outcome of acromegaly induced by ectopic secretion of growth hormone-releasing hormone (GHRH): a French nationwide series of 21 cases. J Clin Endocrinol Metab 2012;97:2093–104.

56. Maton PN, Gardner JD, Jensen RT. Cushing's syndrome in patients with the Zollinger-Ellison syndrome. N Engl J Med 1986;315:1–5.

57. Doppman JLK, Nieman LK, Cutler GB Jr, et al. Adrenocorticotropic hormone-secreting islet cell tumors: are they always malignant? Radiology 1994;190: 59–64.

58. Maragliano R, Vanoli A, Albarello L, et al. ACTH-secreting pancreatic neoplasms associated with Cushing syndrome: clinicopathologic study of 11 cases and review of the literature. Am J Surg Pathol 2015;39:374–82.

59. Srirajaskanthan R, McStay M, Toumpanakis C, et al. Parathyroid hormone-related peptide-secreting pancreatic neuroendocrine tumours: case series and literature review. Neuroendocrinology 2009;89:48–55.

60. Kanakis G, Kaltsas G, Granberg D, et al. Unusual complication of a pancreatic neuroendocrine tumor presenting with malignant hypercalcemia. J Clin Endocrinol Metab 2012;97:E627–31.

61. Waisberg J, de Matos LL, Dos Santos HV, et al. Pancreatic carcinoid: a rare cause of diarrheogenic syndrome. Clinics (Sao Paulo) 2006;61:175–8.

62. Mao C, El Attar A, Domenico DR, et al. Carcinoid tumors of the pancreas. Status report based on two cases and review of the world's literature. Int J Pancreatol 1998;23:153–64.

63. Reid MD, Balci S, Saka B, et al. Neuroendocrine tumors of the pancreas: current concepts and controversies. Endocr Pathol 2014;25:65–79.

State-of-the-art Imaging of Pancreatic Neuroendocrine Tumors

Eric P. Tamm, MD[a],*, Priya Bhosale, MD[a], Jeffrey H. Lee, MD[b], Eric M. Rohren, MD, PhD[c]

KEYWORDS

- Pancreatic neuroendocrine tumor • Computed tomography • Dual energy • MRI
- PET/CT • Octreotide • Endoscopic ultrasonography • Imaging

KEY POINTS

- Knowledge of the type of functional tumor (eg, gastrinoma versus insulinoma) is important in choosing appropriate imaging strategies to identify primary lesions and their metastases.
- Fluorodeoxyglucose PET/computed tomography (CT) has poor sensitivity for well-differentiated pancreatic neuroendocrine tumors but good sensitivity for poorly differentiated types, and therefore has a complementary role with octreotide scanning.
- To optimize treatment planning, it is important to inspect all potential sites of disease, particularly with regard to the extent of liver and nodal involvement, and potential distant metastases to lung and bone.
- Metastatic adenopathy can show enhancement similar to adjacent vasculature structures and can be difficult to detect on CT. MRI, particularly diffusion-weighted imaging, and nuclear medicine studies can be helpful.

INTRODUCTION

Pancreatic neuroendocrine tumors (PNETs) account for only 3% of pancreatic malignancies, but have an increasing incidence, currently 0.3 to 0.4 per 100,000.[1–3] They are notably more common in multiple endocrine neoplasia type I (MEN-I), von Hippel-Lindau syndrome, neurofibromatosis type I, and tuberous sclerosis.[4,5] PNETs can be divided into 2 groups: functional tumors, usually subcentimeter, that manifest

Disclosure: The authors have nothing to disclose.
[a] Diagnostic Radiology, University of Texas MD Anderson Cancer Center, Unit 1473, PO Box 301402, Houston, TX 77230-1402, USA; [b] Department of Gastroenterology, Hepatology and Nutrition, T. Boone Pickens Academic Tower (FCT13.6028), 1515 Holcombe Boulevard, Unit 1466, Houston, TX 77030, USA; [c] Department of Nuclear Medicine, T. Boone Pickens Academic Tower (FCT16.6012), 1515 Holcombe Boulevard, Unit 1483, Houston, TX 77030, USA
* Corresponding author.
E-mail address: etamm@mdanderson.org

because of the symptoms caused by the hormones they produce; and nonfunctional tumors, usually several centimeters, that manifest secondary to mass effect.

State-of-the-art imaging plays a central role in the identification, diagnosis, and staging of PNETs. Computed tomography (CT) and MRI are often used initially to detect and stage these lesions, and evolving nuclear medicine techniques provide improved specificity and whole-body assessments for distant disease. A multimodality approach may be necessary to identify potentially very small primary tumors and to identify all sites of metastatic disease to optimize treatment planning.

IMAGING TECHNIQUES
Computed Tomography

CT is often used for the initial evaluation of patients with abdominal pain or to identify suspected small functional PNETs because of its speed, resolution, and robustness. Recent advances allow detailed multiplanar reconstructions, and new low-kilovoltage imaging or multispectral imaging may improve the conspicuity of PNETs.

A typical abdominal multidetector CT examination for PNET is multiphasic (**Figs. 1** and **2**).[6] Unenhanced images may be obtained to help identify calcifications or hemorrhage. At our institution, patients are then imaged following injection of iodinated intravenous contrast at 4 to 5 mL per second for an injection duration of approximately 30 seconds, with abdominal imaging obtained first at 40 to 45 seconds after the start of contrast injection for the late arterial phase of enhancement, and then 60 to 70 seconds after the start of contrast injection for the portal venous phase (see **Figs. 1** and **2**). Images are created at a slice thickness of 2 to 3 mm for diagnostic review, and at 0.625 mm for creating coronal and sagittal multiplanar reconstructions to facilitate problem solving. CT was reported in a 2009 consensus statement to have a mean

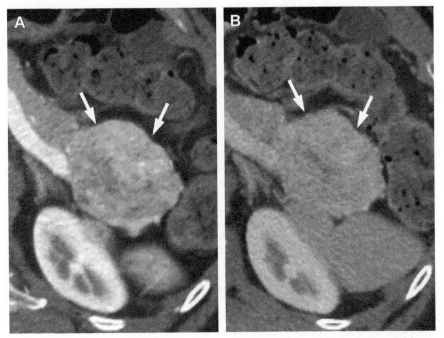

Fig. 1. Pancreatic tail neuroendocrine tumor (*white arrows*) on multiphasic CT is (*A*) hyperdense to background on the arterial phase and (*B*) isodense on the portal venous phase.

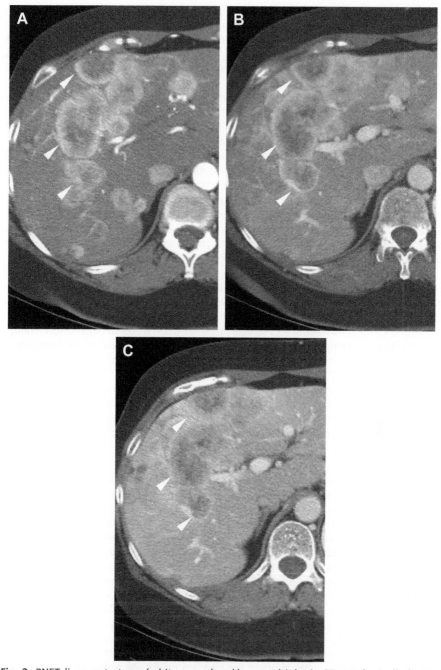

Fig. 2. PNET liver metastases (*white arrowheads*) on multiphasic CT are classically hyperdense to background on (*A*) early and (*B*) late arterial phases and either isodense or hypodense on (*C*) portal venous phase, but they can be variable.

sensitivity of 73% and specificity of 96%.[7] Sensitivities for small functional tumors, such as insulinomas, vary by phase: approximately 83% to 88% for the arterial phase versus 11% to 76% for portal venous phase imaging, although a small study of 13 patients evaluating the late arterial phase (pancreatic parenchymal phase) showed a sensitivity of 100% for that phase.[8–11] Detection is optimized by close evaluation of all phases.

New multispectral CT may improve detection of subtle differences in enhancement between lesions and background. Conventional multidetector CT uses a single polychromatic energy beam (eg, 120 kV peak [kVp]). Multispectral imaging uses either 2 polychromatic beams of high and low strengths (eg, 80 kVp and 140 kVp) or a dual-layer detector that can discriminate between photons of high and low energy.[12,13] Multispectral imaging uses these additional data to mathematically create new types of images (**Figs. 3** and **4**), two of the most common being monochromatic energy images (the equivalent of theoretically being scanned at a discrete single energy level), and material density or material decomposition images (semiquantitative images based on decomposing image data into representative amounts of just 2 or more materials to mimic the actual behavior at each image voxel).[12] The precise makeup of material decomposition images varies between vendors.

Low-energy monochromatic images (ie, 40–50 keV) improve the conspicuity of contrast enhancement. A small study investigating the detection of insulinoma compared 16 patients scanned with conventional dual-phase multidetector CT with 23 patients scanned with rapid switching single-source dual-energy dual-phase multidetector CT.[14] A sensitivity of 95.7% was obtained when a combination of low-energy monochromatic energy images and iodine (minus water) material decomposition images were used, compared with a sensitivity of 68.8% for conventional dual-phase multidetector CT.[14]

Another related approach has been the use of a low polychromatic kVp (ie, 80 kVp) technique, which improved contrast to noise results compared with conventional 140-kVp imaging for overall pancreatic tumor imaging but did not statistically improve tumor detection.[15] To our knowledge, no assessment has been published of this technique for PNETs.

MRI

MRI offers several advantages for the imaging of PNETs, including multiple different sequences that provide opportunities to differentiate tumor from normal pancreas. A typical abdominal protocol at our institution includes fat-suppressed T2-weighted; fat-suppressed precontrast and post-contrast dynamically obtained T1-weighted, in-phase and out-of-phase T1-weighted images; diffusion-weighted images with multiple b values and apparent diffusion coefficient (ADC) maps; and fat-suppressed true fast imaging with steady-state precession (FISP) or fast imaging employing steady-state acquisition (FIESTA) images (**Fig. 5**). An effective slice thickness of 3 to 6 mm is used to minimize volume averaging artifact and improve sensitivity. The overall sensitivity of MRI published in a consensus report was 93%, with specificity of 88%.[7] Limitations of MRI include greater frequency of motion-related artifacts and a longer imaging time compared with CT. Benefits include good sensitivity even in the absence of administration of an intravenous contrast agent (making it a useful alternative for patients with renal impairment or allergy to iodine-based CT contrast agents) and the absence of ionizing radiation, which is of particular concern in young patients who may require surveillance. Recent studies of advances in diffusion-weighted imaging suggest potential for improving detection,[16] differentiating accessory spleen from small islet cell tumors,[17] differentiating near-solid serous cystadenomas from neuroendocrine tumors,[18]

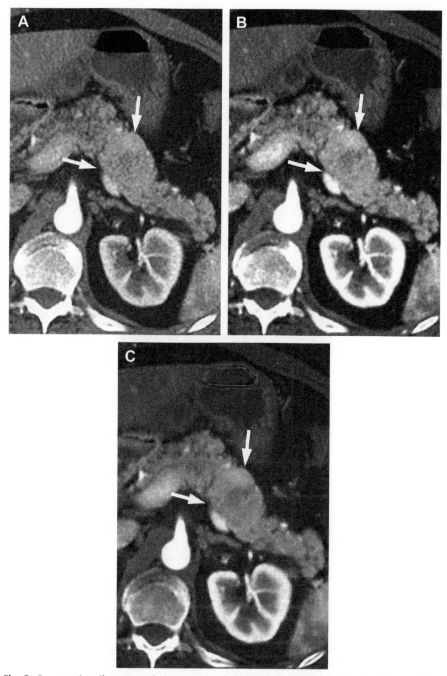

Fig. 3. Pancreatic tail neuroendocrine tumor (*white arrows*) seen on late arterial phase CT, as seen (*A*) conventionally at 140 kVp, and more conspicuously at dual-energy CT (DECT) (*B*), low-energy 50-keV, and (*C*) iodine (minus water) material density images.

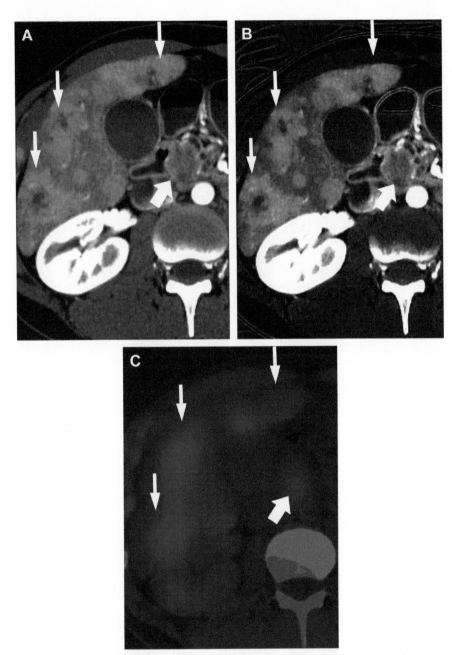

Fig. 4. PNET metastases to liver (*white arrows*) and nodes (*thick white arrow*) seen on DECT late arterial phase at (*A*) 70 keV and (*B*) more conspicuously on iodine (minus water) material density images. Uptake in these sites on (*C*) octreotide images is highly specific to neuroendocrine tumors.

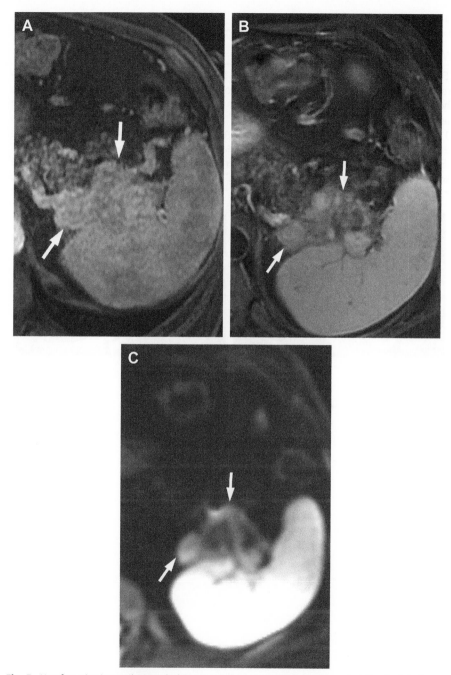

Fig. 5. Nonfunctioning tail PNET (*white arrows*) seen on MRI on dynamic (*A*) arterial phase, (*B*) T2, and (*C*) diffusion-weighted imaging. Diffusion imaging improves contrast, although resolution is less than in other series.

and potentially in evaluating tumor grade.[19,20] MRI also offers potential advantages compared with CT in the detection of liver metastases, which is discussed later.

Nuclear Medicine

The primary nuclear medicine imaging tool for PNET is somatostatin receptor scintigraphy performed with a radiolabeled somatostatin analogue. Somatostatin is a peptide hormone for which 5 types of receptors have been identified. Octreotide, a somatostatin analogue, binds to receptors type 2 and 5.[21] Octreotide is typically labeled with indium-111, administered intravenously, and patients are then imaged 4 hours and 24 hours after tracer administration using both planar imaging and single-photon emission CT (SPECT).[22] At our institution, and in many centers, a CT study is performed concurrently with SPECT on a dedicated hybrid SPECT/CT camera, allowing more precise anatomic localization of octreotide uptake (**Figs. 6–8**).[22] Overall sensitivity for ^{111}In-octreotide for

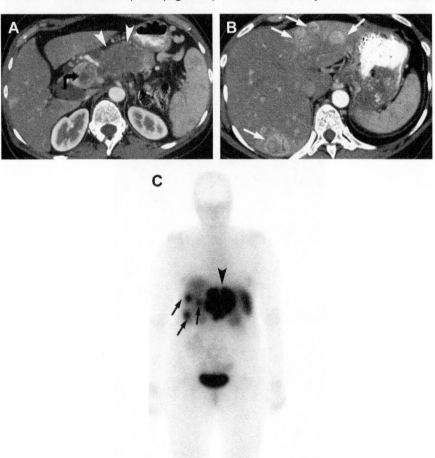

Fig. 6. Patient with increased gastrin levels and large pancreatic gastrinoma (*white arrowheads*) on multiphasic CT in (*A*) arterial phase with invasion and marked distention of the portal vein (*curved black arrow*) and (*B*) multiple liver metastases (*white arrows*). Octreotide scan (*C*) projection images show intense uptake in primary gastrinoma (*black arrowhead*), and liver metastases (*black arrows*).

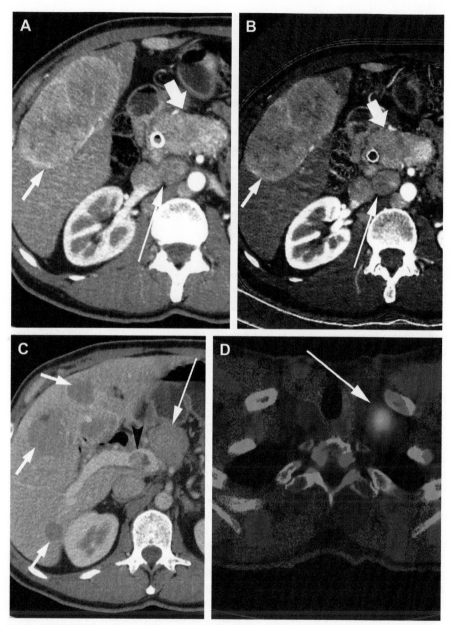

Fig. 7. PNET (*thick white arrow*), adenopathy (*long white arrow*), liver metastases (*white arrow*), and tumor thrombus in vein (*black arrowhead*) as seen on arterial phase (*A*) 70 keV, (*B*) iodine material density, and (*C*) portal venous phase imaging, the last showing metastases and portal vein thrombus. Octreotide fused SPECT CT (*D*), as a whole-body study, identifies distant metastatic left supraclavicular node. Note the similarity of some adenopathy to adjacent vessels.

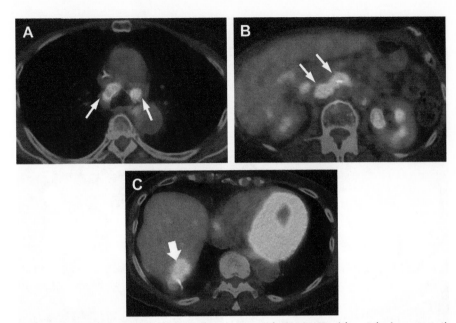

Fig. 8. Metastatic PNET on whole-body fused octreotide SPECT/CT with uptake in metastatic nodal disease (*white arrows*) in (*A*) mediastinum, (*B*) retroperitoneum, and (*C*) liver metastasis (*thick white arrow*).

PNET is approximately 70% to 90% but varies with tumor type and diminishes particularly for subcentimeter lesions.[22,23] Sensitivity for insulinoma, which typically expresses receptor type 3, is notably limited (**Fig. 9**), at 50% to 70%.[24]

Although fluorodeoxyglucose (FDG)-PET/CT would offer potentially greater precision, PNET's don't typically demonstrate sufficient uptake unless they are poorly differentiated. FDG-PET/CT is therefore used as a complementary technique (**Fig. 10**) to SPECT/CT octreotide, which shows poor uptake in poorly differentiated tumors.[22] New PET/CT agents that have been developed include gallium labeled somatostatin analogs such as DOTA-tyrosine-3-octreotide (DOTA-TOC), which has a higher affinity for somatostatin receptor type 2, and DOTA-1-Nal-octreotide (DOTA-NOC), which demonstrates a higher affinity for subtypes 2, 3, and 5 (**Fig. 11**).[24] Although these PET somatostatin radiotracers have faced many regulator barriers in the United States, the somatostatin analogue, DOTA-octreotate (DOTA-TATE, GaTate), has recently been given orphan drug status by the US Food and Drug Administration (FDA). Somatostatin receptor imaging using positron-emitting isotopes is attractive because of the improved spatial resolution of PET imaging compared with SPECT.[25] A recent meta-analysis of 22 studies of the broad category of somatostatin receptor PET/CT, including more than 2100 patients, showed a sensitivity of 93% and specificity of 95%.[26] The radiation dose to the patient is often lower with PET agents compared with conventional ^{111}In-labeled radiotracers. Although Ga-68 has been used extensively, other radioisotopes are under investigation for imaging of neuroendocrine tumors, including Cu-64 and F-18. Using the approach of theranostics, a therapeutic radioisotope (such as Y-90 or Lu-177) can be paired to the somatostatin-binding pharmaceuticals to deliver a high-dose radioisotope therapy to eligible patients, and trials are currently underway in the

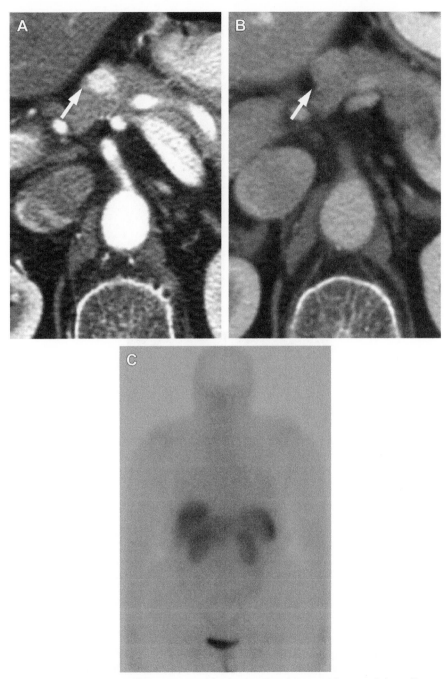

Fig. 9. Small pancreatic insulinoma on multiphasic CT and octreotide scan. (*A*) Insulinoma (*white arrow*) here is uniformly hyperdense on late arterial phase but (*B*) near isodense to background on portal venous phase. On octreotide scan (*C*), it is not seen (normal uptake in liver, spleen, and kidneys).

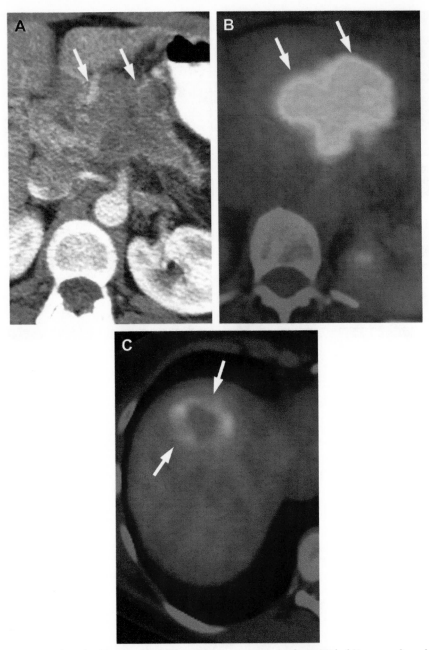

Fig. 10. Nonfunctioning poorly differentiated pancreatic body PNET (*white arrows*) on (*A*) axial late arterial phase CT, and (*B*) showing intense uptake on PET/CT fused image, as is (*C*) a liver metastasis.

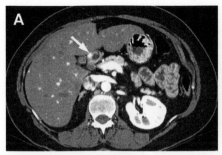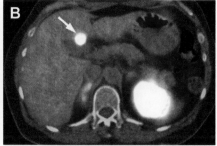

Fig. 11. Proximal duodenal histopathologically proven gastrinoma (*white arrow*) on (*A*) 50-keV dual-energy CT, late arterial phase, and (*B*) 68Ga-DOTA-NOC fused PET/CT images has a hypervascular appearance on CT and shows intense uptake of tracer. Water was used as negative contrast on CT.

United States to achieve regulatory approval. In addition, metabolic pathways are being explored as a means to image PNET tumors, including PET imaging with amino acid precursors such as F-18 dihydroxyphenylalanine (DOPA), and C-11–labeled hydroxytryptophan (5-HTP).[27]

Endoscopic Ultrasonography

Endoscopic ultrasonography (EUS) reportedly has a mean detection rate for neuroendocrine tumors of 90%.[7] EUS-guided fine-needle aspiration (FNA) has been reported to result in overall diagnostic accuracy of 90.1%.[28] Endoscopic ultrasonography (**Fig. 12**) is particularly helpful for gastrinomas because many are located within bowel, a region that is poorly evaluated by both CT and MRI.[29] The primary limitations of EUS are that it depends on the skill and experience of the operator, requires sedation, and the technique is invasive.[29]

A recent development is that of intravenous contrast agents, namely blood-pool contrast agents (microbubbles) for ultrasonography imaging, currently approved in the United States by the FDA for cardiac imaging but not abdominal imaging, although they have been approved for use more widely in other parts of the world.[30] A study of 37 insulinomas, using one such microbubble agent, sulfur hexafluoride lipid-type A microspheres, reportedly showed an improvement from a sensitivity of 24% for transabdominal unenhanced ultrasonography to 87% to 89% following the administration of intravenous contrast.[30] To our knowledge, only limited information is available regarding its use in the setting of pancreatic EUS. The already high sensitivity of EUS and the high specificity of EUS-guided FNA likely account for contrast enhancement not being more widely used.

IMAGING FINDINGS

The appearance of PNETs can vary considerably, even within the same patient, and differs markedly between functional tumors, which are typically small, and nonfunctional tumors, which are typically several centimeters in size.

Functional Pancreatic Neuroendocrine Tumors

Because they manifest with systemic symptoms, functional pancreatic tumors are usually 1 to 2 cm in diameter at the time of imaging but can be smaller.[8,31,32] The most common types are insulinoma (see **Fig. 9**) and gastrinoma (see **Figs. 6** and **11**; **Fig. 13**).

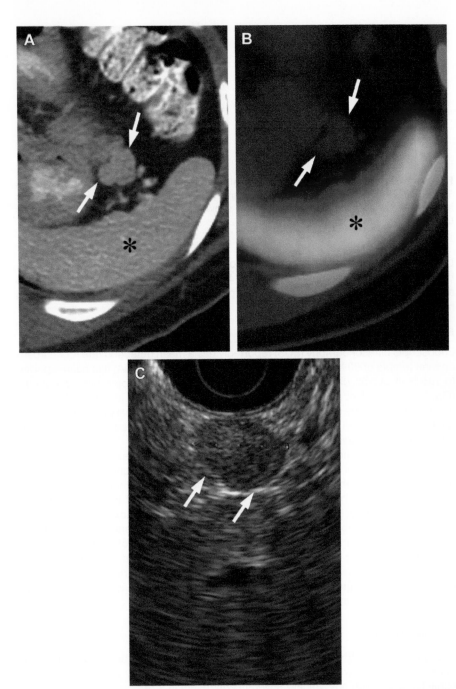

Fig. 12. Incidentally identified pancreatic tail mass (*white arrows*) on CT (*A*) similar to spleen (*black asterisk*) on multiphasic imaging, showed (*B*) no uptake of technetium sulfur colloid (therefore not an accessory spleen). (*C*) EUS with FNA showed well-defined slightly hypoechoic mass and PNET on histopathology.

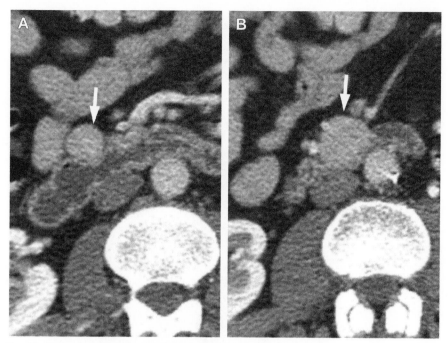

Fig. 13. Peripancreatic adenopathy as site of gastrinoma. Portal venous phase CT shows enhancing adenopathy (*white arrow*) (*A*) anterior to transverse duodenum and (*B*) near the aortocaval space, similar to aorta and opacified bowel loops.

Their incidence is increased in syndromes such as the autosomally dominant MEN-I, and von Hippel-Lindau disease.[4,5]

Their classic appearance is of a uniformly hypervascular, well-defined lesion (see **Figs. 9** and **11**) that is most notably prominent on arterial phases of contrast enhancement.[8,31,33] Studies that have evaluated phases of contrast enhancement have shown a sensitivity of 83% to 88% for arterial phase imaging versus 11% to 76% for later portal venous phase imaging.[8,9,34,35] However, lesions may be seen on only 1 of these 2 phases.

Cystic changes are typically seen with larger lesions,[33] but even marked cystic transformation can occur with smaller lesions (**Fig. 14**). The presence of a hypervascular rim, sometimes very subtle, can be helpful in suggesting the diagnosis of PNET.[36] Features such as heterogeneity, calcifications, and necrosis become more notable with increasing tumor size.[33]

Insulinomas

Knowledge of the suspected tumor type (eg, insulinoma or gastrinoma) is important to guide assessment of the images. Insulinomas are typically solitary, 97% occur within the pancreas, are typically smaller than other functioning tumors at initial evaluation (40% are <1 cm), and only 10% are malignant, with malignancy usually seen in lesions larger than 3 cm.[32,37,38] Insulinomas are much more likely to be multiple in the setting of syndromes, notably MEN-I.[37,39] CT and MRI are often used initially in this setting given their good sensitivity for intrapancreatic lesions and lack of invasiveness, and the poor sensitivity of octreotide as well as PET/CT.

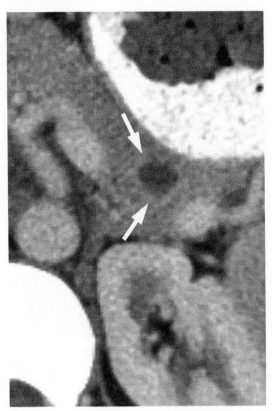

Fig. 14. Cystic pancreatic tail lesion (*white arrows*) on CT shows subtle peripheral enhancement. EUS FNA confirmed PNET.

Invasive techniques such as arterial stimulation and venous sampling, and transhepatic portal venous sampling, can be used to increase the likelihood of detection[37] but may be controversial because intraoperative assessment has been reported to have high sensitivity.[37,40,41] Noninvasive techniques such as CT and MRI, when able to localize lesions, can provide information that may be helpful in guiding decisions regarding surgery, such as the extent of primary tumor, potential metastatic nodal involvement, or the identification of liver metastases.[32]

Gastrinomas

Gastrinomas (see **Figs. 6**, **11**, and **13**) have a very different pattern of presentation from insulinomas. Only 60% are located within the pancreas, with the remainder most commonly located in the duodenum or peripancreatic nodes; overall about 90% are identified within the so-called gastrinoma triangle bounded by the cystic duct junction with the common bile duct, the pancreatic neck, and the junction of the second and third portions of the duodenum.[8,32] Rarely, lesions have been reported in the stomach and jejunum.[8] Although gastrinomas within the pancreas are typically 3 to 4 cm and usually within the head,[42] those within the duodenum are usually within the wall, multiple, and subcentimeter in size, making assessment by CT and MRI difficult.[42] For this reason, EUS is particularly useful for identifying gastrinomas preoperatively and to biopsy suspicious nodes.[8] Because of the nature and high concentration of their somatostatin receptor expression, these lesions are more amenable to evaluation with nuclear medicine octreotide scanning.[8] Unlike insulinomas, 60% of gastrinomas show malignant behavior at presentation, requiring careful inspection for all sites of disease and close evaluation for potential liver metastases.[8] Gastrinomas are the most common functioning PNET in the MEN-I syndrome, in which they are most likely to manifest with multifocal duodenal involvement.[8]

NONFUNCTIONING PANCREATIC NEUROENDOCRINE TUMORS

Nonfunctioning PNETs (see **Fig. 5**; **Fig. 15**), typically manifest because of symptoms caused by mass effect, such as pain and weight loss, and as such typically present at a larger size.[8,33] These nonfunctioning tumors often secrete hormones, such as pancreatic polypeptide, but without causing an apparent clinical syndrome. Being larger, these lesions also more commonly manifest as heterogeneously enhancing lesions, may contain areas of necrosis/cystic change that can be markedly extensive, and can contain foci of calcification.[33] They are also more likely to be metastatic (see **Fig. 3**) at presentation (60%–80% of cases), most often to liver and lymph nodes (see **Fig. 7**).[32,37,43] The presence of calcifications is a useful indicator for potential malignancy.[31] Duct obstruction can be seen secondary to mass effect, and occasionally tumor can be seen to have spread within a distended duct.[8,31,44] In a study of 88 patients with nonfunctioning tumors, 33% had venous tumor thrombus (see **Fig. 15**), identification of which can alter

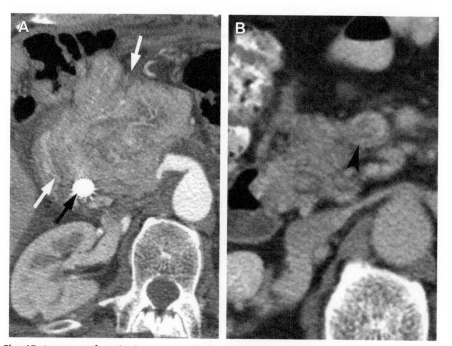

Fig. 15. Large nonfunctioning pancreatic head PNET on CT. (*A*) Late arterial phase shows tumor (*white arrows*) extending anterior to a metallic biliary stent (*black arrow*), and (*B*) infiltrating (*black arrowhead*) the superior mesenteric vein.

surgical planning, and is a useful distinguishing feature from pancreatic ductal adenocarcinoma.[44]

Although most often solitary, nonfunctional PNET can be multiple in familial syndromes, and is the most common pancreatic endocrine tumor in patients with MEN-I and von Hippel-Lindau disease.[8] With the growing use generally of cross-sectional imaging, up to 35% of nonfunctional PNETs are now found incidentally, which often portends a better prognosis.[43]

POORLY DIFFERENTIATED PANCREATIC ENDOCRINE TUMORS

An important criterion is poorly versus well-differentiated PNETs. The former are more likely associated with nodal and/or liver metastases, have few somatostatin receptors, and are therefore poorly visualized on octreotide studies, but are more likely to be visualized (see **Fig. 10**) on FDG-PET/CT studies.[8,44,45]

Recent studies have attempted to identify imaging biomarkers of aggressiveness. A study of 60 PNETs showed on dual-phase imaging (arterial/portal venous) that atypical enhancement, namely persistent enhancement on portal venous phase imaging or increasing enhancement on later phase compared with typical early enhancement followed by washout on portal venous phase (**Fig. 16**), was more likely to be carcinoma on histopathologic examination.[46] A study that evaluated similar characteristics and diffusion-weighted imaging on MRI also showed that malignant features were more likely to be hypovascular on the arterial phase of imaging, and also showed lower ADC values.[18] In one study, the presence of multiple factors, such as poorly defined margin, upstream pancreatic duct dilatation, vascular invasion, tumor size, and enhancement features, were significant in predicting histopathologic grading of tumors,[47] whereas another study found that only identification of ill-defined boundaries between tumor and peripancreatic tissues or vessels was significantly associated with World Health Organization 2010 pathologic classification.[48]

STAGING

The 2 most commonly used staging systems are the European Neuroendocrine Tumor Society system (ENETS, 2006) and the American Joint Committee on Cancer (AJCC)/ Union for International Cancer Control (UICC) 2009 system. Their differences are primarily in T staging, as shown in **Table 1**.

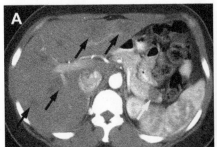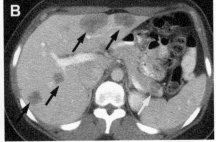

Fig. 16. A PNET (*white arrow*) and its liver metastases (*black arrows*) that are atypically hypodense on CT on (*A*) late arterial and (*B*) portal venous phases, which mimics pancreatic ductal adenocarcinoma.

Table 1
T staging of PNETs: AJCC versus ENETS

Stage	AJCC/UICC 2009	ENETS 2006
T1	Pancreatic confined primary tumor <2 cm	Pancreatic confined primary tumor <2 cm
T2	Pancreatic confined primary tumor >2 cm	Pancreatic confined primary tumor 2–4 cm
T3	Pancreatic tumor extending beyond pancreas without major vessel involvement	Pancreatic tumor >4 cm in size or extending beyond pancreas with invasion limited to duodenum or bile duct
T4	Pancreatic tumor extending to involve major vessels such as celiac or superior mesenteric artery	Pancreatic tumor invading major vessels or invasion of adjacent organs other than duodenum or bile duct

Adapted from Rindi G, Klöppel G, Alhman H, et al. TNM staging of foregut (neuro)endocrine tumors: a consensus proposal including a grading system. Virchows Arch 2006;449(4):395–401; and Available at: https://cancerstaging.org/references-tools/quickreferences/Documents/PancreasSmall.pdf.

Primary Tumor

As noted earlier, the type of tumor being considered (ie, insulinoma vs gastrinoma) and differentiation (well vs poorly differentiated) can have significant implications regarding the imaging modalities being chosen (nuclear medicine octreotide study, FDG-PET/CT, EUS/CT/MRI).

The 2 primary modalities for assessing local extent of disease, including involvement of adjacent organs and vasculature, are MRI and CT. CT has the advantages of relative insensitivity to motion and submillimeter slice thickness, and therefore can produce detailed reconstructions useful for evaluating the relationship of tumors to adjacent structures (**Fig. 17**). MRI can image directly in multiple planes with good soft tissue contrast even when intravenous contrast agents cannot be administered.

Disease Beyond the Pancreas: Nodal and Distant Metastatic

Nodal disease

It is important to identify potential metastatic nodal sites of PNET preoperatively to improve the likelihood of resecting all sites of disease. The most commonly used techniques are CT, MRI, and octreotide scanning (see **Figs. 7** and **8**; **Fig. 18**), with octreotide scanning being the most specific. However, only limited information is available on nodal staging. As noted previously, CT provides high-resolution imaging with few artifacts. A recent study of 181 patients undergoing pancreatic resection with curative intent showed a sensitivity and specificity of CT for detecting nodal metastases of 35% and 91% respectively.[49] PNET nodal metastases can be prominently hypervascular and therefore more conspicuous on the arterial phase of dynamic imaging.[35] In our experience, such enhancement can also be similar to, and therefore difficult to distinguish from, adjacent vasculature. In this context, T2-weighted and diffusion-weighted MR imaging can be helpful, because vessels are typically black on images obtained with these techniques because of flow phenomena, whereas nodes (both metastatic and benign) are characteristically bright on both T2-weighted and diffusion imaging (see **Fig. 18**). However, both CT and MRI are insensitive for micrometastases. Using size criteria of greater than 1 cm in short axis to identify adenopathy is fairly insensitive but somewhat specific. Octreotide scanning with SPECT with fusion with unenhanced CT images can be helpful for identifying small, avid liver, node, and bone metastases but is also insensitive for micrometastases.[8,24] A very recent study of Ga-DOTA-TOC

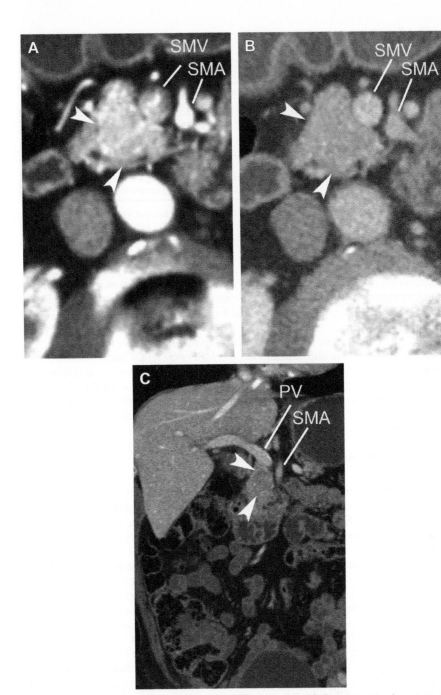

Fig. 17. Staging of pancreatic head NET (*white arrowheads*) showing superior mesenteric vein (SMV) abutment on late arterial phase CT (*A*). Although PNET is not as well seen on (*B*) portal venous phase images, the SMV is clearly free of thrombus, and coronal reconstruction (*C*) shows PNET not involving the portal vein (PV) and separate from the superior mesenteric artery (SMA).

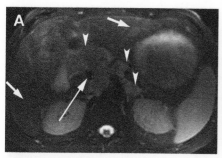 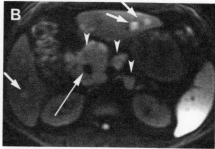

Fig. 18. Metastatic PNET with liver metastases (*short white arrows*) and nodal disease (*white arrowheads*) appear bright on typical (*A*) T2 fat-suppressed imaging and (*B*) diffusion-weighted imaging with B value of 500. Unlike on CT, the portal vein (*long white arrow*) is black, clearly distinguishable from nodes. Note that metastatic and reactive nodes appear similar on both techniques.

PET/MRI with gadoxetate disodium compared with Ga-DOTA-TOC PET/CT showed an advantage for PET/CT for evaluation of involved lymph nodes.[50] As noted previously, conventional FDG-PET/CT may be advantageous compared with octreotide scanning for identifying metastatic sites for poorly differentiated PNET.

Liver metastases

Multiphasic imaging on CT is also useful for liver metastases, which have a variable appearance requiring careful inspection of all dynamic phases. The classic appearance (see **Fig. 2**) is of a hypervascular metastasis seen best on the arterial phase of imaging. However, metastases can also be hypoenhancing on all phases, portending a worse prognosis.[51] A study of 64 patients in 2005 compared SPECT octreotide scanning, spiral CT, and MRI. SPECT octreotide identified 200 liver metastases, CT identified 325, and MRI identified 394 lesions.[52] Newer developments since then include MRI diffusion-weighted imaging, and the development of liver-specific agents. A study of MRI in 59 patients, 41 patients with 162 liver metastases from neuroendocrine tumors and 18 control subjects with no liver metastases, showed sensitivities of 72% for diffusion-weighted, 57.2% for T2-weighted, and 48% for conventional intravenous gadolinium dynamic multiphasic imaging with decreasing sensitivities for decreasing size of metastases.[53] Gadoxetate disodium, a liver-specific agent retained by normal liver parenchyma, washes out of liver metastases, making them notably conspicuous on 20-minute delayed images (**Fig. 19**).[54,55] Although very limited information is available regarding PNET liver metastases, a study has shown greater detection of colorectal liver metastases with gadoxetate disodium MRI than triphasic CT.[56] An interesting recent development has been combined Ga-DOTA-TOC PET/MRI with gadoxetate disodium.[50]

Other Distant Metastases

PNET can also metastasize to bone and lung. Although CT has excellent sensitivity for assessing lung metastases, it is less capable at assessing bone metastases. MRI is useful for characterizing and assessing limited regions of the skeleton, whereas nuclear medicine studies provide the benefit of a whole-body assessment.

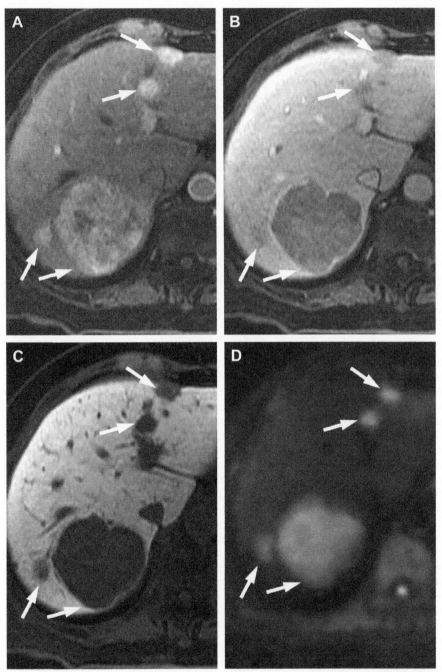

Fig. 19. PNET liver metastases (*white arrows*) on MRI on (*A*) arterial phase of dynamic, (*B*) portal venous phase, (*C*) 20-minute delayed post–gadoxetate disodium, and (*D*) diffusion-weighted imaging. Conspicuity of liver metastases can vary greatly between arterial/portal venous images but, because they lack hepatocytes, metastases are usually distinctly dark and well defined on (*C*) delayed gadobenate dimeglumine images. Diffusion-weighted imaging also shows lesions well.

SUMMARY

State-of-the-art imaging for PNET continues to evolve with developments such as dual-energy CT, new MRI techniques such as diffusion-weighted imaging, the increasing use of EUS for solid pancreatic lesions, and the evolving use of PET/CT, including the role of FDG-PET for poorly differentiated tumors and new PET agents that promise greater utility than conventional octreotide nuclear medicine imaging. Optimal use of imaging techniques (focused abdominal imaging and complementary whole-body imaging) depends on such issues as functional versus nonfunctional tumors and well versus poorly differentiated tumors. Insulinomas, which are almost always confined to the pancreas, are typically best imaged by a combination of cross-sectional imaging techniques, such as CT or MRI, with cautious use of whole-body nuclear medicine conventional octreotide imaging, given the often poor uptake of octreotide by this tumor. In contrast, gastrinomas, which are frequently extrapancreatic and octreotide avid, are best managed by a combination of CT or MRI, whole-body octreotide imaging, and EUS to evaluate for pancreatic and intraluminal lesions. In contrast, the typically large size of nonfunctional tumors is such that these are often best managed by cross-sectional imaging, CT or MRI, to provide detail with regard to staging with the type of whole-body imaging depending on whether tumor is well differentiated (in which case whole-body octreotide is used and FDG-PET/CT has only limited utility) versus poorly differentiated (in which case octreotide scanning often performs poorly, but FDG-PET can provide a useful whole-body assessment).

REFERENCES

1. Fraenkel M, Kim MK, Faggiano A, et al. Epidemiology of gastroenteropancreatic neuroendocrine tumours. Best Pract Res Clin Gastroenterol 2012;26(6):691–703.
2. Lawrence B, Gustafsson BI, Chan A, et al. The epidemiology of gastroenteropancreatic neuroendocrine tumors. Endocrinol Metab Clin North Am 2011; 40(1):1–18, vii.
3. Zhou J, Enewold L, Stojadinovic A, et al. Incidence rates of exocrine and endocrine pancreatic cancers in the United States. Cancer Causes Control 2010; 21(6):853–61.
4. Baur AD, Pavel M, Prasad V, et al. Diagnostic imaging of pancreatic neuroendocrine neoplasms (pNEN): tumor detection, staging, prognosis, and response to treatment. Acta Radiol 2015. [Epub ahead of print].
5. Jensen RT, Berna MJ, Bingham DB, et al. Inherited pancreatic endocrine tumor syndromes: advances in molecular pathogenesis, diagnosis, management, and controversies. Cancer 2008;113(7 Suppl):1807–43.
6. Ichikawa T, Peterson MS, Federle MP, et al. Islet cell tumor of the pancreas: biphasic CT versus MR imaging in tumor detection. Radiology 2000;216(1):163–71.
7. Sundin A, Vullierme MP, Kaltsas G, et al. ENETS consensus guidelines for the standards of care in neuroendocrine tumors: radiological examinations. Neuroendocrinology 2009;90(2):167–83.
8. Lewis RB, Lattin GEJM, Paal E. Pancreatic endocrine tumors: radiologic-clinicopathologic correlation. Radiographics 2010;30(6):1445–64.
9. Fidler JL, Fletcher JG, Reading CC, et al. Preoperative detection of pancreatic insulinomas on multiphasic helical CT. AJR Am J Roentgenol 2003;181(3): 775–80.
10. Gouya H, Vignaux O, Augui J, et al. CT, endoscopic sonography, and a combined protocol for preoperative evaluation of pancreatic insulinomas. AJR Am J Roentgenol 2003;181(4):987–92.

11. Rockall AG, Reznek RH. Imaging of neuroendocrine tumours (CT/MR/US). Best Pract Res Clin Endocrinol Metab 2007;21(1):43–68.
12. Silva AC, Morse BG, Hara AK, et al. Dual-energy (spectral) CT: applications in abdominal imaging. Radiographics 2011;31(4):1031–46 [discussion: 1047–50].
13. Faby S, Kuchenbecker S, Sawall S, et al. Performance of today's dual energy CT and future multi energy CT in virtual non-contrast imaging and in iodine quantification: a simulation study. Med Phys 2015;42(7):4349.
14. Lin XZ, Wu ZY, Tao R, et al. Dual energy spectral CT imaging of insulinoma–Value in preoperative diagnosis compared with conventional multi-detector CT. Eur J Radiol 2012;81(10):2487–94.
15. Marin D, Nelson RC, Barnhart H, et al. Detection of pancreatic tumors, image quality, and radiation dose during the pancreatic parenchymal phase: effect of a low-tube-voltage, high-tube-current CT technique–preliminary results. Radiology 2010;256(2):450–9.
16. Brenner R, Metens T, Bali M, et al. Pancreatic neuroendocrine tumor: added value of fusion of T2-weighted imaging and high b-value diffusion-weighted imaging for tumor detection. Eur J Radiol 2012;81(5):e746–9.
17. Kang BK, Kim JH, Byun JH, et al. Diffusion-weighted MRI: usefulness for differentiating intrapancreatic accessory spleen and small hypervascular neuroendocrine tumor of the pancreas. Acta Radiol 2014;55(10):1157–65.
18. Jang KM, Kim SH, Song KD, et al. Differentiation of solid-type serous cystic neoplasm from neuroendocrine tumour in the pancreas: value of abdominal MRI with diffusion-weighted imaging in comparison with MDCT. Clin Radiol 2015;70(2):153–60.
19. Jang KM, Kim SH, Lee SJ, et al. The value of gadoxetic acid-enhanced and diffusion-weighted MRI for prediction of grading of pancreatic neuroendocrine tumors. Acta Radiol 2014;55(2):140–8.
20. Hwang EJ, Lee JM, Yoon JH, et al. Intravoxel incoherent motion diffusion-weighted imaging of pancreatic neuroendocrine tumors: prediction of the histologic grade using pure diffusion coefficient and tumor size. Invest Radiol 2014;49(6):396–402.
21. Tamm EP, Kim EE, Ng CS. Imaging of neuroendocrine tumors. Hematol Oncol Clin North Am 2007;21(3):409–32, vii.
22. Balachandran A, Bhosale PR, Charnsangavej C, et al. Imaging of pancreatic neoplasms. Surg Oncol Clin N Am 2014;23(4):751–88.
23. Kwekkeboom DJ, Krenning EP. Somatostatin receptor imaging. Semin Nucl Med 2002;32(2):84–91.
24. Rufini V, Calcagni ML, Baum RP. Imaging of neuroendocrine tumors. Semin Nucl Med 2006;36(3):228–47.
25. Hofman MS, Lau WF, Hicks RJ. Somatostatin receptor imaging with 68Ga DOTATATE PET/CT: clinical utility, normal patterns, pearls, and pitfalls in interpretation. Radiographics 2015;35(2):500–16.
26. Geijer H, Breimer LH. Somatostatin receptor PET/CT in neuroendocrine tumours: update on systematic review and meta-analysis. Eur J Nucl Med Mol Imaging 2013;40(11):1770–80.
27. Kauhanen S, Seppanen M, Minn H, et al. Clinical PET imaging of insulinoma and beta-cell hyperplasia. Curr Pharm Des 2010;16(14):1550–60.
28. Atiq M, Bhutani MS, Bektas M, et al. EUS-FNA for pancreatic neuroendocrine tumors: a tertiary cancer center experience. Dig Dis Sci 2012;57(3):791–800.
29. Zimmer T, Scherubl H, Faiss S, et al. Endoscopic ultrasonography of neuroendocrine tumours. Digestion 2000;62(Suppl 1):45–50.

30. An L, Li W, Yao KC, et al. Assessment of contrast-enhanced ultrasonography in diagnosis and preoperative localization of insulinoma. Eur J Radiol 2011;80(3): 675–80.

31. Sahani DV, Bonaffini PA, Fernandez-Del Castillo C, et al. Gastroenteropancreatic neuroendocrine tumors: role of imaging in diagnosis and management. Radiology 2013;266(1):38–61.

32. Heller MT, Shah AB. Imaging of neuroendocrine tumors. Radiol Clin North Am 2011;49(3):529–48, vii.

33. Buetow PC, Miller DL, Parrino TV, et al. Islet cell tumors of the pancreas: clinical, radiologic, and pathologic correlation in diagnosis and localization. Radiographics 1997;17(2):453–72 [quiz: 472A–B].

34. King AD, Ko GT, Yeung VT, et al. Dual phase spiral CT in the detection of small insulinomas of the pancreas. Br J Radiol 1998;71(841):20–3.

35. Stafford Johnson DB, Francis IR, Eckhauser FE, et al. Dual-phase helical CT of nonfunctioning islet cell tumors. J Comput Assist Tomogr 1998;22(1):59–63.

36. Ligneau B, Lombard-Bohas C, Partensky C, et al. Cystic endocrine tumors of the pancreas: clinical, radiologic, and histopathologic features in 13 cases. Am J Surg Pathol 2001;25(6):752–60.

37. Mansour JC, Chen H. Pancreatic endocrine tumors. J Surg Res 2004;120(1): 139–61.

38. Ectors N. Pancreatic endocrine tumors: diagnostic pitfalls. Hepatogastroenterology 1999;46(26):679–90.

39. Balachandran A, Tamm EP, Bhosale PR, et al. Pancreatic neuroendocrine neoplasms: diagnosis and management. Abdom Imaging 2012;38(2):342–57.

40. Brown CK, Bartlett DL, Doppman JL, et al. Intraarterial calcium stimulation and intraoperative ultrasonography in the localization and resection of insulinomas. Surgery 1997;122(6):1189–93 [discussion: 1193–4].

41. Doppman JL, Chang R, Fraker DL, et al. Localization of insulinomas to regions of the pancreas by intra-arterial stimulation with calcium. Ann Intern Med 1995; 123(4):269–73.

42. Horton KM, Hruban RH, Yeo C, et al. Multi-detector row CT of pancreatic islet cell tumors. Radiographics 2006;26(2):453–64.

43. Gullo L, Migliori M, Falconi M, et al. Nonfunctioning pancreatic endocrine tumors: a multicenter clinical study. Am J Gastroenterol 2003;98(11):2435–9.

44. Balachandran A, Tamm EP, Bhosale PR, et al. Venous tumor thrombus in nonfunctional pancreatic neuroendocrine tumors. AJR Am J Roentgenol 2012;199(3):602–8.

45. Binderup T, Knigge U, Loft A, et al. 18F-fluorodeoxyglucose positron emission tomography predicts survival of patients with neuroendocrine tumors. Clin Cancer Res 2010;16(3):978–85.

46. Cappelli C, Boggi U, Mazzeo S, et al. Contrast enhancement pattern on multidetector CT predicts malignancy in pancreatic endocrine tumours. Eur Radiol 2014; 25(3):751–9.

47. Takumi K, Fukukura Y, Higashi M, et al. Pancreatic neuroendocrine tumors: correlation between the contrast-enhanced computed tomography features and the pathological tumor grade. Eur J Radiol 2015;84(8):1436–43.

48. Luo Y, Dong Z, Chen J, et al. Pancreatic neuroendocrine tumours: correlation between MSCT features and pathological classification. Eur Radiol 2014; 24(11):2945–52.

49. Partelli S, Gaujoux S, Boninsegna L, et al. Pattern and clinical predictors of lymph node involvement in nonfunctioning pancreatic neuroendocrine tumors (NF-PanNETs). JAMA Surg 2013;148(10):932–9.

50. Hope TA, Pampaloni MH, Nakakura E, et al. Simultaneous Ga-DOTA-TOC PET/MRI with gadoxetate disodium in patients with neuroendocrine tumor. Abdom Imaging 2015;40(6):1432–40.

51. Denecke T, Baur AD, Ihm C, et al. Evaluation of radiological prognostic factors of hepatic metastases in patients with non-functional pancreatic neuroendocrine tumors. Eur J Radiol 2013;82(10):e550–5.

52. Dromain C, de Baere T, Lumbroso J, et al. Detection of liver metastases from endocrine tumors: a prospective comparison of somatostatin receptor scintigraphy, computed tomography, and magnetic resonance imaging. J Clin Oncol 2005;23(1):70–8.

53. d'Assignies G, Fina P, Bruno O, et al. High sensitivity of diffusion-weighted MR imaging for the detection of liver metastases from neuroendocrine tumors: comparison with T2-weighted and dynamic gadolinium-enhanced MR imaging. Radiology 2013;268(2):390–9.

54. Ringe KI, Husarik DB, Sirlin CB, et al. Gadoxetate disodium-enhanced MRI of the liver: part 1, protocol optimization and lesion appearance in the noncirrhotic liver. AJR Am J Roentgenol 2010;195(1):13–28.

55. Cruite I, Schroeder M, Merkle EM, et al. Gadoxetate disodium-enhanced MRI of the liver: part 2, protocol optimization and lesion appearance in the cirrhotic liver. AJR Am J Roentgenol 2010;195(1):29–41.

56. Patel S, Cheek S, Osman H, et al. MRI with gadoxetate disodium for colorectal liver metastasis: is it the new "imaging modality of choice"? J Gastrointest Surg 2014;18(12):2130–5.

Surgical Management of Pancreatic Neuroendocrine Tumors

Amareshwar Chiruvella, MD, David A. Kooby, MD*

KEYWORDS

- Carcinoid • Neuroendocrine tumor • Pancreatic neoplasm • Pancreatectomy
- Hepatectomy • Pancreatic neoplasm • Gastrinoma • Insulinoma

KEY POINTS

- Pancreatic neuroendocrine tumors (pancNETs) comprise 2% to 4% of all detected pancreatic tumors; they can be indolent, and yet their malignant potential is often underestimated.
- The management of this disease poses a challenge because of the heterogeneous clinical presentation and varying degree of aggressiveness.
- Surgical therapy remains the most efficient approach and offers the longest lasting benefits for patients with pancNETs.
- Clinical management of pancNETs involves benefits substantially from a multidisciplinary approach.

INTRODUCTION

Pancreatic neuroendocrine tumors (pancNETs) are uncommon tumors with an estimated incidence of 1 to 1.5 per 100,000 and a prevalence of 35 per 100,000 in the United States. They originate from the embryonic endodermal cells that give rise to the islets of Langerhans. These cells are specialized cells that produce, store, and secrete peptides and biogenic amines and were formerly known as the amine precursor uptake and decarboxylation cells or APUD cells.[1]

PancNETs comprise 2% to 4% of all pancreatic neoplasms, and peak incidence is found between the sixth to the eighth decades. Data from the SEER (Surveillance, Epidemiology, and End Results) registry have shown an increase in incidence from 0.17 in 1970 to 0.43 in 2007, with the lowest 5-year survival compared with other gastrointestinal neuroendocrine tumors (NETs) (**Fig. 1**).

Disclosure Statement: The authors have nothing to disclose.
Department of Surgery, Winship Cancer Institute, Emory University School of Medicine, 1365 C Clifton Road, Northeast, 2nd Floor, Atlanta, GA 30322, USA
* Corresponding author.
E-mail address: dkooby@emory.edu

Surg Oncol Clin N Am 25 (2016) 401–421
http://dx.doi.org/10.1016/j.soc.2015.12.002
1055-3207/16/$ – see front matter © 2016 Elsevier Inc. All rights reserved.

surgonc.theclinics.com

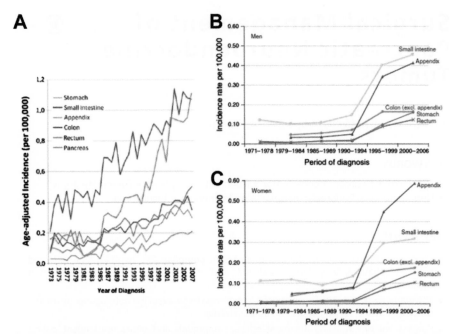

Fig. 1. Rising incidence of NETs in (*A*) all patients, (*B*) men, and (*C*) women. (*Data from* [*A*] US National Cancer Institute. SEER Database. Available at: http://seer.cancer.gov/. Accessed April, 2015; and *From* [*B*, *C*] Ellis L, Shale MJ, Coleman MP. Carcinoid tumors of the gastro-intestinal tract: trends in incidence in England since 1971. Am J Gastroenterol 2010;105: 2566; with permission.)

PancNETs are often classified as functional (F) or nonfunctional (NF) based on the presence or absence of clinically evident hormone production. NF tumors are more common than functional tumors. Functional tumors secrete one or more biologically active peptides, which may result in systemic clinical symptoms (**Table 1**). NF is likely a misnomer because these tumors often secrete various peptides, albeit in the absence of a clinical syndrome (see **Table 1**).

Efforts have been made to create a universal classification system of these tumors from a prognostic and therapeutic standpoint. In 2000, under the auspices of the World Health Organization (WHO), a NET classification was proposed with 3 categories: well-differentiated tumors with benign or uncertain behavior; well-differentiated carcinoma with malignant characteristics; and poorly differentiated carcinoma[2,3] (**Table 2**). This classification, updated in 2010, takes into account the anatomic location, mitotic activity, and the Ki67 proliferative index. This classification was then incorporated into the seventh edition of the American Joint Committee on Cancer staging manual and into the National Comprehensive Cancer Network (NCCN) guidelines.[4,5]

GENERAL FEATURES OF PANCREATIC NEUROENDOCRINE TUMORS

There are 10 different commonly recognized pancNETs, of which 9 are associated with a clinical syndrome, including gastrinomas, insulinomas, glucagonomas, VIPomas, GRFomas, ACTHomas, somatostatinomas, pancNETs causing carcinoid syndrome, and pancNETs causing hypercalcemia. Amounts of 60% to 100% of NF pancNETs secrete various peptides such as chromogranin A, neuron-specific

Table 1
Established pancreatic neuroendocrine tumor subtypes and syndromes (most frequent)

pNET	Syndrome Name	Primary Location(s)	Incidence (No. of New/100,000/y)	Malignancy (%)	Hormone-Causing Syndrome
Functional pNETs					
Gastrinoma	ZES	Pancreas (30%), duodenum (60%–70%), other (5%–10%)	0.5–1.5	60–90 (30–560)	Gastrin
Insulinoma	Insulinoma	Pancreas (100%)	1–3	5–15	Insulin
VIPoma	Verner-Morrison, Pancreatic cholera, WDHA	Pancreas 85%–95%, other (neural, periganglionic, adrenal) (10%)	0.05–0.2	70–90	Vasoactive intestinal peptide
Glucagonoma	Glucagonoma	Pancreas (100%)	0.01–0.1	60–75	Glucagon
Somatostastinoma	Somatostastinoma	Pancreas (50%–60%), duodenal/jejunal (40%–50%)	<0.1%, uncommon	40–60	Somatostatin
GRFoma	GRFoma	Pancreas (30%), lung (54%), jejunal (75%), other (adrenal, foregut, retroperitoneal) (13%)	Unknown	30–50	Growth hormone–releasing factor
ACTHoma	ACTHoma	4%–25% of all ectopic Cushing syndrome	<0.1%, uncommon	95	ACTH
PET causing carcinoid syndrome	PET causing carcinoid syndrome	Pancreas (100%) (<1% of all carcinoid syndrome)	Uncommon (<50 cases)	60–90	Serotonin, tachykinins
PET causing hypercalcemia	PTHrPoma	Pancreas (100%)	<0.1%, uncommon	>85	PTHrP, other unknown
NF pNET	PPomas NF-PET	Pancreas (100%)	1–5	60–90	None secrete pancreatic polypeptide (PP) (60%–85%), chromogranin A but cause no symptoms

Abbreviations: ACTH, adrenocorticotropic hormone; GRF, growth hormone releasing factor; pNET, pancreatic neuroendocrine tumor subtypes and syndromes; PP, pancreatic polypeptide; PPoma-pNET, secreting pancreatic polypeptide; PTHrP, parathyroid hormone–related peptide; WDHA, watery diarrhea, hypokalemia, and achlorhydria.

Table 2
Evolution of World Health Organization classification of neuroendocrine tumors

WHO 1980	WHO 2000	WHO 2010
I. Carcinoid	1. Well-differentiated endocrine tumor	1. NET G1
II. Mucocarcinoid		2. NET G2[a]
III. Mixed forms carcinoid-adenocarcinoma	2. Well-differentiated endocrine carcinoma	3. NEC G3 (large cell or small cell)
IV. Pseudotumor lesions	3. Poorly differentiated endocrine carcinoma	4. Mixed adenoneuroendocrine carcinoma
	4. Mixed exocrine-endocrine carcinoma	5. Hyperplastic and preneoplastic lesions
	5. Tumorlike lesions	

Abbreviations: G, grade; NEC, neuroendocrine carcinoma; NET, neuroendocrine tumor.
[a] G2 NET may include WDET or WDEC of the WHO 2000 classification.

enolase, pancreatic polypeptide, ghrelin, neurotensin, motilin, or subunits of human chorionic gonadotropin, all of which cause no obvious clinical syndrome.[6–9] Insulinomas, gastrinomas, and nonfunctioning pancNETs were previously reported as representing about a third of all pancNETS, respectively. More recent reports suggest pancNETs occur with increasing frequency, making up twice the above percentage of pancNETs, often discovered when still asymptomatic and without advanced disease.[10,11]

Some pancNETs are part of 1 of 4 different inherited syndromes: multiple endocrine neoplasia type-1 (MEN-1), von Hippel-Lindau disease (VHL), von Recklinghausen disease neurofibromatosis 1, and tuberous sclerosis[12] (**Table 3**). These tumors frequently differ in clinical presentation, prognosis, and management from sporadic pancNETs. Of these, MEN-1 is the most important inherited pancNET because 20% to 80% of all patients with this autosomal-dominant disorder develop a clinically relevant NET. MEN-1 is found in 20% to 25% of patients with gastrinomas, 4% with insulinomas, and less than 3% with other pancNETs. Almost all patients with MEN-1 have multifocal, asymptomatic NF-pancNETs, whereas symptomatic pancNETs occur in less than 10% of this group of patients.[12,13]

Diagnosis of pancNETs is often delayed for months to years, given their indolent nature and relatively nonspecific symptoms, even for patients with functional tumors. Around 60% to 70% of patients have metastatic disease at presentation, most commonly involving the liver and less frequently the bones.[14] With the exception of insulinomas, where fewer than 10% are considered malignant, pancNETs typically demonstrate malignant behavior in at least 50% of cases.

Preoperative imaging and localization are essential before considering surgical resection of these tumors. The imaging modalities most commonly used are triple-phase multidetector computed tomography (CT) scan and MRI with gadolinium contrast. PancNETs are usually hyperenhancing masses in the arterial phase of the scan (both primary and metastatic lesions) due to their hypervascular nature (**Fig. 2**). Contrast-enhanced ultrasound is used more frequently in Europe than in the United States and may be useful in monitoring response to treatment with peptide receptor radionuclide therapy (PRRT) and locoregional ablation of liver metastases.[15,16] As most pancNETs (excluding insulinomas) express a high density of somatostatin receptors (specifically subtypes 2 and 5), indium-111-labeled somatostatin receptor scintigraphy (SRS) is an effective localizing tool in this disease.[17,18] There is evidence that

Table 3
Association of multiple endocrine neoplasia type 1 with pancreatic neuroendocrine tumors

Syndrome	Frequency	Location/Type of Genetic Abnormality	Altered Protein Function(s)	Frequency of PETs, %	Type of PETs (%)
MEN-1 (Wermer syndrome)	Prevalence, 1–10 per 100,000	11q13; encodes 610 amino acid protein (menin)	Nuclear location; exact function unclean interacts with JunD, NF-kB, SMAD signaling pathways; effects cell cycle, growth, genomic stability, and apoptosis	80–100 (microscopic), 20–80 (clinical)	NF-PET, microscopic; > functional (20–80)
VHL	Prevalence, 2–3 per 100,000	3p25: encodes 232 amino acid protein (pVHL)	Interacts with elongins, which act as transcriptional regulators that degrade HIF, regulates cell cycle, VEGF	10–17	NF (>98)
Von Recklinghausen disease (neurofibromatosisl [NF-1])	Prevalence, 1 per 4000–5000	17q11.2: encodes 2485 amino acid protein (neurofibromin)	Ras GTPase-activating activity, binds microtubules, modulates adenylate cyclase, mTor-regulates growth, cell cytoskeleton	0–10 (uncommon)	Duodenal somatostatinomas, rare PETs
Tuberous sclerosis (Bourneville disease)	Prevalence, 1 per 10,000	9q34 (TSC1): encodes 1164 amino acid protein (hamartin); 16p13 (TSC2): encodes 1807 amino acid protein (tuberin)	Interacts with PI3K signaling pathway regulating GTPase and mTor, which play a key role in growth, energy regulation, response to hypoxia, nutrients	Uncommon	Rarely develop functional, NF-PETs

Abbreviations: HIF, hypoxia inducible factor; VEGF, vascular endothelial growth factor; VHL, von hippel lindau syndrome.

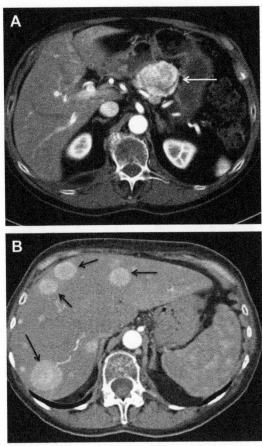

Fig. 2. CT imaging of pancreatic neuroendocrine primary tumor (*A, arrow*) and metastatic disease (*B, arrows*).

SRS informs us of tumor receptor status, and that this may be useful for guiding therapeutic use of somatostatin analogues. Recent development of PET scanning with gallium-68-labeled somatostatin analogues (DOTATOC, DOTANOC, and DOTATATE) may be more sensitive than CT, MRI, and octreoscan in detecting NETs (100% vs 75%).[19,20]

Management steps for pancNETs include establishing diagnosis, localizing tumor, assessing for underlying inherited disorder, controlling hormonal excess when present, removing and/or ablating tumor if possible and appropriate, and considering alternative forms of therapy (regional and/or medical). Depending on the situation, pancNETs can either be enucleated or removed with formal organ resection. The former approach is considered in cases of smaller tumors with presumed indolent behavior, assuming pancreatic duct disruption can be avoided. Intraoperative ultrasound (IOUS) is an integral part of resection of these tumors. If the above criteria are not met, formal resection, such as pancreaticoduodenectomy, distal pancreatectomy, and the less commonly performed central pancreatectomy, is considered.

SURGICAL MANAGEMENT OF LOCALIZED PANCREATIC NEUROENDOCRINE TUMORS
Insulinoma

Insulinoma is the most common form of F-pancNET encountered. It can be sporadic or associated with MEN-1. It is more commonly found in women (F:M = 2:1) in the fifth or sixth decade and can present in the third decade of life in patients with MEN-1. Sporadic insulinomas are usually unifocal, but those associated with MEN-1 may present with multifocal disease. Clinical presentation is characterized by the Whipple triad constituted by hypoglycemia after a fast or exercise, neuroglycopenic symptoms, and immediate relief with oral or intravenous glucose administration.[21] Most patients also present with hyperphagia and new-onset weight gain.

The diagnostic criteria for insulinoma are established during a 72-hour fast or until symptoms develop with a blood glucose less than 50 mg/dL, elevated insulin, C-peptide, and proinsulin, in the absence of urine or plasma sulfonylureas, and relief of symptoms after an oral glucose load (**Box 1**); 99% of insulinomas can be detected in this manner. Approximately 80% to 90% of insulinomas are small (<2 cm), solitary, benign tumors that are equally distributed among the head, body, and tail of the pancreas. The remaining 10% occur as multiple tumors in the setting of MEN-1.[22,23] Most insulinomas are less than 2 cm in diameter and are benign, with a brick-red appearance due to increased vascularity. Given their small size, preoperative localization remains a challenge. CT scanning can detect approximately two-thirds of all lesions on arterial phase imaging. MRI is typically performed as a second-line imaging modality after CT, although the sensitivity for detecting these tumors may be higher than that of a CT scan. The sensitivity of endoscopic ultrasound (EUS) varies with tumor location (92.6%, 78.9%, and 40.0% for the head, body, and tail of the pancreas, respectively) and with user experience.[24] SRS for this type of tumor is limited because only 30% possess somatostatin type 2 receptors.[25] Intra-arterial calcium stimulation (selective infusion of calcium into branches of the celiac axis and superior mesenteric artery) with hepatic venous sampling for insulin can be a sensitive localizing modality, but carries some risk of complications,[26] and is typically used when the tumor or tumors are not localized with other forms of imaging (**Fig. 3**).

Despite this, 20% to 50% of insulinomas remain undetected at the time of surgery. Some evidence suggests that preoperative localizing studies for the primary tumor may not be necessary.[27,28] This finding is based on the observation that a combination of surgical exploration and IOUS can detect more than 90% of insulinomas.

Definitive treatment of insulinomas is surgical resection; however, presurgical medical therapy is provided to alleviate symptoms, including eating small, frequent meals

---

Box 1
Diagnostic criteria for insulinoma

Monitored fast for less than 48 hours with documented blood glucose less than 50 mg/dL with hypoglycemic symptoms

Relief of symptoms after oral glucose load

Elevated insulin level (>5–10 μU/mL)

Increased serum proinsulin level (>22 pmol)

Absence of urinary or plasma sulfonylureas

Elevated C-peptide levels

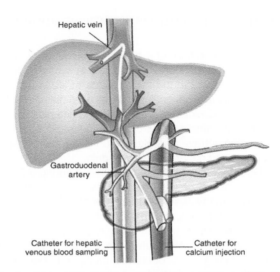

Fig. 3. Schematic of calcium stimulation testing for localization of insulinomas. Catheters are placed in the arterial system for calcium injection and in the venous system for sampling. (*From* Vanderveen K, Grant C. Insulinoma. In: Morita SY, Dackiw APB, Zeiger MA, editors. Endocrine surgery. Chapter 17. McGraw-Hill Manual; 2010; with permission.)

and using insulin antisecretagogues, such as diazoxide or octreotide, both of which work only 40% to 60% of the time.[29,30] Before proceeding to surgery, the presence of MEN-1 must be excluded by testing for other components such as hyperparathyroidism and pituitary tumors. Intraoperative glucose monitoring is essential to avoid hypoglycemia, and dextrose infusion must be stopped before surgical resection to permit intraoperative glucose measurements as an indicator of biochemical cure. Many sporadic adenomas are amenable to enucleation. Surgical exploration commences by gaining access to the pancreas in the lesser sac and traversing the gastrocolic omentum. A wide kocherization of the duodenum is essential for tumor involving the pancreatic head. This wide kocherization enables palpation to be combined with IOUS, which in experienced hands can detect up to 98% of insulinomas.[31] It also helps to detect the location of the pancreatic duct to ascertain safety during enucleation and prevent a pancreatic fistula. Once the insulinoma is enucleated, a thorough examination must be performed to evaluate for a ductal leak, in the presence of which a suture repair can be attempted along with surgical drainage (**Fig. 4**). Rates of pancreatic fistula reported after enucleation are higher than those after a formal resection, in the range of 18% to 38%.[32]

In MEN-1 patients, these tumors are multiple and subcentimeter and usually coalesce. If multiple tumors are found throughout the pancreas, judicious use of surgical resection must be considered because total pancreatectomy should be avoided for insulinomas in most cases. If the lesion is not found, a pancreatic biopsy specimen should be obtained to rule out nesidioblastosis (a condition characterized by diffuse β-cell proliferation), in which case a subtotal pancreatectomy can improve symptoms.

No follow-up is necessary in the case of benign insulinomas unless symptoms recur. For malignant insulinomas and those associated with MEN-1, follow-up is every 3 to 12 months with biomarkers, CT/MRI, and octeroscan/PET.

The treatment of malignant/metastatic pancNETs is discussed in a separate section.

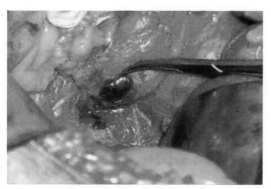

Fig. 4. Enucleation of insulinoma: a salmon-colored tumor being dissected out from the pancreatic parenchyma. (*From* Shah S, Patel A, Prajapati J, et al. Insulinoma: a commonly misdiagnosed pancreatic tumour. Internet J Gastroenterol 2009;9(1):2; with permission.)

Gastrinoma

Gastrinomas are the second most common functional islet cell tumor of the pancreas. Mean age at diagnosis is 50 years with a slight male predominance. Although slow growing in nature, more than 60% demonstrate malignant behavior. Because of their indolent growth pattern, 10-year patient survival approaches 90% even in the presence of metastatic disease. Two-thirds of all gastrinomas are sporadic, with the remainder associated with MEN-1. Individuals with gastrinomas associated with MEN-1 may have a better 20-year survival rate than individuals with sporadic gastrinomas.[33] As with other pancNETs, gastrinomas in the setting of MEN-1 tend to be multifocal, and as many as 50% of patients have distant metastases at the time of presentation.[34]

The clinical syndrome associated with gastrinoma (Zollinger-Ellison syndrome [ZES]) arises principally from dysregulated hypergastrinemia and subsequent luminal hyperacidity resulting in development of intractable gastrointestinal ulcers. Diarrhea, heartburn, nausea, and weight loss are the typical constellation of symptoms at presentation. With the advent and widespread use of antisecretory medications, patients may or may not present with intractable ulcer disease at the time of diagnosis. Given the nonspecificity of symptoms and relative rarity of this disorder, the mean time to diagnosis is around 5.9 years.[35,36] The diagnostic criteria (**Table 4**) include an increased basal acid output in the presence of a fasting gastrin level (FSG) >100 pg/mL or >10-fold the upper limit of normal. Proton pump inhibitors (PPIs) are stopped at least a week prior and H2 antagonists 2 days before testing. Because almost two-thirds of patients with ZES have equivocal FSG levels, secretin stimulation testing or

Table 4 Diagnostic criteria for gastrinoma	
Fasting gastrin level	>100 pg/mL or >10 times higher than upper limit of normal
Basic acid output level	>15 mEq/h
Secretin stimulation testing	Increase of >200 pg/mL
Calcium infusion provocative testing	Rise >395 pg/mL

Patients should not take antisecretory agents a minimum of 3 to 7 days.

calcium provocative testing can be useful in establishing the diagnosis. An increase of 200 pg/mL in the serum gastrin level following secretin administration is consistent with ZES. Higher serum gastrin levels are seen with pancreatic rather than duodenal primaries and in patients with tumors larger than 3 cm and/or those with liver metastases.[35]

Modalities for localizing gastrinomas are similar to those used for insulinomas and include CT, MRI, EUS, SRS, and angiography with selective hepatic venous sampling after intra-arterial secretin injection. SRS is considered the imaging modality of choice for both primary and metastatic gastrinomas with a sensitivity and specificity of more than 90% compared with 30% to 50% with CT or MRI.[37,38]

The goals of surgery are 2-fold: resection of primary tumor for potential cure and prevention of malignant progression. Most gastrinomas (80%) are found in the gastrinoma triangle, as described by Stabile and colleagues[39] (**Fig. 5**). The gastrinoma triangle is defined by a line that joins the confluence of the cystic and common bile ducts superiorly, the junction of the second and third portions of the duodenum inferiorly, and the junction of the neck and body of the pancreas medially. Historically, ZES patients were offered total gastrectomy to control acid production; however, with the advent of PPIs, this is no longer performed. A complete exploration of the gastrinoma triangle is performed intraoperatively and starts with an extended Kocher maneuver to mobilize the duodenum and gain exposure of the pancreas in the lesser sac. Bimanual palpation and use of IOUS is a key step in identifying small lesions and multifocal tumors. Irrespective of the presence of pancreatic tumors, a routine duodenotomy is advocated by some experts in all patients undergoing operative exploration for ZES.[40,41] Several studies have shown that a routine duodenotomy doubles the cure rate from 30% to 60%.[40,41] Pancreatic tumors that are small and away from the pancreatic duct can be enucleated; however, large, unencapsulated tumors, deep within the pancreas and close to the pancreatic duct, require formal resection. Duodenal tumors less than 0.5 cm can be enucleated but larger tumors require a full-thickness excision of the duodenal wall. In about 5% of cases, the surgeon is unable to localize these tumors, in which case, a highly selective vagotomy may be considered to decrease postoperative requirement of antisecretory medications.

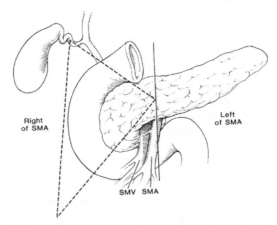

Right of SMA

Left of SMA

SMV SMA

Fig. 5. Gastrinoma triangle. This region is bound by the junction of cystic/common bile ducts, junction of the second and third parts of the duodenum, and the junction of the neck and body of the pancreas. SMA, superior mesenteric artery; SMV, superior mesenteric vein. (*From* Howard TJ, Sawicki M, Lewin KJ, et al. Pancreatic polypeptide immunoreactivity in sporadic gastrinoma: relationship to intra-abdominal location. Pancreas 1993;11:351; with permission.)

There exists some controversy regarding the management of MEN-1-associated gastrinomas. Because more than 50% of these patients have metastatic and multifocal disease at presentation, MEN-1 patients are rarely cured by surgery (**Fig. 6**). Hence, the goal of surgery in this group of patients is to reduce the risk of metastases and improve survival. Bartsch and colleagues[42] showed that patients with tumors less than 1 cm have only a 4% likelihood of having liver metastases compared with 60% of those with a tumor size greater than 3 cm. Most centers now observe patients with tumors smaller than 2 cm, and recommendations are to resect the primary tumor if size is greater than 2 cm. Controversy still exists about the use of a Whipple procedure in management of pancreatic head tumors in MEN-1 patients. For now, this approach is recommended for young patients and those who have large isolated pancreatic head tumors.[40,43] In the case of MEN-1 with primary hyperparathyroidism and ZES,

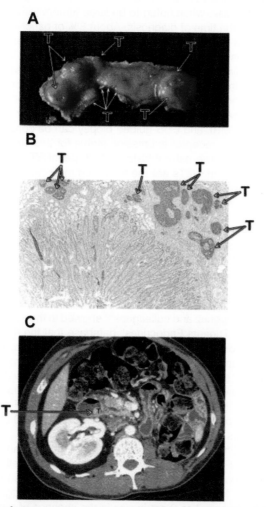

Fig. 6. Multifocality of MEN-1 gastrinomas. (*A*) Multifocal tumor (T) in a pancreatic resection gross specimen. (*B*) Multifocal tumor deposits (T) in a low-power photomicrograph. (*C*) Duodenal primary tumor (T). (*From* Huang LC, Poultsides GA, Norton JA. Surgical management of neuroendocrine tumors of the gastrointestinal tract. Oncology 2011;25(9):794–803.)

studies have shown that successful neck exploration for resection of parathyroid hyperplasia can reduce end organ effects of hypergastrinemia.[44] In these patients, parathyroidectomy must be performed before attempting a resection for the gastrinoma.[45]

Surgical treatment of sporadic gastrinomas has a high cure rate with a 20-year disease-free survival of 98% compared with 74% in nonoperated cases. Patients are followed yearly with fasting serum gastrin and chromogranin levels. A secretin provocation test is used if the patient is on PPIs. Imaging studies are less indicated if the above biochemical studies remain normal.

Nonfunctional Pancreatic Neuroendocrine Tumors

More than 75% of pancreatic endocrine tumors are NF-pancNETs.[46] They are so named because they lack a clinical syndrome of hormonal overproduction. Because the symptoms of NF-pancNETs are nonspecific, they are usually diagnosed late in the course of their disease, when noted to be large tumors with a high rate (60%) of metastatic disease at the time of diagnosis. About 8% of pancNETs occur in association with MEN-1, and in patients with MEN-1, 55% of tumors are NF-pancNETs.[47]

These tumors are usually discovered on routine radiographic imaging for nonspecific abdominal complaints. With compression of surrounding structures, many patients complain of pain or obstruction. Presence of these tumors is ascertained by measuring inert tumor markers such as chromogranin, pancreatic polypeptide, neuron-specific enolase, protein S, and neurotensin. Given their larger size, they are easily detected by CT/MRI, and EUS-guided biopsy can be considered. SRS is recommended to determine receptor expression status for postsurgical treatment with somatostatin analogues. The natural history of NF-pancNETs in MEN-1 is not well established. Malignant pancNETs are the most common cause of death in patients with MEN-1. They are the most common enteropancreatic NET associated with MEN-1 and confer a worse prognosis than functioning tumors such as insulinoma and gastrinoma.

Treatment of sporadic NF-pancNETs is surgical resection that is geared toward cure. The approach to surgery in MEN-1 patients, however, remains controversial. The goal of treatment here is to reduce morbidity and mortality because of metastatic disease while preserving as much pancreatic tissue as possible. MEN-1 patients tend to have a field defect that makes the entire pancreas at risk for neoplastic disease; therefore, resection of a primary lesion does not necessarily prevent recurrence in the remaining gland. Triponez and colleagues[48] showed in their analysis of the French "Groupe d' Etude des Tuneurs Endocrines" database that the risk of lymph node or distant metastases correlates directly with primary tumor size. In this study, only 3% of patients with tumors less than 2 cm had synchronous lymph nodes or distant metastases, and their survival was similar to patients with MEN-1 who had no pancreaticoduodenal involvement. Another study by the same group reported the presence of synchronous metastases in 43% of patients with NF-pancNETs of more than 3 cm, in 18% of patients with tumors between 2.1 and 3.0 cm, and in only 4% of patients with tumors less than 1 cm.[49]

Currently, several different recommendations exist for the management of MEN-1 patients with small NF-pancNETs. The clinical practice guidelines for MEN-1 by Thakker and colleagues[50] suggest considering surgical resection for tumors larger than 1 cm in size. The NCCN guidelines in the United States suggest a more conservative approach for tumors 1 to 2 cm in size in the absence of rapid progression on serial imaging. There seems to be consensus for a conservative stance toward tumors less than 1 cm and for resection for tumors greater than 2 cm. The management of tumors between 1 and 2 cm remains a matter of debate. Surgical resection is also recommended for lesions that have significant growth, such as doubling of tumor size over a 3- to 6-month interval for tumors of any size.

Other Functional Pancreatic Neuroendocrine Tumors

Glucagonomas are rare tumors that present in the fifth or sixth decade of life. They are frequently large (usually greater than 4 cm) at diagnosis, and 60% to 70% are malignant. Association with MEN-1 is rare. Clinical manifestations encompass what is commonly known as the "4 D syndrome," which includes diabetes mellitus type 2, dermatitis (necrolytic migratory erythema), deep vein thrombosis, and depression.[51] Other symptoms include weight loss, anemia, painful glossitis, and pulmonary emboli.

Biochemical diagnosis is made by measuring elevated plasma levels of glucagon to greater than 500 pg/mL and decreased levels of amino acids. Because most patients present with large tumors, CT scan with contrast is sufficient to detect 86% of tumors. SRS has also been shown to be useful in locating tumors and for long-term follow-up of patients.[52] These tumors cluster in the pancreatic tail and often present with synchronous liver metastases that may be amenable to distal pancreatectomy with or without partial hepatectomy in a staged or simultaneous fashion. A complete, margin-negative resection is typically achieved in only 30% of cases.[53] Somatostatin analogues should be considered preoperatively because their use can markedly diminish circulating levels of glucagon controlling its catabolic effects. Like other metastatic pancNETs, liver metastases have been treated with resection, ablation, hepatic artery embolization, and liver transplantation.

Somatostatinomas represent only 1% of all pancNETs and present clinically with steatorrhea, cholelithiasis, diabetes mellitus type 2, and hypochlorhydria that together comprise the somatostatinoma syndrome.[54] Most patients present with solitary lesions that are around 5 to 6 cm in size, and these clinical manifestations are rarely observed with lesions arising in the duodenum. Most somatostatinomas are malignant at presentation, and more than 75% have evidence of metastases at the time of surgical exploration particularly in tumors greater than 2 cm in size.[55]

Most are located in the head of the pancreas, and resection usually involves pancreaticoduodenectomy. Some surgeons perform a cholecystectomy at the same time because of the high incidence of symptomatic cholelithiasis in these patients. In patients without metastatic disease, the median 5-year survival can be 100% versus 60% in patients who undergo pancreatectomy and debulking of metastatic disease.[53]

MANAGEMENT OF NEUROENDOCRINE LIVER METASTASES

Hepatic metastases occur in more than 50% of patients with NETs. In contrast to exocrine pancreatic cancers, patients with endocrine tumors may warrant aggressive treatment and may benefit from reoperation for resectable recurrences or metastatic disease due to their indolent nature. Debulking of metastatic disease, even in situations wherein not all of the tumor can be removed, may still hold value in cases wherein patients are symptomatic from hormonal activity relating to the disease burden. Neuroendocrine liver metastases (NELMs) can progress without raising suspicion, until symptoms associated with pain, mass effect, or hormone overproduction occur. The rationale for cytoreductive surgery is (1) to improve quality of life in patients with bulky, symptomatic tumors; (2) to reduce volume to prevent further metastases; (3) to improve symptom-free survival.[56] The estimated 5-year survival in patients treated medically ranges from 0% to 40%. Studies have shown extended survival and symptom control with aggressive cytoreduction.[14,57]

A retrospective study by Chamberlain and colleagues[14] in 2000 at Memorial Sloan-Kettering Cancer Center reviewed records of 85 patients with hepatic NET metastases between 1992 and 1998. In this study, 41 patients had carcinoids, 26 were NF-pancNETs, and 18 were F-pancNETs. Eighty-four percent of patients had bilobar metastases. Thirty-three patients underwent hepatic artery embolization (HAE), and 34 underwent hepatic resection. Eighteen patients were treated with best medical treatment (BMT). The 1-, 3-, and 5-year survival rates for patients treated by HAE are 94%, 83%, and 51%, respectively, and the 1-, 3-, and 5-year survivals for patients treated operatively were 94%, 83%, and 76%, which was far superior to the 0% to 40% 5-year survival rate on BMT alone. The authors of this report concluded that hepatic metastases from NETs are best managed through a multidisciplinary approach, and that although surgical resection of NELMs may prolong survival, it is rarely curative. In 2003, Sarmiento and colleagues,[58] using data from the Mayo Clinic, published a retrospective review of 170 patients with NELMs who were identified between 1977 and 1998. Primary sites were carcinoid of the small bowel and pancNETs. Resection was classified as complete (75 patients) or incomplete (palliative intent, 95 patients). When done for palliation, all patients had at least 90% of their disease resected. Overall survival was 61% at 5 years with a median survival of 81 months, and recurrence rate was 84% at 5 years. No difference was found in recurrence rates between carcinoids and islet cell tumors (82% vs 88%). No difference was found in overall survival either. Recurrence rates were lower for patients with a complete resection compared with those who underwent an incomplete resection (76% vs 91% at 5 years with median time to recurrence being 30 months vs 16 months). The conclusion drawn from this study was that, in the case of resectable lesions and good operative candidacy, aggressive resection for NET metastases definitely improved survival. Recurrence was high within 5 years of resection.

More recently, Mayo and colleagues[59] reported 339 patients who underwent surgical management of NELMs at 8 major hepatobiliary centers. Most had a pancreatic (40%) or a small bowel (25%) primary tumor. Seventy-eight percent of patients underwent hepatic resection; 3% underwent ablation alone, and 19% underwent both ablation and resection. Forty-six patients underwent a second liver-directed procedure. Median survival after surgery in this study was 125 months, with overall 5-year and 10-year survival rates of 74% and 51%, respectively (**Fig. 7**). Patients whose metastatic burden was confined to the liver had a median survival of 148 months following surgery compared with 85 months in patients with extrahepatic disease also. Looking at patients who underwent a repeat resection, median survival in this subset also was significant at 82.9 months. As with the Mayo Clinic study, the recurrence rate was still 94% at 5 years with a median time to recurrence of 15.2 months. On performing a multivariate analysis, 2 other factors that impacted survival aside from presence of extrahepatic disease were nonfunctional NET and synchronous disease, with increased recurrence found in these subsets of patients. Using this information, the investigators plotted Kaplan-Meier survival curves stratified by margin status and functionality of the tumor. They found that patients with functional tumors who had an R0/R1 resection had greater survival than the nonfunctional tumors (see **Fig. 7**). Thus, this study, like the others before it, showed that although cytoreduction definitely improves survival despite a high recurrence rate, it serves a better purpose in patients with functional NELMs who undergo R0/R1 resections than the nonfunctional tumors, in which case other liver-directed therapies may have to be considered.

Although patients with symptomatic disease are often offered cytoreduction to help palliate symptoms, the role of surgery for asymptomatic and nonfunctional NELMs is more controversial and needs to be highly individualized. Most patients with NELMs

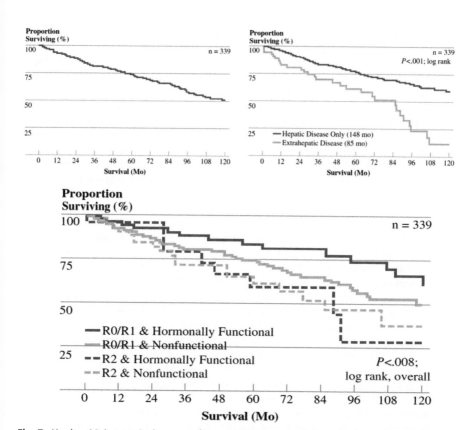

Fig. 7. Kaplan-Meier survival curves after surgical resection of NELMs. (*Data from* Mayo SC, Herman JM, Cosgrove D, et al. Emerging approaches in the management of patients with neuroendocrine liver metastasis: role of liver-directed and systemic therapies. J Am Coll Surg 2013;216(1):123–34.)

will present with bilobar disease, and achieving an R0 resection appears to be significantly lower compared with resections performed for colorectal metastases.[60–62] The literature supports the notion that patients in whom more than 75% of the liver is involved have a poor prognosis, and surgery alone should be avoided[14]; this is the reason in most centers, that NELM resection is usually combined with ablation to treat the hepatic tumor burden. Also, less than 20% of recurrences are amenable to reoperative surgery, and hence, other liver-directed therapies must be considered.

Ablation has thus been used (1) for deeper lesions that are less than 4 cm and less than 8 to 10 in number to minimize volume of resection; (2) in patients with recurrence following a prior resection; (3) as an adjunct to resection in patients with bilobar disease; (4) to palliate symptoms in patients with inoperable tumors. Several modalities are available, such as radiofrequency ablation (RFA, most common), microwave, laser, and cryotherapy. RFA is the dominant ablative modality used and is done in a percutaneous, open, or laparoscopic fashion. Several studies have shown a reduction in local and hormonal symptoms in 70% to 80% of patients for 1 year with a 50% reduction of tumor markers in a similar number of patients. Mazzaglia and colleagues[63] reported on the largest series of laparoscopic RFA, involving 63 patients with NELMs. All had resectable disease on imaging. Sixty-three patients were treated for 452 liver metastases without resection. Twenty-two percent of them had repeat ablations for progression of disease.

Fifty-seven percent of patients in this study were symptomatic, and 94% of them achieved symptom relief after the procedure. Median duration of symptom control was 11 months. The 5-year survival after RFA was 48% with a median survival of 3.9 years, which was higher than their medically treated counterparts. Breaking up survival based on number of ablations, patients who underwent single ablations had a survival of 5.2 years compared with 2.9 years for patients who underwent multiple ablations. Unfortunately, progressive liver disease was demonstrated on surveillance imaging in 80% of patients. Given this high rate of recurrence with surgery and ablation, many investigators suggested that the use of intra-arterial therapy (IAT) might be better suited for treating NELMs.

The concept of IAT stems from the fact that NELMs, unlike most hepatic metastases, derive their blood supply from the hepatic artery. Embolization of the feeding vessels to the tumor thus deprives them of their blood supply and helps retard tumor progression and palliate symptoms. IAT consists of (1) transarterial chemoembolization (TACE); (2) transarterial bland embolization (TAE); (3) chemoembolization with drug-eluting beads; and (4) radioembolization using Y90 spheres. Detailed discussion on IAT is beyond the scope of this topic; however, the authors will present one of the largest studies to date comparing surgery versus IAT for treatment of NELMs by Mayo and colleagues.[59] They compared 753 patients who underwent either surgery (339) or IAT/TACE (414) from 1985 to 2010. However, there were statistically significant differences in the baseline characteristics of the patient populations. For example, IAT patients were more likely to have an unknown primary, extrahepatic disease, bilobar disease, and higher disease burden (>25% liver involvement)—all of which were independent predictors of decreased survival in univariate analyses. Median survival with surgery was 123 months with a 5-year survival of 74% versus 33.5 months and 30% for IAT. An issue here was patient selection, because there was higher disease burden and worse biology for patients in the IAT arm. Using propensity score methodology, a subgroup of 118 patients (66 surgery and 52 IAT) were identified who were matched on similar clinicopathologic features. Analyzing this subgroup, the median survival was 84 months versus 38.9 months for surgery versus IAT. Additional analysis of this cohort, based on symptoms and tumor burden, revealed that high-volume, symptomatic patients benefited most from surgical management. Asymptomatic patients, on the other hand, fared better with IAT, although this difference did not reach statistical significance (16.7 months with surgery vs 18 months with IAT). Hence, this study concluded that surgery should be reserved for low-volume disease or high-volume functional disease, without compromising the functional liver remnant. In contrast, patients with a high burden of hepatic disease, especially those with asymptomatic disease, are probably best served with locoregional IAT than a surgical resection.

ROLE OF LIVER TRANSPLANTATION IN TREATMENT OF NEUROENDOCRINE LIVER METASTASES

Orthotopic liver transplantation (OLT) for patients with NELMs who have unresectable disease remains controversial and is performed only at a few centers. Reasons cited by advocates for OLT are (1) relative indolent nature of NETs; (2) propensity for liver-only metastases; and (3) high risk of intrahepatic recurrence after resection.[59] In Europe, NELMs account for only 0.4% of liver transplants. There have been no meaningful published data that show an improvement in life expectancy after transplant compared with spontaneous survival, that is, 20% to 30% at 5 years. To date, the largest series examining the role of OLT for NELMs was a multicenter French study by Le Treut and colleagues.[64] This study included 85 patients who underwent liver transplantation for NELMs from 1989 to 2005. In 40 cases, the primary tumor was located in the pancreas or the duodenum, digestive tract in 26 cases, and the bronchial tree in 5 cases. In the remaining 14 cases, the primary was undetermined. The investigators reported an in-hospital mortality of 14% and an overall survival rate of 47%. Factors associated with a poor prognosis were hepatomegaly and a primary NET arising from the duodenum or pancreas. Twenty-three patients who had both unfavorable prognostic factors had a 5-year survival rate of 12% versus 68% for the 55 patients presenting with one or neither factor. The study concluded that liver transplant can benefit selected patients with nonresectable NELMs. However, patients presenting with pancreaticoduodenal primaries in association with hepatomegaly are poor indications for liver transplantation. Mazzaferro and colleagues[65] developed criteria analogous to the Milan criteria for HCC. The inclusion criteria include low-grade NET histology, primary tumor drained by the portal system removed with a curative resection pretransplantation, less than 50% hepatic involvement by tumor, stable disease for at least 6 months during the pretransplantation period, and age 55 years or younger.

As of 2012, the NCCN practice guidelines consider transplantation for NELM to be investigational and not part of routine care at this time.[59]

SUMMARY

With the advent of various medical treatment options for these tumors, including somatostatin analogues, cytotoxic agents, mTOR inhibitors, and PRRT, the management of pancNETs and NELMs has truly become multimodal. Although the discussion regarding medical management of pancNETs using these modalities can be found in the article by Jennifer A. Chan and Matthew H. Kulke: Medical Management of Pancreatic Neuroendocrine Tumors: Current and Future Therapy, in this issue, surgical resection still plays a significant role with regards to improved survival and symptom control. Although liver-directed therapy such as ablation and IAT has been studied in tandem, and in comparison with surgery, further research is required to analyze the use of medical treatment options in concert with surgical resection in both the adjuvant and neoadjuvant settings to improve patient outcomes.

REFERENCES

1. Kloppel G, Heitz PU. Classification of normal and neoplastic neuroendocrine cells. Ann N Y Acad Sci 1994;733:19–23.
2. Rindi G, Capella C, Solcia E. Introduction to a revised clinicopathological classification of neuroendocrine tumors of the gastroenteropancreatic tract. Q J Nucl Med 2000;44(1):13–21.
3. Rindi G, Klöppel G, Alhman H, et al. TNM staging of foregut (neuro)endocrine tumors: a consensus proposal including a grading system. Virchows Arch 2006; 449(4):395–401.
4. American Joint Commission on Cancer, American Cancer Society. AJCC cancer staging manual. 7th edition. New York: Springer; 2010.
5. The NCCN Clinical Practice Guidelines in Oncology (NCCN Guidelines) Neuroendocrine tumors. 2012.
6. Ito T, Igarashi H, Jensen RT. Therapy of metastatic pancreatic neuroendocrine tumors (PancNETs): recent insights and advances. J Gastroenterol 2012;47(9): 941–60.

7. Jensen RT, Cadiot G, Brandi ML, et al. ENETS Consensus Guidelines for the management of patients with digestive neuroendocrine neoplasms: functional pancreatic endocrine tumor syndromes. Neuroendocrinology 2012;95(2):98–119.

8. Kulke MH, Anthony LB, Bushnell DL, et al. NANETS treatment guidelines: well-differentiated neuroendocrine tumors of the stomach and pancreas. Pancreas 2010;39(6):735–52.

9. Metz DC, Jensen RT. Gastrointestinal neuroendocrine tumors: pancreatic endocrine tumors. Gastroenterology 2008;135(5):1469–92.

10. Gullo L, Migliori M, Falconi M, et al. Nonfunctioning pancreatic endocrine tumors: a multicenter clinical study. Am J Gastroenterol 2003;98(11):2435–9.

11. Ito T, Sasano H, Tanaka M, et al. Epidemiological study of gastroenteropancreatic neuroendocrine tumors in Japan. J Gastroenterol 2010;45(2):234–43.

12. Jensen RT, Berna MJ, Bingham DB, et al. Inherited pancreatic endocrine tumor syndromes: advances in molecular pathogenesis, diagnosis, management, and controversies. Cancer 2008;113(7 Suppl):1807–43.

13. Pipeleers-Marichal M, Somers G, Willems G, et al. Gastrinomas in the duodenums of patients with multiple endocrine neoplasia type 1 and the Zollinger-Ellison syndrome. N Engl J Med 1990;322(11):723–7.

14. Chamberlain RS, Canes D, Brown KT, et al. Hepatic neuroendocrine metastases: does intervention alter outcomes? J Am Coll Surg 2000;190(4):432–45.

15. Hoeffel C, Job L, Ladam-Marcus V, et al. Detection of hepatic metastases from carcinoid tumor: prospective evaluation of contrast-enhanced ultrasonography. Dig Dis Sci 2009;54(9):2040–6.

16. Massironi S, Conte D, Sciola V, et al. Contrast-enhanced ultrasonography in evaluating hepatic metastases from neuroendocrine tumours. Dig Liver Dis 2010; 42(9):635–41.

17. de Herder WW, Kwekkeboom DJ, Valkema R, et al. Neuroendocrine tumors and somatostatin: imaging techniques. J Endocrinol Invest 2005;28(11 Suppl International):132–6.

18. Kwekkeboom DJ, Krenning EP, Scheidhauer K, et al. ENETS Consensus Guidelines for the Standards of Care in Neuroendocrine Tumors: somatostatin receptor imaging with (111)In-pentetreotide. Neuroendocrinology 2009;90(2):184–9.

19. Ambrosini V, Campana D, Bodei L, et al. 68Ga-DOTANOC PET/CT clinical impact in patients with neuroendocrine tumors. J Nucl Med 2010;51(5):669–73.

20. Frilling A, Sotiropoulos GC, Radtke A, et al. The impact of 68Ga-DOTATOC positron emission tomography/computed tomography on the multimodal management of patients with neuroendocrine tumors. Ann Surg 2010;252(5):850–6.

21. Grama D, Eriksson B, Mårtensson H, et al. Clinical characteristics, treatment and survival in patients with pancreatic tumors causing hormonal syndromes. World J Surg 1992;16(4):632–9.

22. Park BJ, Alexander HR, Libutti SK, et al. Operative management of islet-cell tumors arising in the head of the pancreas. Surgery 1998;124(6):1056–61 [discussion: 1061–2].

23. Sheppard BC, Norton JA, Doppman JL, et al. Management of islet cell tumors in patients with multiple endocrine neoplasia: a prospective study. Surgery 1989; 106(6):1108–17 [discussion: 1117–8].

24. Sotoudehmanesh R, Hedayat A, Shirazian N, et al. Endoscopic ultrasonography (EUS) in the localization of insulinoma. Endocrine 2007;31(3):238–41.

25. Kisker O, Bartsch D, Weinel RJ, et al. The value of somatostatin-receptor scintigraphy in newly diagnosed endocrine gastroenteropancreatic tumors. J Am Coll Surg 1997;184(5):487–92.

26. Guettier JM, Kam A, Chang R, et al. Localization of insulinomas to regions of the pancreas by intraarterial calcium stimulation: the NIH experience. J Clin Endocrinol Metab 2009;94(4):1074–80.

27. Hashimoto LA, Walsh RM. Preoperative localization of insulinomas is not necessary. J Am Coll Surg 1999;189(4):368–73.

28. Lo CY, Lam KY, Kung AW, et al. Pancreatic insulinomas. A 15-year experience. Arch Surg 1997;132(8):926–30.

29. Arnold R, Wied M, Behr TH. Somatostatin analogues in the treatment of endocrine tumors of the gastrointestinal tract. Expert Opin Pharmacother 2002;3(6):643–56.

30. Boukhman MP, Karam JH, Shaver J, et al. Insulinoma–experience from 1950 to 1995. West J Med 1998;169(2):98–104.

31. Norton JA, Cromack DT, Shawker TH, et al. Intraoperative ultrasonographic localization of islet cell tumors. A prospective comparison to palpation. Ann Surg 1988;207(2):160–8.

32. Nikfarjam M, Warshaw AL, Axelrod L, et al. Improved contemporary surgical management of insulinomas: a 25-year experience at the Massachusetts General Hospital. Ann Surg 2008;247(1):165–72.

33. Weber HC, Venzon DJ, Lin JT, et al. Determinants of metastatic rate and survival in patients with Zollinger-Ellison syndrome: a prospective long-term study. Gastroenterology 1995;108(6):1637–49.

34. Andersen DK. Current diagnosis and management of Zollinger-Ellison syndrome. Ann Surg 1989;210(6):685–703.

35. Berna MJ, Hoffmann KM, Long SH, et al. Serum gastrin in Zollinger-Ellison syndrome: II. Prospective study of gastrin provocative testing in 293 patients from the National Institutes of Health and comparison with 537 cases from the literature. evaluation of diagnostic criteria, proposal of new criteria, and correlations with clinical and tumoral features. Medicine (Baltimore) 2006;85(6):331–64.

36. Roy PK, Venzon DJ, Shojamanesh H, et al. Zollinger-Ellison syndrome. Clinical presentation in 261 patients. Medicine (Baltimore) 2000;79(6):379–411.

37. Klose KJ, Heverhagen JT. Localisation and staging of gastrin producing tumours using cross-sectional imaging modalities. Wien Klin Wochenschr 2007; 119(19–20):588–92.

38. Noone TC, Hosey J, Firat Z, et al. Imaging and localization of islet-cell tumours of the pancreas on CT and MRI. Best Pract Res Clin Endocrinol Metab 2005;19(2): 195–211.

39. Stabile BE, Morrow DJ, Passaro E Jr. The gastrinoma triangle: operative implications. Am J Surg 1984;147(1):25–31.

40. Morrow EH, Norton JA. Surgical management of Zollinger-Ellison syndrome; state of the art. Surg Clin North Am 2009;89(5):1091–103.

41. Norton JA, Alexander HR, Fraker DL, et al. Does the use of routine duodenotomy (DUODX) affect rate of cure, development of liver metastases, or survival in patients with Zollinger-Ellison syndrome? Ann Surg 2004;239(5):617–25 [discussion: 626].

42. Bartsch DK, Langer P, Rothmund M. Surgical aspects of gastrinoma in multiple endocrine neoplasia type 1. Wien Klin Wochenschr 2007;119(19–20):602–8.

43. Fendrich V, Langer P, Waldmann J, et al. Management of sporadic and multiple endocrine neoplasia type 1 gastrinomas. Br J Surg 2007;94(11):1331–41.

44. Norton JA. Gastrinoma: advances in localization and treatment. Surg Oncol Clin N Am 1998;7(4):845–61.

45. Norton JA, Cornelius MJ, Doppman JL, et al. Effect of parathyroidectomy in patients with hyperparathyroidism, Zollinger-Ellison syndrome, and multiple endocrine neoplasia type I: a prospective study. Surgery 1987;102(6):958–66.

46. Halfdanarson TR, Rabe KG, Rubin J, et al. Pancreatic neuroendocrine tumors (PANCNETs): incidence, prognosis and recent trend toward improved survival. Ann Oncol 2008;19(10):1727–33.

47. Thomas-Marques L, Murat A, Delemer B, et al. Prospective endoscopic ultrasonographic evaluation of the frequency of nonfunctioning pancreaticoduodenal endocrine tumors in patients with multiple endocrine neoplasia type 1. Am J Gastroenterol 2006;101(2):266–73.

48. Triponez F, Goudet P, Dosseh D, et al. Is surgery beneficial for MEN1 patients with small (< or = 2 cm), nonfunctioning pancreaticoduodenal endocrine tumor? An analysis of 65 patients from the GTE. World J Surg 2006;30(5):654–62 [discussion: 663–4].

49. Triponez F, Dosseh D, Goudet P, et al. Epidemiology data on 108 patients from the GTE with isolated nonfunctioning tumors of the pancreas. Ann Surg 2006; 243(2):265–72.

50. Thakker RV, Newey PJ, Walls GV, et al. Clinical practice guidelines for multiple endocrine neoplasia type 1 (MEN1). J Clin Endocrinol Metab 2012;97(9): 2990–3011.

51. Norton JA. Neuroendocrine tumors of the pancreas and duodenum. Curr Probl Surg 1994;31(2):77–156.

52. Lipp RW, Schnedl WJ, Stauber R, et al. Scintigraphic long-term follow-up of a patient with metastatic glucagonoma. Am J Gastroenterol 2000;95(7):1818–20.

53. Abood GJ, Go A, Malhotra D, et al. The surgical and systemic management of neuroendocrine tumors of the pancreas. Surg Clin North Am 2009;89(1): 249–66, x.

54. Krejs GJ, Orci L, Conlon JM, et al. Somatostatinoma syndrome. Biochemical, morphologic and clinical features. N Engl J Med 1979;301(6):285–92.

55. Tanaka S, Yamasaki S, Matsushita H, et al. Duodenal somatostatinoma: a case report and review of 31 cases with special reference to the relationship between tumor size and metastasis. Pathol Int 2000;50(2):146–52.

56. Maithel SK, Fong Y. Hepatic ablation for neuroendocrine tumor metastases. J Surg Oncol 2009;100(8):635–8.

57. Norton JA, Kivlen M, Li M, et al. Morbidity and mortality of aggressive resection in patients with advanced neuroendocrine tumors. Arch Surg 2003;138(8):859–66.

58. Sarmiento JM, Heywood G, Rubin J, et al. Surgical treatment of neuroendocrine metastases to the liver: a plea for resection to increase survival. J Am Coll Surg 2003;197(1):29–37.

59. Mayo SC, Herman JM, Cosgrove D, et al. Emerging approaches in the management of patients with neuroendocrine liver metastasis: role of liver-directed and systemic therapies. J Am Coll Surg 2013;216(1):123–34.

60. de Jong MC, Mayo SC, Pulitano C, et al. Repeat curative intent liver surgery is safe and effective for recurrent colorectal liver metastasis: results from an international multi-institutional analysis. J Gastrointest Surg 2009;13(12):2141–51.

61. de Jong MC, Pulitano C, Ribero D, et al. Rates and patterns of recurrence following curative intent surgery for colorectal liver metastasis: an international multi-institutional analysis of 1669 patients. Ann Surg 2009;250(3):440–8.

62. Pawlik TM, Vauthey JN. Surgical margins during hepatic surgery for colorectal liver metastases: complete resection not millimeters defines outcome. Ann Surg Oncol 2008;15(3):677–9.

63. Mazzaglia PJ, Berber E, Milas M, et al. Laparoscopic radiofrequency ablation of neuroendocrine liver metastases: a 10-year experience evaluating predictors of survival. Surgery 2007;142(1):10–9.

64. Le Treut YP, Grégoire E, Belghiti J, et al. Predictors of long-term survival after liver transplantation for metastatic endocrine tumors: an 85-case French multicentric report. Am J Transplant 2008;8(6):1205–13.

65. Mazzaferro V, Pulvirenti A, Coppa J. Neuroendocrine tumors metastatic to the liver: how to select patients for liver transplantation? J Hepatol 2007;47(4):460–6.

Medical Management of Pancreatic Neuroendocrine Tumors: Current and Future Therapy

 CrossMark

Jennifer A. Chan, MD, MPH*, Matthew H. Kulke, MD, MMSc

KEYWORDS

- Pancreatic neuroendocrine tumor • Somatostatin analogue • mTOR • Everolimus
- Sunitinib • Temozolomide

KEY POINTS

- Low- and intermediate-grade pancreatic neuroendocrine tumors (NETs) are characterized by variable but most often indolent biological behavior.
- Somatostatin analogues decrease hormone production in functional NETs and improve progression-free survival.
- The tyrosine kinase inhibitor sunitinib and the mechanistic target of rapamycin inhibitor everolimus improve progression-free survival in patients with progressive pancreatic NETs.
- Pancreatic NETs may respond to alkylating agents, including streptozocin and temozolomide.
- Studies to evaluate the optimal timing, sequence, and combination of therapies and to identify predictors of response are warranted.

INTRODUCTION

Well-differentiated neuroendocrine tumors (NETs) are a rare and heterogeneous group of neoplasms that arise from neuroendocrine cells located throughout the body. These tumors can be broadly classified as either pancreatic NETs or carcinoid tumors, which include NETs arising in other sites, including the thymus, lung, and gastrointestinal (GI) tract. They are characterized by variable but most often indolent biological behavior and are also classically characterized by their ability to secrete peptides resulting in distinctive hormonal syndromes.

Disclosure Statements: Dr J.A. Chan has received institutional research funding from Novartis and Sanofi-Aventis. She has served as an advisor for Ipsen and Novartis and holds stock in Merck. Dr M.H. Kulke has served as an advisor for Ipsen and Novartis.
Department of Medical Oncology, Dana-Farber Cancer Institute, Dana 1220, 450 Brookline Avenue, Boston, MA 02215, USA
* Corresponding author.
E-mail address: jang@partners.org

Surg Oncol Clin N Am 25 (2016) 423–437
http://dx.doi.org/10.1016/j.soc.2015.11.009
1055-3207/16/$ – see front matter © 2016 Elsevier Inc. All rights reserved.

surgonc.theclinics.com

Pancreatic NETs compose approximately 1% to 2% of all pancreatic neoplasms. Although NETs have been considered rare, recent studies suggest that they are more common than previously suspected. Analysis of the Surveillance, Epidemiology, and End Results database has demonstrated a significant increase in the incidence of NETs over time, with an age-adjusted annual incidence of pancreatic NETs in the United States of 0.3 cases per 100,000 population.[1] The increase in incidence is likely attributable to increasing awareness, improved diagnostic strategies, and possibly other undetermined environmental and genetic factors.

When pancreatic NETs are diagnosed at an early stage, surgical resection is often curative. Unfortunately, curative surgery is rarely an option for patients with metastatic disease. Until recently, systemic treatment options for patients with advanced pancreatic NETs were limited. However, improvements in our understanding of signaling pathways involved in the pathogenesis, growth, and spread of NETs have translated into an expansion of treatment options. Treatment approaches with somatostatin analogues, agents targeting the vascular endothelial growth factor (VEGF) signaling pathway and the mechanistic target of rapamycin (mTOR), provide therapeutic options for these patients. Cytotoxic chemotherapy may also benefit some patients, particularly those with high disease burden. The aim of this article is to summarize the current and future systemic therapy options for patients with advanced pancreatic NETs.

CLASSIFICATION OF PANCREATIC NEUROENDOCRINE TUMORS

Several histologic and anatomic classification systems for NETs have been proposed. Although there are differences in the specific criteria for grading tumors, the classification systems reflect the observation that NETs consist of a spectrum of diseases ranging from indolent well-differentiated, low-grade tumors to aggressive poorly differentiated, high-grade tumors (**Table 1**). In general, tumors with a high histologic grade represent aggressive neuroendocrine carcinomas that have a different natural history and response to treatment compared with low-grade, well-differentiated NETs.[2-4] In the 2010 World Health Organization (WHO) classification, neuroendocrine neoplasms of the digestive system are categorized as low grade (G1), intermediate grade (G2), and high grade (G3) based on the mitotic count and proliferative (Ki-67) index.[2] High-grade carcinomas have a more aggressive biology and are generally treated with platinum-based chemotherapy regimens used to treat small cell lung cancer. In contrast, well-differentiated, low- and intermediate-grade NETs have lower measures of cell proliferation and a more indolent biology.

Notably, there is a subset of patients with NETs that seem histologically well differentiated or moderately differentiated but have Ki-67 proliferation indices greater than 20% that fall into the high-grade range.[5] The most appropriate therapy for this heterogeneous subgroup of patients has not been well established. In a retrospective study of 305 patients with G3 neuroendocrine carcinomas of the GI tract (23% with pancreatic primary site), patients with a Ki-67 less than 55% had significantly longer median survival compared with patients with higher Ki-67 indices (14 months vs 10 months).[6] Response rates to platinum-based chemotherapy were lower in patients with a Ki-67 less than 55% (15% vs 42%). Because sensitivity to platinum-based chemotherapy seems to be associated with higher Ki-67 proliferation rates, other cytotoxic agents, such as temozolomide, or targeted agents, such as mTOR inhibitors or VEGF pathway inhibitors, may play a role in the management of well- to moderately differentiated high-grade disease.

Pancreatic NETs are also classified according to their functional status. Functional tumors, which account for approximately 30% of pancreatic NETs, are associated

Table 1
Nomenclature and classification for NETs

Differentiation	Grade	Mitotic Count[a]	Ki-67 Index[b] (%)	Traditional	ENETS,[65,66] WHO[2]
Well differentiated	Low grade (G1)	<2 per 10 HPF	≤2	Carcinoid, islet cell, pancreatic NET	NET, grade 1
	Intermediate grade (G2)	2–20 per 10 HPF	3–20	Carcinoid, atypical carcinoid[c], islet cell, pancreatic NET	NET, grade 2
Poorly differentiated	High grade (G3)	>20 per 10 HPF	>20	Small cell carcinoma	Neuroendocrine carcinoma, grade 3, small cell
				Large cell neuroendocrine carcinoma	Neuroendocrine carcinoma, grade 3, large cell

Abbreviations: ENETS, European Neuroendocrine Tumor Society; HPF, high power field.

[a] Counted in 10 high power fields. High power field = 2 mm^2 at least 40 fields (at 40× magnification) evaluated in areas of highest mitotic density. Cutoffs per AJCC seventh edition.[67]

[b] MIB1 antibody; percentage of 2000 tumor cells in areas of highest nuclear labeling. Cutoffs per AJCC seventh edition.[67]

[c] The term *atypical carcinoid* only applies to intermediate-grade NETs of the lung.

with clinical syndromes related to hormone secretion.[7] These tumors, including insulinoma, gastrinoma, glucagonoma, and vasoactive intestinal peptide (VIPoma), are named according to the hormone that is secreted. In contrast, nonfunctional tumors include those that are not associated with a specific clinical syndrome related to hormone secretion.

GENETIC BASIS OF NEUROENDOCRINE TUMORS
Inherited Neuroendocrine Tumor Syndromes

Most pancreatic NETs occur as nonfamilial (sporadic) tumors. However, several autosomal dominant genetic syndromes, including multiple endocrine neoplasia type 1 (MEN1), von Hippel-Lindau syndrome (VHL), neurofibromatosis type 1 (NF-1), and tuberous sclerosis (TS), have been associated with the development of NETs. MEN1 is caused by inactivating mutations of the *MEN1* gene. VHL results from germline mutations in the *VHL* gene, which functions as a tumor suppressor gene that regulates hypoxia-induced cell proliferation and angiogenesis. NF-1 and TS are caused by inactivating mutations in the tumor suppressor genes *NF1* and *TSC1* and *TSC2*, respectively.[8] *NF1* encodes the protein neurofibromin, which regulates *TSC1* and *TSC2*.[9] TSC1 and TSC2 form a tumor suppressor heterodimer that inhibits *mTOR*. Although most NETs are sporadic, the molecular genetics of these tumor susceptibility syndromes provide insight into the genetic mechanisms of this disease.

Recent efforts have also focused on the genetic basis of sporadic, nonfamilial pancreatic NETs. In a study involving exome sequencing of nonfamilial pancreatic NETs, Jiao and colleagues[10] found that the most frequently mutated genes encoded proteins involved in chromatin remodeling. Forty-four percent of tumors had somatic inactivating mutations in *MEN1*, and 43% had mutations in genes encoding either death-domain-associated protein (*DAXX*) or α thalassemia/mental retardation syndrome X-linked (*ATRX*). Mutations in genes in the mTOR pathway occurred in 14% of tumors. Furthermore, mutations in *MEN1* and *DAXX/ATRX* genes may identify a biologically distinct subgroup of pancreatic NETs with a favorable prognosis. Mutations in *MEN1, DAXX/ATRX*, or the combination of these genes were associated with improved survival; 100% of patients with mutations in both *MEN1* and *DAXX/ATRX* survived at least 10 years in contrast to death within 5 years of diagnosis for 60% of patients without these mutations.[10] Studies are ongoing to investigate whether the mutational profile is a predictive response to chemotherapy or targeted agents, including mTOR inhibitors.

SYSTEMIC TREATMENT OF ADVANCED PANCREATIC NEUROENDOCRINE TUMORS

Multiple options are available for the management of patients with advanced, metastatic pancreatic NETs, including surgical resection, liver-directed therapies, and systemic therapy. Because of the heterogeneity of disease biology and presentation, a multidisciplinary approach to management is critical. The goals of therapy are to improve symptoms related to hormone hypersecretion, slow disease progression, and improve survival. Systemic therapy options include somatostatin analogue therapy, cytotoxic chemotherapy, and targeted agents, including everolimus and sunitinib.

Somatostatin Analogues

Somatostatin is a natural 14-amino acid peptide that binds to G-protein-coupled somatostatin receptors (SSTRs) that are expressed on most NETs.[11] Of the 5 different SSTR subtypes, SSTR-2 is expressed in approximately 80% of pancreatic NETs, with the exception of insulinomas, which express SSTR-2 in less the 50% of cases.[12]

By binding to somatostatin receptors, somatostatin analogues, including octreotide and lanreotide, have both antisecretory and antiproliferative effects.

Somatostatin analogues and control of symptoms from hormone secretion
Patients with metastases from functional pancreatic NETs often become symptomatic from hormone hypersecretion rather than from tumor bulk. Symptoms related to hormone secretion can often be well controlled with somatostatin analogues. The role of somatostatin analogues has been best established for patients with VIPoma and glucagonoma.[13,14] Overproduction of vasoactive intestinal peptide can result in severe secretory diarrhea and hypokalemia. These tumors are very responsive to administration of somatostatin analogues, which can reduce VIP levels and improve symptoms.[15,16] In patients with glucagonoma, reduction in glucagon levels and improvement in the characteristic rash (necrolytic migratory erythema) are observed in most patients with the use of somatostatin analogues.[17,18]

Although insulinomas and gastrinomas represent the most common types of functioning pancreatic NETs, the role of somatostatin analogues in controlling hormone-related symptoms for these tumor types is less well established. In patients with gastrinoma, high-dose proton pump inhibitors can effectively control hypergastrinemia-related gastric acid production and remain a mainstay of treatment in these patients. In patients with insulinoma, only 50% of patients express SSTR-2. In patients without SSTR-2 expression, hypoglycemia may paradoxically worsen because of inhibition of glucagon secretion caused by somatostatin analogue therapy. Therefore, patients with insulinoma need to be closely monitored when initiating therapy with somatostatin analogue therapy.

Somatostatin analogues and disease control
The antiproliferative effects of somatostatin analogues occur through both direct and indirect mechanisms. Binding of somatostatin analogues to SSTR-2 and SSTR-5 can lead to arrest of mitosis and cell cycle and may also induce apoptosis. The indirect antiproliferative effects of somatostatin analogues may be mediated through decreased production of circulating growth factors and inhibition of angiogenesis via reduction in production and release of proangiogenic factors.[19–21]

Although objective tumor shrinkage with somatostatin analogues is rare, tumor growth may be slowed. In the PROMID study, 85 patients with inoperable or metastatic well-differentiated midgut NETs were randomized to receive octreotide LAR 30 mg monthly or placebo.[22] Median time to tumor progression was significantly longer for patients receiving octreotide (14.3 vs 6.0 months). A limitation of this study, however, was that it did not include patients with pancreatic NETs.

More recently, however, support for the antiproliferative effect of somatostatin analogues in pancreatic NETs was provided by the phase III CLARINET trial, which compared lanreotide versus placebo in 204 patients with advanced well- or moderately differentiated, nonfunctioning GI and pancreatic (45%) NETs.[23] Patients were randomly assigned to receive either 120 mg lanreotide Autogel or placebo every 4 weeks for 96 weeks or until progressive disease or death. All patients had avid disease on SSTR scintigraphy. Most patients (96%) had no tumor progression in the 3 to 6 months before randomization. Compared with placebo, lanreotide was associated with significantly prolonged progression-free survival (PFS), with a similar effect seen across major subgroups. At a time point of 2 years following initiation of treatment, the median PFS was not reached with lanreotide compared with 18 months with placebo (hazard ratio [HR] for progression or death 0.45; 95% confidence interval [CI] 0.30–0.73). Based on these data, lanreotide has been approved in the United

States for the treatment of patients with unresectable, well- or moderately differentiated, locally advanced or metastatic gastroenteropancreatic NETs.

TARGETED THERAPY
Mechanistic Target of Rapamycin Inhibitors

The mTOR (also referred to as mammalian target of rapamycin) is an intracellular serine/threonine kinase that regulates key cell functions involved in cell survival, proliferation, and metabolism. Signaling through the PI3K (phosphatidylinositide 3-kinase)/AKT/mTOR pathway leads to increased translation of proteins regulating cell cycle progression and metabolism.[24] mTOR mediates downstream signaling from several pathways, including VEGF and insulin-like growth factor (IGF), that are implicated in NET growth.[25] Several observations support the importance of the mTOR pathway in the pathogenesis of NET. First, although most NETs arise sporadically, NETs can arise within the context of several familial cancer syndromes, including NF-1 and TSC, that are due to inactivating mutation in tumor suppressor genes leading to activation of the mTOR pathway. Additionally, gene expression analyses have demonstrated altered expression of genes in the mTOR pathway, and recent gene sequencing studies of pancreatic NETs have revealed mutations in genes in the mTOR pathway in 14% of tumors.[10,26]

Everolimus monotherapy was compared with best supportive care alone in the placebo-controlled RADIANT-3 trial, which included 410 patients with advanced pancreatic NETs (**Table 2**).[27] Approximately 40% of patients also received somatostatin analogue therapy. Everolimus was associated with a significant prolongation in median PFS (11.0 vs 4.6 months, HR for progression 0.35, 95% CI 0.27–0.45). Confirmed objective partial radiographic responses were observed in 5% of patients receiving everolimus compared with 2% of those receiving placebo. The rate of tumor stabilization was high, 73% among patients receiving everolimus versus 51% in the placebo group. Based on this result, everolimus was approved by the Food and Drug Administration (FDA) for patients with progressive pancreatic NETs.

Table 2
Clinical trials of mTOR inhibitors in pancreatic NET tumors

Study	Agent	No. Patients	Tumor Response Rate (%)	Median TTP (T) or PFS (P)	Reference
Phase II studies					
RADIANT-1	Everolimus	115	9	9.7 mo[P]	Yao et al,[61] 2010
	Everolimus + octreotide	45	4	16.7 mo[P]	
	Temsirolimus[a]	15	7	10.6 mo[T]	Duran et al,[68] 2006
	Temsirolimus + bevacizumab	58	41	13.2 mo[P]	Hobday et al,[58] 2014
Phase III studies					
RADIANT-3	Everolimus	207	5	11.0 mo[P]	Yao et al,[27] 2011
	Placebo	203	2	4.6 mo[P]	
CALGB 80701	Everolimus	75	12	14.0 mo[P]	Kulke et al,[59] 2015
	Everolimus + bevacizumab	75	31	16.7 mo[P]	

Abbreviations: CALGB, Cancer and Leukemia Group B; PFS, progression-free survival; TTP, time to progression.
[a] Data from the subset of patients with pancreatic NET in this phase II study of unselected patients with NET are presented.

Drug-related adverse events included stomatitis, rash, diarrhea, and fatigue.[27] The most common grade 3 or 4 drug-related adverse events were stomatitis (7%), anemia (6%), and hyperglycemia (5%). Although rare, everolimus has been associated with serious adverse events, including pneumonitis.

Everolimus causes hyperglycemia, particularly in those with preexisting hyperglycemia. In the RADIANT-3 trial, the frequency of severe (grade 3 or 4) hyperglycemia was higher in those with preexisting diabetes mellitus or baseline hyperglycemia (15% vs 3% in those without diabetes or baseline hyperglycemia).[28] Because of this effect, everolimus may be of particular value in patients with hypoglycemia related to insulinoma.[29,30] An objective tumor response may lead to improvements in insulin secretion, and it is also possible that everolimus may have a direct effect on insulin production and/or release or an effect on peripheral insulin sensitivity.

Vascular endothelial growth factor pathway inhibitors

A key role for angiogenesis and VEGF pathway signaling in NET is suggested by clinical observations that NETs are vascular tumors. Expression of VEGF has been demonstrated in carcinoid and pancreatic NETs.[31,32] Increased expression of VEGF receptor-2 (VEGFR-2) has been demonstrated in tissue from GI carcinoid tumors and a carcinoid cell line.[33,34] Additionally, pancreatic NETs show widespread expression of VEGFR-2 and -3 in addition to platelet-derived growth factor receptors α and β, stem-cell factor receptor (c-kit).[35–37]

Sunitinib was evaluated in a multi-institutional phase II study enrolling 109 patients with advanced NETs (**Table 3**).[38] Partial responses were observed in 16% of the pancreatic neuroendocrine cohort. Based on evidence of activity in this study, an international randomized phase III study to confirm the activity of sunitinib in pancreatic NETs was undertaken. After enrolling 171 patients, the study was halted before a planned interim analysis. Treatment with sunitinib was associated with a median PFS of 11.4 months, as compared with 5.5 months for placebo (HR 0.42, 95% CI 0.26–0.66).[39] Based on this result, sunitinib was approved by the FDA for patients with progressive pancreatic NETs. The most common grade 3 or 4 drug-related adverse events were neutropenia (12%), hypertension (10%), fatigue (5%), and diarrhea (5%).

Table 3 Clinical trials of VEGF pathway inhibitors in pancreatic NET tumors					
Study	Agent	No. Patients	Tumor Response Rate (%)	Median TTP or PFS	Reference
Phase II studies	Sunitinib[a]	66	17	7.7 mo[T]	Kulke et al,[38] 2008
	Sorafenib[a]	43	11	11.9 mo[P]	Hobday et al,[40] 2007
	Pazopanib[a]	32	22	14.4 mo[P]	Phan et al,[41] 2015
	Bevacizumab	22	9	13.6 mo[P]	Hobday et al,[42] 2015
	Temsirolimus + bevacizumab	58	41	13.2 mo[P]	Hobday et al,[58] 2014
Phase III studies	Sunitinib	86	9	11.4 mo[P]	Raymond et al,[39] 2011
	Placebo	85	0	5.5 mo[P]	
CALGB 80701	Everolimus	75	12	14 mo[P]	Kulke et al,[59] 2015
	Everolimus + bevacizumab	75	31	16.7 mo[P]	

Abbreviations: P, median PFS; PFS, progression-free survival; T, median time to progression; TTP, time to progression.
  [a] Data from the subset of patients with pancreatic NET in these phase II studies of unselected patients with NET are presented.

Other tyrosine kinase inhibitors with activity against VEGFR have been evaluated in prospective trials of patients with advanced pancreatic NETs (see **Table 3**). In a preliminary report of a phase II study examining the activity of sorafenib in the treatment of NETs, responses were seen 11% of 43 patients with pancreatic NETs.[40] Pazopanib has been evaluated in a phase II study that enrolled 52 patients with advanced NETs, including 32 with pancreatic NETs. Seven (22%) of the patients with pancreatic NETs achieved an objective response. Notably, 6 (29%) of the 21 patients with pancreatic NETs who had progressive disease at study entry showed objective responses. The median PFS and overall survival (OS) in the cohort with pancreatic NETs were 14.4 months and 25.0 months, respectively.[41]

Bevacizumab, a monoclonal antibody against VEGF, has also been evaluated as monotherapy in patients with advanced pancreatic NETs. In a phase II study of 22 patients with progressive well- or moderately differentiated pancreatic NETs, treatment with bevacizumab was associated with a confirmed partial response rate of 9% and median PFS of 13.6 months.[42]

Cytotoxic Chemotherapy

Various studies have demonstrated that pancreatic NETs are responsive to cytotoxic chemotherapy. Because of the higher response rates associated with chemotherapy compared with somatostatin analogues and targeted agents, chemotherapy is often used in patients who are symptomatic from tumor bulk or who have more rapidly progressive disease.

Streptozocin-containing regimens

In an early randomized trial, streptozocin plus doxorubicin had a combined biochemical and radiologic response rate of 69% and a median survival of 2.2 years.[43] The FDA subsequently approved streptozocin as a treatment of patients with pancreatic NETs. The very high response rates reported in this study may derive in part from the use of nonstandard response criteria. A large retrospective analysis of 84 patients with either locally advanced or metastatic pancreatic endocrine tumors receiving a 3-drug regimen of streptozocin, fluorouracil, and doxorubicin showed that this regimen was associated with an overall response rate of 39% and a median survival duration of 37 months.[44] Despite the demonstrated efficacy of streptozocin-based regimens, concerns about toxicity, together with a cumbersome 5-consecutive-day infusion schedule, has precluded their more widespread use.

Dacarbazine- and temozolomide-containing regimens

Like streptozocin, dacarbazine is an alkylating agent with activity against pancreatic NETs. In an Eastern Cooperative Oncology Group (ECOG) phase II trial of dacarbazine in 42 patients with advanced pancreatic NETs, the objective response rate was 33%.[45] As with streptozocin, concerns regarding toxicity have limited use of dacarbazine. Temozolomide is a less toxic orally active analogue of dacarbazine. Recent prospective and retrospective studies have suggested that temozolomide-based regimens may be comparable in efficacy with streptozocin-based regimens and that these regimens may also be more tolerable (**Table 4**). In retrospective series, temozolomide-based therapy has been associated with overall response rates of 8% to 70%.[46–48] Temozolomide has been evaluated prospectively in combination with thalidomide, bevacizumab, and everolimus, with overall response rates of 33% to 45%.[49–51] In a retrospective series of 30 patients who were treated with temozolomide plus capecitabine, the response rate was 70%.[48] Although temozolomide-based therapy is clearly active in pancreatic NETs, neither the optimal dosing regimen nor the relative benefits of combination

Table 4
Clinical trials of temozolomide-based therapy in pancreatic NET tumors

Regimen	N	Tumor Response Rate (%)	PFS (mo)	Reference
Retrospective studies				
Temozolomide	12	8	NR	Ekeblad et al,[46] 2007
Temozolomide + capecitabine	30	70	18.0	Strosberg et al,[48] 2011
Temozolomide (various regimens)	53	34	13.6	Kulke et al,[47] 2009
Prospective trials				
Temozolomide + thalidomide	11	45	NR	Kulke et al,[49] 2006
Temozolomide + bevacizumab	15	33	14.3	Chan et al,[50] 2012
Temozolomide + everolimus	40	40	15.4	Chan et al,[51] 2013

Abbreviations: PFS, progression-free survival; NR, not reported.
[a] Data shown are limited to results for pancreatic NET in studies that may have included both pancreatic NET and carcinoid.

therapy has been clearly established. An ongoing trial by ECOG is evaluating the activity of the combination of temozolomide plus capecitabine compared with temozolomide alone (National Clinical Trial [NCT] NCT01824875).

FUTURE DIRECTIONS
Peptide Receptor Radionuclide Therapy

The high rate of SSTR expression in NETs provides the rationale for peptide receptor radionuclide therapy (PRRT) as a treatment modality for patients with inoperable or metastatic disease. Somatostatin analogues with high receptor affinity are conjugated with chelators and a radionuclide to deliver a tumoricidal dose of radiation. The most frequently used radionuclides include the β-emitting radionuclide ^{90}yttrium (^{90}Y) and β- and γ-emitting ^{177}lutetium (^{177}Lu).[52,53] Differences in patient characteristics, tumor types, radionuclides, and cumulative administered doses have made it difficult to compare studies that have reported on the efficacy of PRRT.

In a prospective, phase II study of 90 patients with metastatic carcinoid tumor and symptoms refractory to octreotide treated with ^{90}Y-DOTA-Tyr^3-octreotide, more than 50% of patients had improvement in symptom control. Modest tumor responses were noted, including 4% of patients with a partial radiographic response and 70% stable disease following treatment.[54] In another single-center phase II study of ^{90}Y-DOTA-Tyr^3-octreotide that included 1109 patients, 378 (34%) experienced morphologic response; 172 (16%), biochemical response; and 329 (30%), clinical response. Longer survival was associated with morphologic, biochemical, and clinical responses.[55] Overall, 142 patients (13%) developed severe transient grade 3 to 4 hematologic toxicities. Two patients developed myeloproliferative diseases, and 2 experienced tumor lysis syndrome.

A retrospective analysis of ^{177}Lu-DOTA-Tyr^3-octreotate in the treatment of more than 500 patients with metastatic NET reported efficacy results for 310 patients. Complete and partial tumor remissions were demonstrated in 2% and 28% of patients, respectively. Minor tumor response (decrease in size >25% and <50%) occurred in 16%. The median time to progression was 40 months. The median OS from the start of treatment was 46 months, and the median OS from diagnosis was 128 months.[56] An assessment of toxicity in 504 patients demonstrated acute toxicity, including nausea (25%), vomiting (10%), and abdominal pain (10%). Serious delayed toxicity occurred in 9 patients, including renal insufficiency (n = 2), temporary liver function test abnormalities (n = 3), and myelodysplastic syndrome (n = 4).

Randomized, prospective studies better defining the antitumor activity and long-term toxicity of radiolabeled somatostatin analogues are anticipated. The NETTER-1 study, a multinational randomized phase III study of ^{177}Lu-DOTA-Tyr^3-octreotate compared with high dose octreotide LAR (60 mg monthly) in patients with midgut NET with progressive disease on standard-dose octreotide, completed accrual in early 2015. Results of this study (NCT01578239) will provide additional information on efficacy and safety of PRRT.

Combination therapy
Targeting multiple signaling pathways may provide better tumor control and overcome resistance mechanisms. Combining an mTOR inhibitor of the VEGF pathway, somatostatin analogues, and cytotoxic chemotherapy have been evaluated as treatment strategies for NETs.

Combining mechanistic target of rapamycin inhibitor and vascular endothelial growth factor pathway inhibitor
Several recently completed and ongoing studies have evaluated the combination of an mTOR inhibitor with inhibitors of the VEGF pathway. Combining everolimus with tyrosine kinase inhibitors of VEGFR and other growth factor receptors may be limited by toxicity. In a phase I study of everolimus in combination with sorafenib, dose-limiting toxicity precluding escalation to full doses of each agent was observed.[57] However, combinations of an mTOR inhibitor and bevacizumab seem to be better tolerated and have demonstrated higher levels of activity than would have been expected with single-agent therapy. In a phase II trial of temsirolimus plus bevacizumab in 58 patients with progressive pancreatic NETs, confirmed partial responses were documented in 23 of 56 patients eligible for response assessment (41%) with a median PFS of 13.2 months.[58] Additionally, the Cancer and Leukemia Group B (CALGB) 80701, a randomized phase II trial of 150 patients with advanced pancreatic NETs who received standard-dose octreotide LAR and everolimus with or without bevacizumab, demonstrated superior PFS with everolimus plus bevacizumab compared with everolimus (16.7 vs 14.0 months; HR 0.80, 95% CI 0.55–1.17; $P = .12$).[59] Combination therapy also was associated with a significantly higher response rate (RR) of 31% compared with 12% with everolimus alone ($P = .005$). It should be noted that patients receiving combination therapy had a higher incidence of grade 3/4 adverse events, including hypertension, proteinuria, diarrhea, and electrolyte abnormalities.

Combining mechanistic target of rapamycin inhibitor and somatostatin analogue
Because octreotide has been shown to decrease IGF-1 levels and PI3K/Akt signaling in vitro, it has been postulated that combining an mTOR inhibitor with a somatostatin analogue might result in enhanced antitumor activity.[60] Clinical trial data, however, have not demonstrated a definite benefit. Everolimus has been evaluated in combination with octreotide in several studies, including patients with pancreatic NETs in stratum 2 of the phase II RADIANT-1 trial and patients with carcinoid tumors in the phase III RADIANT-2 trial. In the RADIANT-1 trial, patients with pancreatic NETs receiving octreotide and everolimus had longer PFS compared with patients receiving everolimus monotherapy (**Table 2**).[61] However, the study was not randomized or designed to make this comparison. In the RADIANT-2 trial, although combined therapy with everolimus and octreotide was associated with a significantly longer PFS duration compared with everolimus and placebo based on local investigator radiology review, the improvement in PFS was not statistically significant according to central radiology review.[62]

Pasireotide is a novel somatostatin analog that binds to a broader range of somatostatin receptor subtypes than octreotide. Compared with octreotide, pasireotide has a greater binding affinity to SSTR-1, SSTR-3, and SSTR-5 and less affinity to SSTR-2.[63] The COOPERATE-2 study, a multicenter randomized phase II study, examined the efficacy of everolimus alone or in combination with pasireotide LAR in patients with advanced, progressive pancreatic NETs.[64] The results of this study showed no benefit for the addition of pasireotide with regard to tumor control. Further investigation is needed to determine whether there are specific subsets of patients with advanced NETs who benefit most from combination therapy with somatostatin analogues and targeted agents.

Combining mechanistic target of rapamycin inhibitor and chemotherapy

The combination of temozolomide and everolimus has been evaluated in a phase I/II study of patients with advanced pancreatic NETs.[51] Treatment was associated with known side effects of each drug without evidence of synergistic toxicity. Encouraging evidence of antitumor activity with this combination was observed. Among 40 evaluable patients, 16 (40%) experienced a partial response. The median PFS duration was 15.4 months, which is superior to the reported PFS observed with everolimus alone in the randomized, placebo-controlled RADIANT-3 study. However, these results need to be interpreted with caution because this was a single-arm study. Furthermore, disease progression before study enrollment was not a requirement in this study, as it was in the RADIANT-3 study. Future studies evaluating the relative efficacy of combining chemotherapy with an mTOR inhibitor compared with treatment with either agent alone are warranted.

SUMMARY

Advances in our understanding of the biology of NETs have translated into an expansion of treatment options for patients. Because of the heterogeneity of disease biology and presentation, a multidisciplinary approach to management is critical. Surgical resection remains the mainstay of the treatment of patients with localized disease. Several treatment options are available for patients with advanced pancreatic NETs. These options include hepatic-directed therapies, including surgical resection and hepatic artery embolization. Systemic treatment options include the use of somatostatin analogues for control of hormonal hypersecretion and also disease control. The tyrosine kinase inhibitor sunitinib and the mTOR inhibitor everolimus improve PFS in patients with pancreatic NETs. In patients with low-volume, low- and intermediate-grade disease without symptoms, a period of observation to better understand disease biology can be considered. In the setting of disease progression or development of symptoms related to disease, somatostatin analogue therapy is often initiated as the first-line therapy. Cytotoxic chemotherapy with alkylating agents, including streptozocin and temozolomide, can lead to tumor shrinkage and can be particularly useful for patients with symptoms related to bulk of disease. The optimal timing, sequence, and benefits of combination therapy are not known. Studies to examine these issues and to identify predictors of response may allow us to better tailor personalized treatment of individual patients in the future.

REFERENCES

1. Yao JC, Hassan M, Phan A, et al. One hundred years after "carcinoid": epidemiology of and prognostic factors for neuroendocrine tumors in 35,825 cases in the United States. J Clin Oncol 2008;26(18):3063–72.

2. Rindi G, Arnold R, Bosman FT, et al. Nomenclature and classification of neuroen-docrine neoplasms of the digestive system. In: Bosman TF, Carneiro F, Hruban RH, et al, editors. WHO classification of tumours of the digestive system. Lyon (France): International Agency for Research on Cancer (IARC) Press; 2010. p. 13.

3. Ellison TA, Wolfgang CL, Shi C, et al. A single institution's 26-year experience with nonfunctional pancreatic neuroendocrine tumors: a validation of current staging systems and a new prognostic nomogram. Ann Surg 2014;259(2):204–12.

4. Strosberg J, Gardner N, Kvols L. Survival and prognostic factor analysis in pa-tients with metastatic pancreatic endocrine carcinomas. Pancreas 2009;38(3): 255–8.

5. Velayoudom-Cephise FL, Duvillard P, Foucan L, et al. Are G3 ENETS neuroendo-crine neoplasms heterogeneous? Endocr Relat Cancer 2013;20(5):649–57.

6. Sorbye H, Welin S, Langer SW, et al. Predictive and prognostic factors for treat-ment and survival in 305 patients with advanced gastrointestinal neuroendocrine carcinoma (WHO G3): the NORDIC NEC study. Ann Oncol 2013;24(1):152–60.

7. Rindi G, Falconi M, Klersy C, et al. TNM staging of neoplasms of the endocrine pancreas: results from a large international cohort study. J Natl Cancer Inst 2012;104(10):764–77.

8. Starker LF, Carling T. Molecular genetics of gastroenteropancreatic neuroendo-crine tumors. Curr Opin Oncol 2009;21(1):29–33.

9. Johannessen CM, Reczek EE, James MF, et al. The NF1 tumor suppressor criti-cally regulates TSC2 and mTOR. Proc Natl Acad Sci U S A 2005;102(24):8573–8.

10. Jiao Y, Shi C, Edil BH, et al. DAXX/ATRX, MEN1, and mTOR pathway genes are frequently altered in pancreatic neuroendocrine tumors. Science 2011; 331(6021):1199–203.

11. Rubin J, Ajani J, Schirmer W, et al. Octreotide acetate long-acting formulation versus open-label subcutaneous octreotide acetate in malignant carcinoid syn-drome. J Clin Oncol 1999;17:600–6.

12. Papotti M, Bongiovanni M, Volante M, et al. Expression of somatostatin receptor types 1-5 in 81 cases of gastrointestinal and pancreatic endocrine tumors. A correlative immunohistochemical and reverse-transcriptase polymerase chain re-action analysis. Virchows Arch 2002;440(5):461–75.

13. Harris AG, O'Dorisio TM, Woltering EA, et al. Consensus statement: octreotide dose titration in secretory diarrhea. Diarrhea Management Consensus Develop-ment Panel. Dig Dis Sci 1995;40(7):1464–73.

14. Oberg K, Kvols L, Caplin M, et al. Consensus report on the use of somatostatin analogs for the management of neuroendocrine tumors of the gastroentero-pancreatic system. Ann Oncol 2004;15(6):966–73.

15. Maton PN, O'Dorisio TM, Howe BA, et al. Effect of a long-acting somatostatin analogue (SMS 201-995) in a patient with pancreatic cholera. N Engl J Med 1985;312(1):17–21.

16. Nikou GC, Toubanakis C, Nikolaou P, et al. VIPomas: an update in diagnosis and management in a series of 11 patients. Hepatogastroenterology 2005;52(64): 1259–65.

17. Eldor R, Glaser B, Fraenkel M, et al. Glucagonoma and the glucagonoma syn-drome - cumulative experience with an elusive endocrine tumour. Clin Endocrinol (Oxf) 2011;74(5):593–8.

18. Kindmark H, Sundin A, Granberg D, et al. Endocrine pancreatic tumors with glucagon hypersecretion: a retrospective study of 23 cases during 20 years. Med Oncol 2007;24(3):330–7.

19. Lahlou H, Saint-Laurent N, Esteve JP, et al. sst2 Somatostatin receptor inhibits cell proliferation through Ras-, Rap1-, and B-Raf-dependent ERK2 activation. J Biol Chem 2003;278(41):39356–71.

20. Susini C, Buscail L. Rationale for the use of somatostatin analogs as antitumor agents. Ann Oncol 2006;17(12):1733–42.

21. Pyronnet S, Bousquet C, Najib S, et al. Antitumor effects of somatostatin. Mol Cell Endocrinol 2008;286(1–2):230–7.

22. Rinke A, Muller HH, Schade-Brittinger C, et al. Placebo-controlled, double-blind, prospective, randomized study on the effect of octreotide LAR in the control of tumor growth in patients with metastatic neuroendocrine midgut tumors: a report from the PROMID Study Group. J Clin Oncol 2009;27(28):4656–63.

23. Caplin ME, Pavel M, Cwikla JB, et al. Lanreotide in metastatic enteropancreatic neuroendocrine tumors. N Engl J Med 2014;371(3):224–33.

24. Ma XM, Blenis J. Molecular mechanisms of mTOR-mediated translational control. Nat Rev Mol Cell Biol 2009;10(5):307–18.

25. Wullschleger S, Loewith R, Hall MN. TOR signaling in growth and metabolism. Cell 2006;124(3):471–84.

26. Missiaglia E, Dalai I, Barbi S, et al. Pancreatic endocrine tumors: expression profiling evidences a role for AKT-mTOR pathway. J Clin Oncol 2010;28(2): 245–55.

27. Yao JC, Shah MH, Ito T, et al. Everolimus for advanced pancreatic neuroendocrine tumors. N Engl J Med 2011;364(6):514–23.

28. van der Veldt AA, Kleijn SA. Advances in pancreatic neuroendocrine tumor treatment. N Engl J Med 2011;364(19):1873 [author reply: 1873–5].

29. Kulke MH, Bergsland EK, Yao JC. Glycemic control in patients with insulinoma treated with everolimus. N Engl J Med 2009;360(2):195–7.

30. Fiebrich HB, Siemerink EJ, Brouwers AH, et al. Everolimus induces rapid plasma glucose normalization in insulinoma patients by effects on tumor as well as normal tissues. Oncologist 2011;16(6):783–7.

31. Terris B, Scoazec JY, Rubbia L, et al. Expression of vascular endothelial growth factor in digestive neuroendocrine tumours. Histopathology 1998; 32(2):133–8.

32. Zhang J, Jia Z, Li Q, et al. Elevated expression of vascular endothelial growth factor correlates with increased angiogenesis and decreased progression-free survival among patients with low-grade neuroendocrine tumors. Cancer 2007; 109(8):1478–86.

33. Bowen KA, Silva SR, Johnson JN, et al. An analysis of trends and growth factor receptor expression of GI carcinoid tumors. J Gastrointest Surg 2009;13(10): 1773–80.

34. Silva SR, Bowen KA, Rychahou PG, et al. VEGFR-2 expression in carcinoid cancer cells and its role in tumor growth and metastasis. Int J Cancer 2011;128(5): 1045–56.

35. Fjallskog ML, Hessman O, Eriksson B, et al. Upregulated expression of PDGF receptor beta in endocrine pancreatic tumors and metastases compared to normal endocrine pancreas. Acta Oncol 2007;46(6):741–6.

36. Fjallskog ML, Lejonklou MH, Oberg KE, et al. Expression of molecular targets for tyrosine kinase receptor antagonists in malignant endocrine pancreatic tumors. Clin Cancer Res 2003;9(4):1469–73.

37. Hansel DE, Rahman A, Hermans J, et al. Liver metastases arising from well-differentiated pancreatic endocrine neoplasms demonstrate increased VEGF-C expression. Mod Pathol 2003;16(7):652–9.

38. Kulke MH, Lenz HJ, Meropol NJ, et al. Activity of sunitinib in patients with advanced neuroendocrine tumors. J Clin Oncol 2008;26(20):3403–10.
39. Raymond E, Dahan L, Raoul JL, et al. Sunitinib malate for the treatment of pancreatic neuroendocrine tumors. N Engl J Med 2011;364(6):501–13.
40. Hobday TJ, Rubin J, Holen K, et al. MC044h, a phase II trial of sorafenib in patients (pts) with metastatic neuroendocrine tumors (NET): A Phase II Consortium (P2C) study. J Clin Oncol 2007;25(18S). Abstract 4504.
41. Phan AT, Halperin DM, Chan JA, et al. Pazopanib and depot octreotide in advanced, well-differentiated neuroendocrine tumours: a multicentre, single-group, phase 2 study. Lancet Oncol 2015;16(6):695–703.
42. Hobday TJ, Yun JY, Pettinger A, et al. Multicenter prospective phase II trial of bevacizumab (bev) for progressive pancreatic neuroendocrine tumor (PNET). J Clin Oncol 2015;33(Suppl). Abstract 4096.
43. Moertel C, Lefkopoulo M, Lipsitz S, et al. Streptozocin-doxorubicin, stretpozocin-fluorouracil, or chlorozotocin in the treatment of advanced islet-cell carcinoma. N Engl J Med 1992;326:519–23.
44. Kouvaraki M, Ajani J, Hoff P, et al. Fluorouracil, doxorubicin, and streptozocin in the treatment of patients with locally advanced and metastatic pancreatic endocrine carcinomas. J Clin Oncol 2004;22:4762–71.
45. Ramanathan RK, Cnaan A, Hahn RG, et al. Phase II trial of dacarbazine (DTIC) in advanced pancreatic islet cell carcinoma. Study of the Eastern Cooperative Oncology Group-E6282. Ann Oncol 2001;12(8):1139–43.
46. Ekeblad S, Sundin A, Janson ET, et al. Temozolomide as monotherapy is effective in treatment of advanced malignant neuroendocrine tumors. Clin Cancer Res 2007;13(10):2986–91.
47. Kulke MH, Hornick JL, Frauenhoffer C, et al. O6-methylguanine DNA methyltransferase deficiency and response to temozolomide-based therapy in patients with neuroendocrine tumors. Clin Cancer Res 2009;15(1):338–45.
48. Strosberg JR, Fine RL, Choi J, et al. First-line chemotherapy with capecitabine and temozolomide in patients with metastatic pancreatic endocrine carcinomas. Cancer 2011;117(2):268–75.
49. Kulke MH, Stuart K, Enzinger PC, et al. Phase II study of temozolomide and thalidomide in patients with metastatic neuroendocrine tumors. J Clin Oncol 2006;24(3):401–6.
50. Chan JA, Stuart K, Earle CC, et al. Prospective study of bevacizumab plus temozolomide in patients with advanced neuroendocrine tumors. J Clin Oncol 2012;30(24):2963–8.
51. Chan JA, Blaszkowsky L, Stuart K, et al. A prospective, phase 1/2 study of everolimus and temozolomide in patients with advanced pancreatic neuroendocrine tumor. Cancer 2013;119(17):3212–8.
52. van Vliet EI, Teunissen JJ, Kam BL, et al. Treatment of gastroenteropancreatic neuroendocrine tumors with peptide receptor radionuclide therapy. Neuroendocrinology 2013;97(1):74–85.
53. van der Zwan WA, Bodei L, Mueller-Brand J, et al. GEPNETs update: Radionuclide therapy in neuroendocrine tumors. Eur J Endocrinol 2015;172(1):R1–8.
54. Bushnell DL Jr, O'Dorisio TM, O'Dorisio MS, et al. 90Y-edotreotide for metastatic carcinoid refractory to octreotide. J Clin Oncol 2010;28(10):1652–9.
55. Imhof A, Brunner P, Marincek N, et al. Response, survival, and long-term toxicity after therapy with the radiolabeled somatostatin analogue [90Y-DOTA]-TOC in metastasized neuroendocrine cancers. J Clin Oncol 2011;29(17):2416–23.

56. Kwekkeboom DJ, de Herder WW, Kam BL, et al. Treatment with the radiolabeled somatostatin analog [177 Lu-DOTA 0,Tyr3]octreotate: toxicity, efficacy, and survival. J Clin Oncol 2008;26(13):2124–30.

57. Chan J, Mayer R, Jackson N, et al. Phase I study of sorafenib in combination with everolimus (RAD001) in patients with advanced neuroendocrine tumors (NET). J Clin Oncol 2010;28(Suppl). Abstract 14597.

58. Hobday TJ, Qin R, Reidy-Lagunes D, et al. Multicenter Phase II Trial of Temsirolimus and Bevacizumab in Pancreatic Neuroendocrine Tumors. J Clin Oncol 2014.

59. Kulke MH, Niedzwiecki D, Foster NR, et al. Randomized phase II study of everolimus (E) versus everolimus plus bevacizumab (E+B) in patients (Pts) with locally advanced or metastatic pancreatic neuroendocrine tumors (pNET), CALGB 80701 (Alliance). J Clin Oncol 2015;33(Suppl). Abstract 4005.

60. Bousquet C, Lasfargues C, Chalabi M, et al. Clinical review: Current scientific rationale for the use of somatostatin analogs and mTOR inhibitors in neuroendocrine tumor therapy. J Clin Endocrinol Metab 2012;97(3):727–37.

61. Yao JC, Lombard-Bohas C, Baudin E, et al. Daily oral everolimus activity in patients with metastatic pancreatic neuroendocrine tumors after failure of cytotoxic chemotherapy: a phase II trial. J Clin Oncol 2010;28(1):69–76.

62. Pavel ME, Hainsworth JD, Baudin E, et al. Everolimus plus octreotide long-acting repeatable for the treatment of advanced neuroendocrine tumours associated with carcinoid syndrome (RADIANT-2): a randomised, placebo-controlled, phase 3 study. Lancet 2011;378(9808):2005–12.

63. Schmid HA. Pasireotide (SOM230): development, mechanism of action and potential applications. Mol Cell Endocrinol 2008;286(1–2):69–74.

64. Kulke, M. A Randomized Open-label Phase II Study of Everolimus Alone or in Combination with Pasireotide LAR in Advanced, Progressive Pancreatic Neuroendocrine Tumors (pNET): COOPERATE-2 Trial. in 12th Annual European Neuroendocrine Tumor Society Conference for the Diagnosis and Treatment of Neuroendocrine Tumor Disease. Barcelona, Spain, March 21, 2015.

65. Rindi G, Kloppel G, Alhman H, et al. TNM staging of foregut (neuro)endocrine tumors: a consensus proposal including a grading system. Virchows Arch 2006; 449(4):395–401.

66. Rindi G, Kloppel G, Couvelard A, et al. TNM staging of midgut and hindgut (neuro) endocrine tumors: a consensus proposal including a grading system. Virchows Arch 2007;451(4):757–62.

67. Edge S, Byrd D, Compton C, editors. AJCC Cancer Staging Manual. 7th Edition. New York: Springer; 2010.

68. Duran I, Kortmansky J, Singh D, et al. A phase II clinical and pharmacodynamic study of temsirolimus in advanced neuroendocrine carcinomas. Br J Cancer 2006;95(9):1148–54.

Moving?

Make sure your subscription moves with you!

To notify us of your new address, find your **Clinics Account Number** (located on your mailing label above your name), and contact customer service at:

Email: journalscustomerservice-usa@elsevier.com

800-654-2452 (subscribers in the U.S. & Canada)
314-447-8871 (subscribers outside of the U.S. & Canada)

Fax number: 314-447-8029

Elsevier Health Sciences Division
Subscription Customer Service
3251 Riverport Lane
Maryland Heights, MO 63043

*To ensure uninterrupted delivery of your subscription, please notify us at least 4 weeks in advance of move.

Printed and bound by CPI Group (UK) Ltd, Croydon, CR0 4YY

07/10/2024

01040506-0001